Candidate logbook
Level 3 VRQ

Beauty Therapy

Name: _____

City & Guilds enrolment number: _____

Date registered with City & Guilds: _____

Date enrolled with centre: _____

Centre name: _____

Centre number: _____

Centre address: _____

_____

Centre contact: _____

Assessor name: _____

Internal Verifier name: _____

About City & Guilds
City & Guilds is the UK's leading provider of vocational qualifications, offering over 500 awards across a wide range of industries, and progressing from entry level to the highest levels of professional achievement. With over 8500 centres in 100 countries, City & Guilds is recognised by employers worldwide for providing qualifications that offer proof of the skills they need to get the job done.

Equal opportunities
City & Guilds fully supports the principle of equal opportunities and we are committed to satisfying this principle in all our activities and published material. A copy of our equal opportunities policy statement is available on the City & Guilds website.

Copyright
The content of this document is, unless otherwise indicated, © The City and Guilds of London Institute 2011 and may not be copied, reproduced or distributed without prior written consent.
First edition 2011
Reprinted 2011, 2012 (twice), 2013, 2014 (twice), 2015 (twice), 2016, 2018 (three), 2019

ISBN 978 0 85193 217 0

Please note: National Occupational Standards are © Habia. Please check the conditions upon which they may be copied with Habia.

British Library Cataloguing in Publication Data
A catalogue record for this book is available from the British Library.

Publications
For information about or to order City & Guilds support materials, contact 0844 543 0000 or centresupport@cityandguilds.com. Calls to our 0844 numbers cost 7 pence per minute plus your telephone companys access charge.

Every effort has been made to ensure that the information contained in this publication is true and correct at the time of going to press. However, City & Guilds' products and services are subject to continuous development and improvement and the right is reserved to change products and services from time to time. City & Guilds cannot accept liability for loss or damage arising from the use of information in this publication.

City & Guilds
1 Giltspur Street
London EC1A 9DD
www.cityandguilds.com

City & Guilds would like to sincerely thank the following:

For invaluable Beauty Therapy expertise
Melissa Peacock, Sarah Farrell, Anita Crosland

For providing pictures
Baglioni Spa by SPC (www.baglionispa.co.uk); Balmain; Bev Braisdell; Carlton Group; Carlton Professional; Central Sussex College; Central Training Group; Champneys Health Resorts (www.champneys.com); Cheynes Training; Collin UK; Creative Nail Design; Crystal Clear; Daylesford Day Spa; Decleor; Derby College; Dermalogica; Desmond Murray; Ellisons; Environ; Germaine de Capuccini; Goddess International; Guinot; Hebe Salon; Hertford Regional College; House of Famuir; IIAA College Programme; iStockphoto.com; Jenni Lenard; Kett Cosmetics; Lars Carlsson (Makeup-FX.com); Lash Perfect; London School of Indian Champissage; Maria Retter; Mediscan; Melissa Jenkins; Nail Delights (www.naildelights.com); Nail Systems International; Natural by Nature Oils Ltd (www.naturalbynature.co.uk); naturasun; Natural Health Spa (www.budockvean.co.uk); NSI (UK) Ltd. (www.nsinails,co.uk); Orly; Paul Mitchell; Peeled Orange (www.peeledorange.com); Professionails; Salon System; Science Photo Library; skinbase.co.uk; Spa Find Skincare; Sterex; Su-do Professional – The art of the Sunless Tan (www.su-doprofessional.co.uk); Thalgo; The airbrush co ltd; The Edge Nail & Beauty; The London College of Beauty Therapy; The Sanctuary Spa, Covent Garden; Tisserand (www.tisserand.com); Walsall College; Wella; www.espaonline.com; www.hiveofbeauty.com; www.peteralvey.co.uk; www.therapyessentials.co.uk; Xen-Tan; Youngs Nails

Cover and book design by Purpose
Illustrations by Barking Dog Art
Layout by Select Typesetters Ltd
Edited by Rachel Howells
Printed in the UK by Cambrian Printers Ltd

Front cover Image courtesy of iStockphoto.com/Dodz Larysa

Back cover Image courtesy of Andrew Buckle

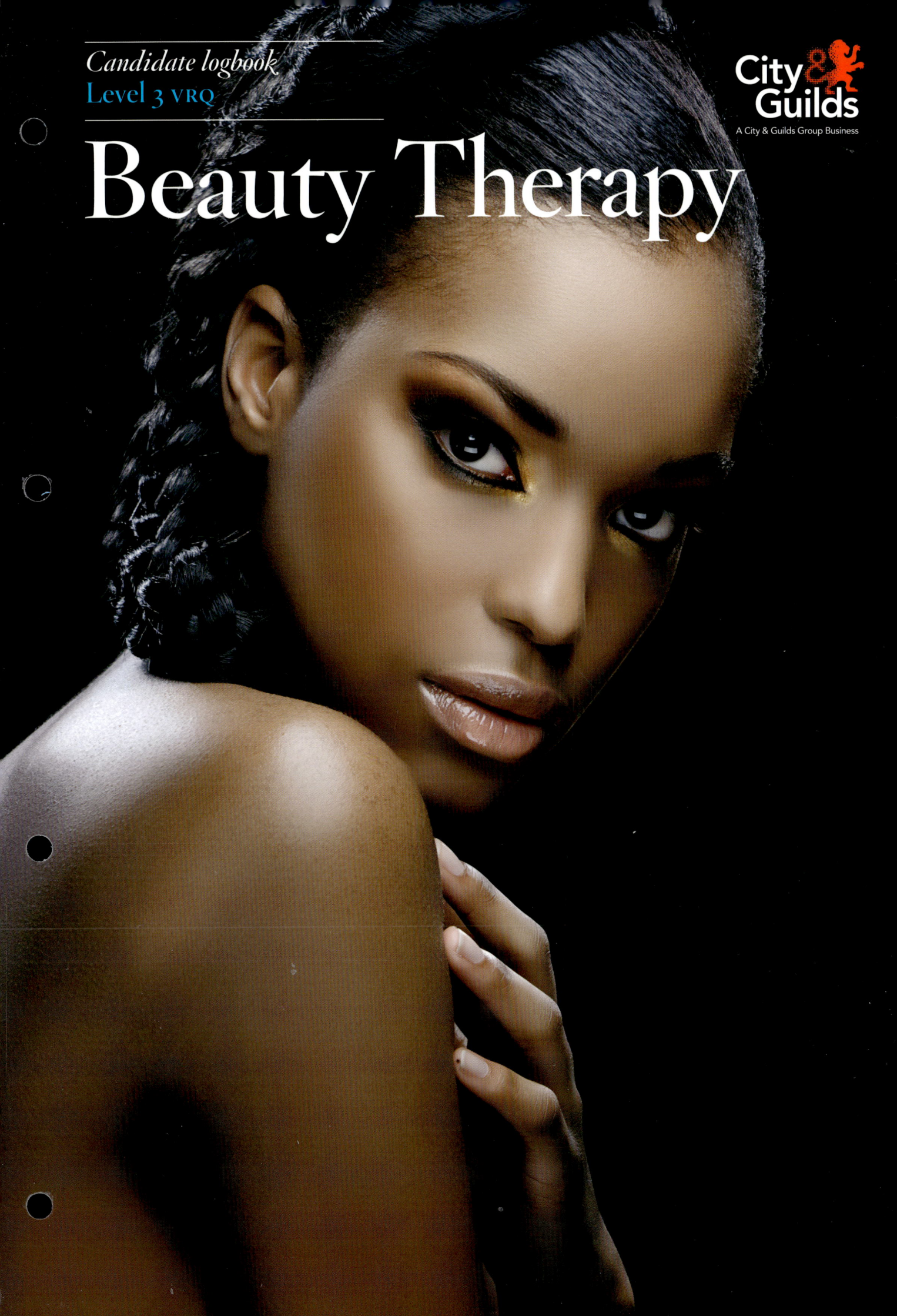

Contents

Summary of unit achievement	5
Credit values	7

Units included in this logbook

301 Working with colleagues within the beauty-related industries	10
302 Monitor and maintain health and safety practice in the salon	20
303 Client care and communication in beauty-related industries	30
304 Promote and sell products and services to clients	42
305 Provide body massage	54
306 Provide facial electrotherapy treatments	68
307 Provide body electrotherapy treatments	82
308 Provide electrical epilation	96
309 Provide massage using pre-blended aromatherapy oils	110
311 Provide Indian head massage	124
313 Provide self tanning	138
314 Apply and maintain nail enhancements	152
316 Creative hairdressing design skills	166
317 Apply individual permanent lashes	178
321 Apply micro-dermabrasion techniques	190
323 Design and apply face and body art	204
324 Fashion and photographic make-up	216
327 Apply airbrush make-up to the face	230
328 Airbrush design for the nails	244
329 Design and apply nail art	258
330 Media make-up	272

Contents (continued)

**Downloadable units
(available at www.cityandguilds.com)**

209 Apply make-up

210 Provide lash and brow treatments

212 Create an image based on a theme within the hair and beauty sector

213 Display stock to promote sales in salon

216 Salon reception duties

226 The art of colouring hair

312 Provide UV tanning

318 Intimate waxing for male clients

319 Intimate waxing for female clients

320 Enhance nails using electrical files

322 Apply stone therapy massage

325 Monitor and maintain spa areas

326 Provide spa treatments

331 Maintain personal health and wellbeing

332 Explore technological developments within hair, beauty and associated areas

333 Camouflage make-up

334 Nail enhancements and advanced hand and nail art techniques

335 Style and fit postiche

336 Provide hair extension services

337 Style and dress hair using a variety of techniques

338 Studio photography

339 Principles of studio photography

Summary of unit achievement

By signing this summary of unit achievement we are confirming that all the performance, knowledge and understanding requirements for these units have been completed and that the evidence is authentic and has been obtained under specified conditions for which certification is now requested.

Candidate name:

Candidate enrolment number:

Centre name:

Centre number:

Start date:

	Date achieved	Grade	Assessor signature	Candidate signature	IV signature (if sampled)
209 Apply make-up					
210 Provide lash and brow treatments					
212 Create an image based on a theme within the hair and beauty sector					
213 Display stock to promote sales in salon					
216 Salon reception duties					
226 The art of colouring hair					
301 Working with colleagues within the beauty-related industries					
302 Monitor and maintain health and safety practice in the salon					
303 Client care and communication in beauty-related industries					
304 Promote and sell products and services to clients					
305 Provide body massage					
306 Provide facial electrotherapy treatments					
307 Provide body electrotherapy treatments					
308 Provide electrical epilation					
309 Provide massage using pre-blended aromatherapy oils					

Continues on next page

Unit	Date achieved	Grade	Assessor signature	Candidate signature	IV signature (if sampled)
311 Provide Indian head massage					
312 Provide UV tanning					
313 Provide self tanning					
314 Apply and maintain nail enhancements					
316 Creative hairdressing design skills					
317 Apply individual permanent lashes					
318 Intimate waxing for male clients					
319 Intimate waxing for female clients					
320 Enhance nails using electrical files					
321 Apply micro-dermabrasion techniques					
322 Apply stone therapy massage					
323 Design and apply face and body art					
324 Fashion and photographic make-up					
325 Monitor and maintain spa areas					
326 Provide spa treatments					
327 Apply airbrush make-up to the face					
328 Airbrush design for the nails					
329 Design and apply nail art					
330 Media make-up					
331 Maintain personal health and wellbeing					
332 Explore technological developments within hair, beauty and associated areas					
333 Camouflage make up					
334 Nail enhancements and advanced hand and nail art techniques					
335 Style and fit postiche					
336 Provide hair extension services					
337 Style and dress hair using a variety of techniques					
338 Studio photography					
339 Principles of studio photography					

Summary of unit achievement Level 3 VRQ Beauty Therapy

Credit values

Unit no.	Unit title	Credits
Units included in this logbook		
301	Working with colleagues within the beauty-related industries	2
302	Monitor and maintain health and safety practice in the salon	4
303	Client care and communication in beauty-related industries	3
304	Promote and sell products and services to clients	4
305	Provide body massage	9
306	Provide facial electrotherapy treatments	11
307	Provide body electrotherapy treatments	11
308	Provide electrical epilation	11
309	Provide massage using pre-blended aromatherapy oils	7
311	Provide Indian head massage	6
313	Provide self tanning	3
314	Apply and maintain nail enhancements	15
316	Creative hairdressing design skills	8
317	Apply individual permanent lashes	4
321	Apply micro-dermabrasion techniques	4
323	Design and apply face and body art	6
324	Fashion and photographic make-up	7
327	Apply airbrush make-up to the face	4
328	Airbrush design for the nails	4
329	Design and apply nail art	5
330	Media make-up	7

Continues on next page

Credit values (continued)

Unit no.	Unit title	Credits
Downloadable units (available at www.cityandguilds.com/logbookoptionalunits)		
209	Apply make-up	5
210	Provide lash and brow treatments	4
212	Create an image based on a theme within the hair and beauty sector	7
213	Display stock to promote sales in salon	3
216	Salon reception duties	3
226	The art of colouring hair	7
312	Provide UV tanning	2
318	Intimate waxing for male clients	4
319	Intimate waxing for female clients	4
320	Enhance nails using electrical files	3
322	Apply stone therapy massage	9
325	Monitor and maintain spa areas	5
326	Provide spa treatments	7
331	Maintain personal health and wellbeing	7
332	Explore technological developments within hair, beauty and associated areas	7
333	Camouflage make-up	7
334	Nail enhancements and advanced hand and nail art techniques	7
335	Style and fit postiche	7
336	Provide hair extension services	5
337	Style and dress hair using a variety of techniques	7
338	Studio photography	10
339	Principles of studio photography	8

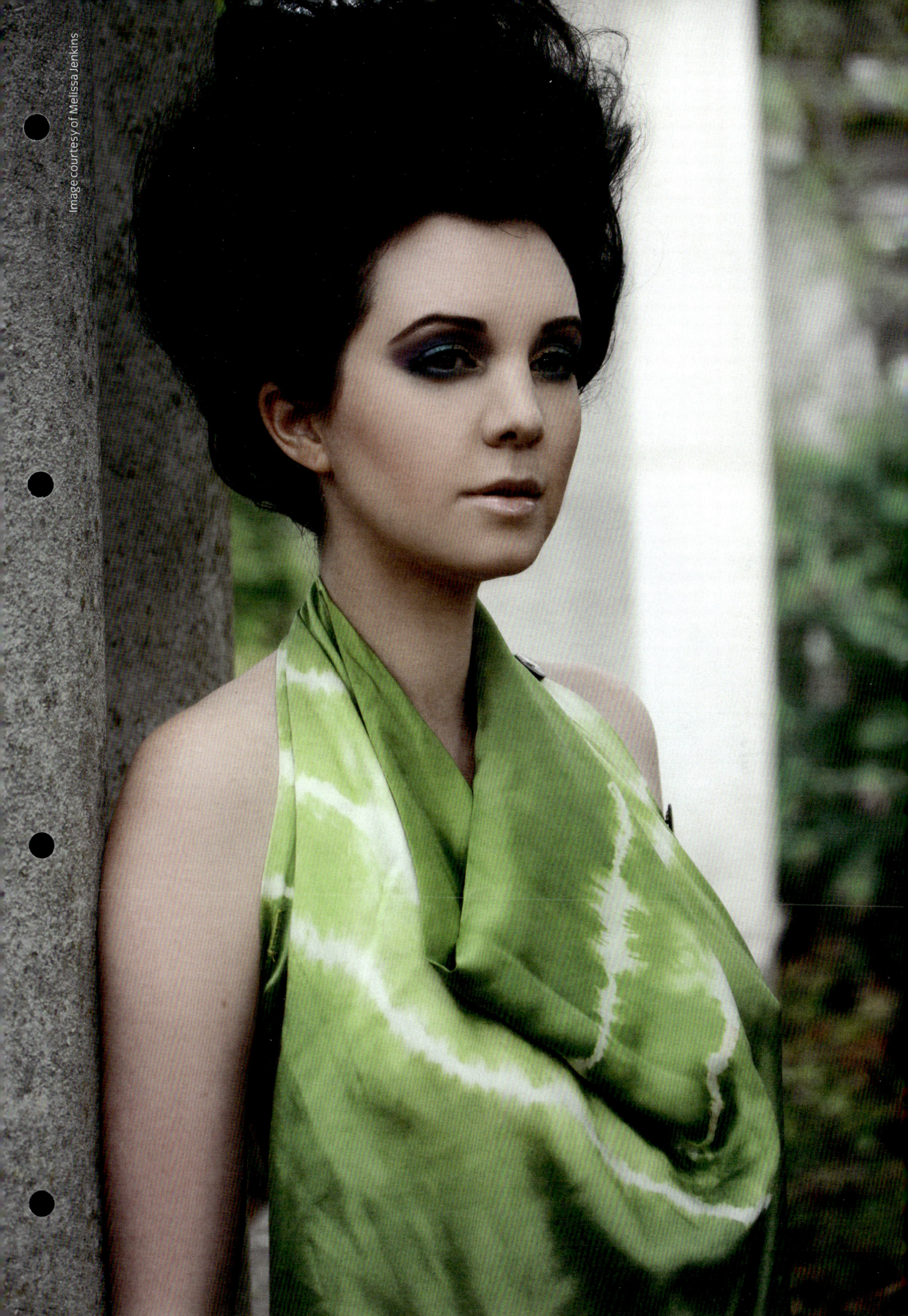
Image courtesy of Melissa Jenkins

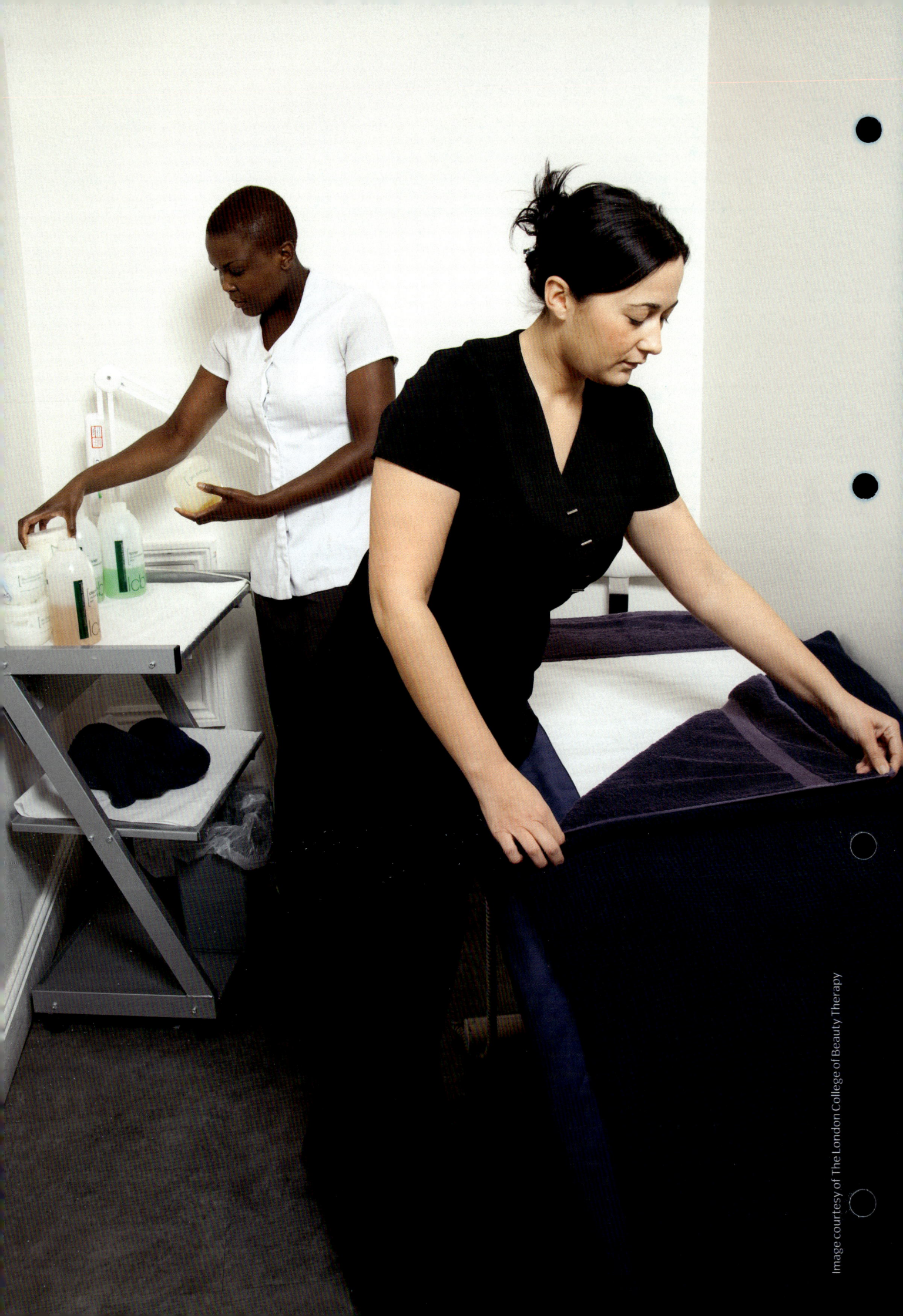

Image courtesy of The London College of Beauty Therapy

301

Working with colleagues within the beauty-related industries

Everyone knows that working well with colleagues is important for businesses, but it can also make the working day more fun! This unit looks at the skills you need to communicate effectively and form good working relationships. Being able to work well with others is a skill that employers will always value, and it will attract and keep clients too!

Assignment mark sheet
Unit 301 Working with colleagues within the beauty-related industries

This page is used to work out your overall grade for the unit. You must pass **all** parts of the tasks to be able to achieve a grade. There are no practical tasks in this unit.

What you must know	Tick when complete
Task 1: produce an information sheet	
Or tick if covered by an online test	

Overall grade

Candidate name:

Candidate signature: Date:

Assessor signature: Date:

Quality assurance co-ordinator signature (where applicable):   Date:

External Verifier signature (where applicable):   Date:

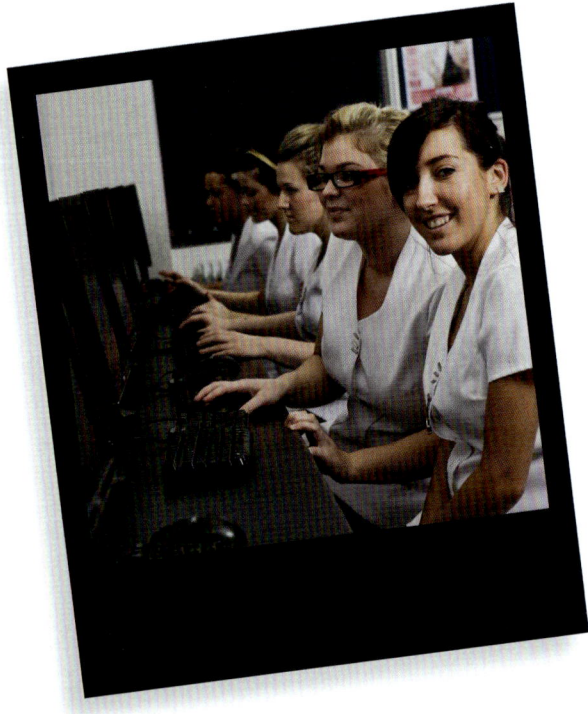

Image courtesy of The London College of Beauty Therapy

What does it mean?
Some useful words are explained below

Active listening
Paying close attention to what is being said.

Beauty-related terminology
A specialised vocabulary used within the beauty-related industries.

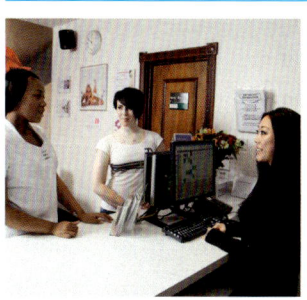

Body language
The way we communicate with our bodies, often without realising. Examples include gestures, facial expressions, eye contact and posture.

Closed questions
Questions that result in a 'yes' or 'no' answer. They are useful when specific, factual information is needed.

Communication
The way we talk to others, ie the giving, receiving and reacting to information. This might be face-to-face, over the phone or through email.

Co-operation
Working together effectively to meet a common objective.

Feedback
Evaluation of a process, activity or performance.

Junior therapist
A therapist qualified up to Level 2 treatments. It may also refer to a newly qualified therapist when they first start work.

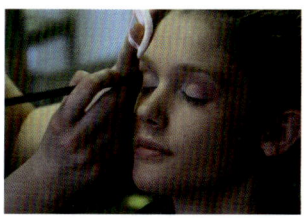

Make-up artist
Someone who uses make-up and specialised techniques to alter or enhance the appearance of others.

Masseur
The term for a male who is qualified in massage.

Open questions
These usually begin with 'who', 'when', 'where', 'why' or 'what'. They are useful when feelings or opinions are needed.

Rapport
A relationship of understanding, trust and agreement between two or more people.

Responsibilities
The duties that a person within a particular job role is expected to perform.

Role
The actions and activities expected of a person within a particular job.

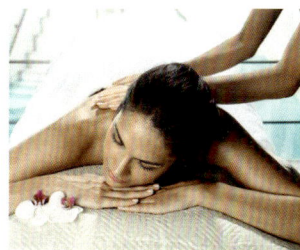

Spa therapist
A therapist who specialises in spa treatments such as hydrotherapy and body wraps.

Team
A group of people who work together.

Team work
The team members working together to achieve a particular aim.

> **Revision tip**
>
> Make the time to observe the body language of others! Look for positive signals as well as negative so you learn to 'read' how people are feeling.

What you must know
You must be able to:

1. Describe roles and responsibilities of team members in a salon
2. Describe the benefits of effective team working and working with colleagues
3. Describe the different methods of communication
4. Describe how to adapt communication techniques for different situations
5. Explain the importance of giving instruction, support and guidance and timely feedback
6. Describe the processes of giving instruction, support and guidance and timely feedback
7. Describe the effects of negative attitude and behaviour on others
8. State when and whom to refer problems to

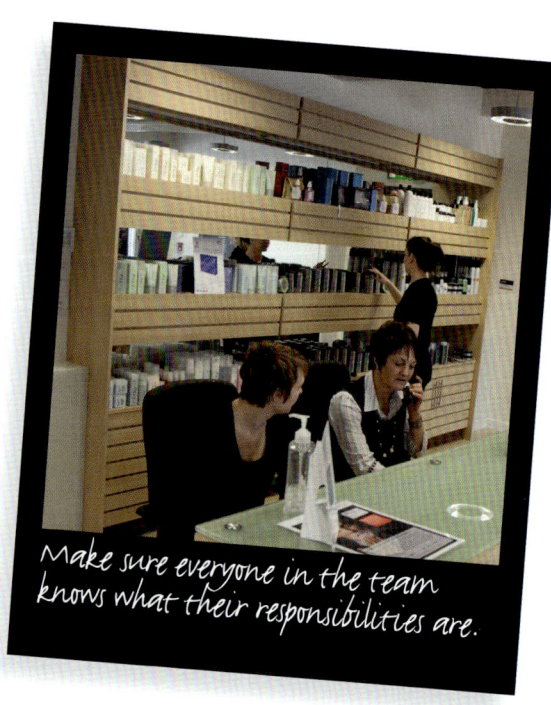

Make sure everyone in the team knows what their responsibilities are.

Image courtesy of Walsall College

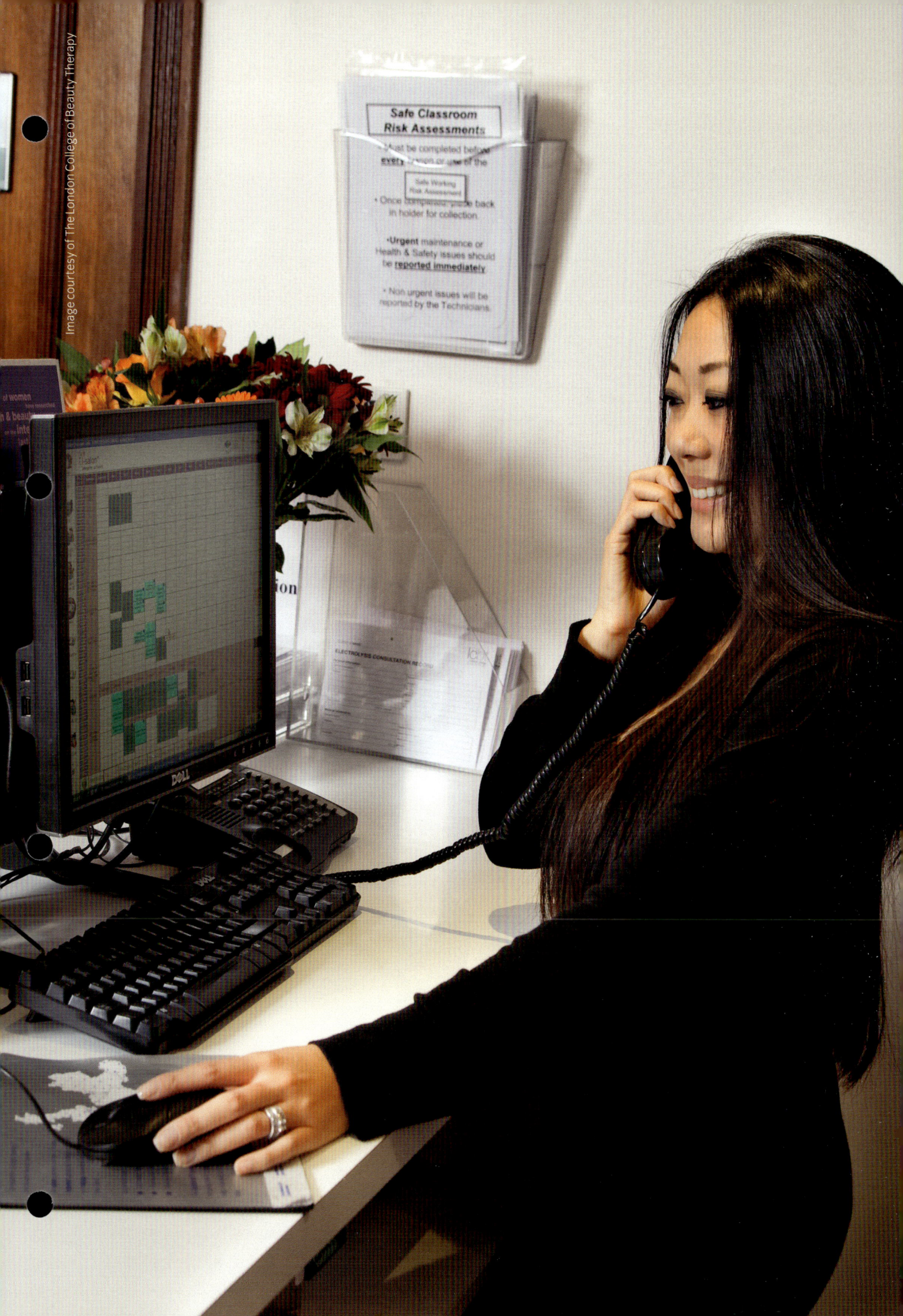

> As well as watching body language, be aware of what your own is saying! Your true feelings may be given away, especially at times when it's important to be professional.

Working

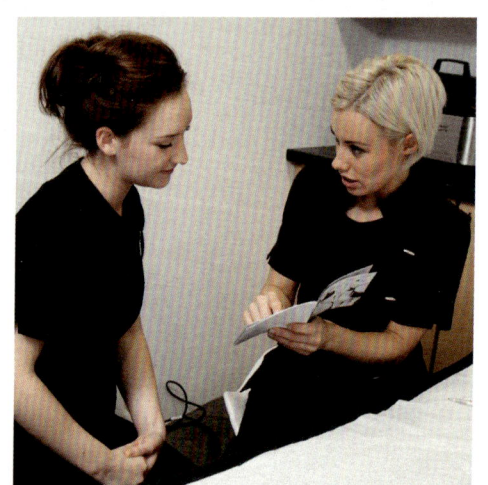

Always ask colleagues or your manager for clarification if you need it.

> Show that you are listening by using appropriate eye contact, concentrating and leaning slightly forward. Don't interrupt the speaker,

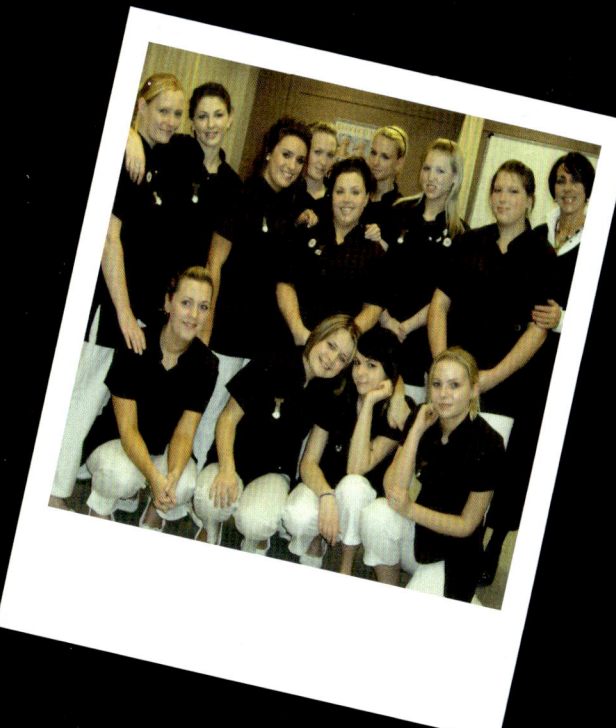

Image courtesy of IIAA College Programme

together

Feedback is only useful if it's constructive. Be honest without being hurtful, and use positive words. Always end on an encouraging note.

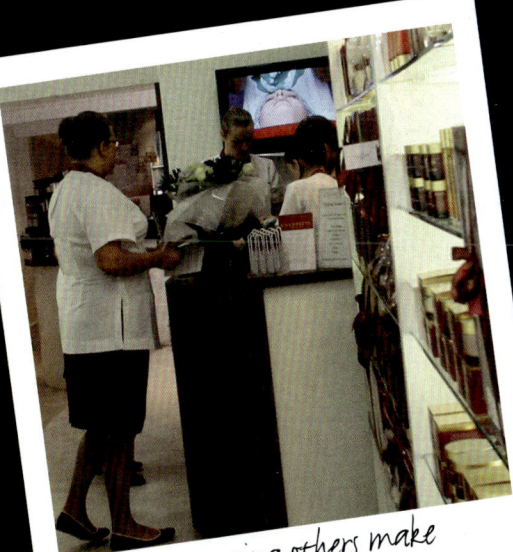

When instructing others make sure they can clearly see what you are doing.

Image courtesy of Champneys Health Resorts (www.champneys.com)

Comment form
Unit 301 Working with colleagues within the beauty-related industries

This form can be used to record comments by you, your client, or your assessor.

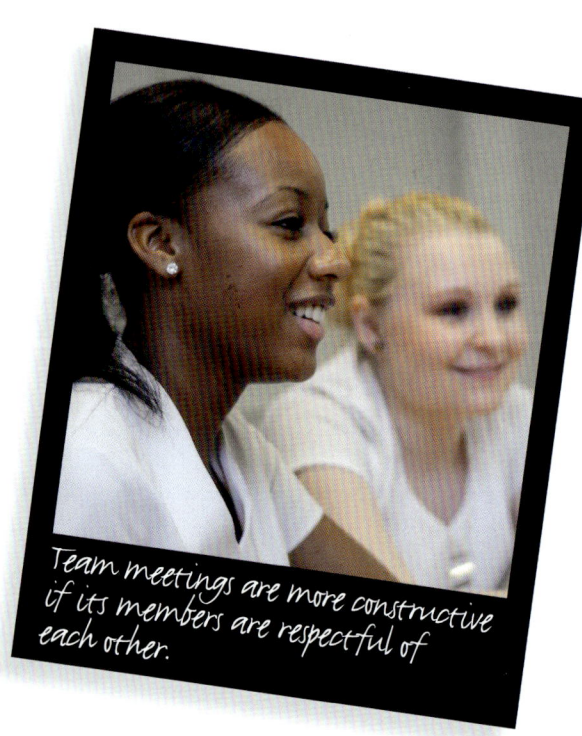

Team meetings are more constructive if its members are respectful of each other.

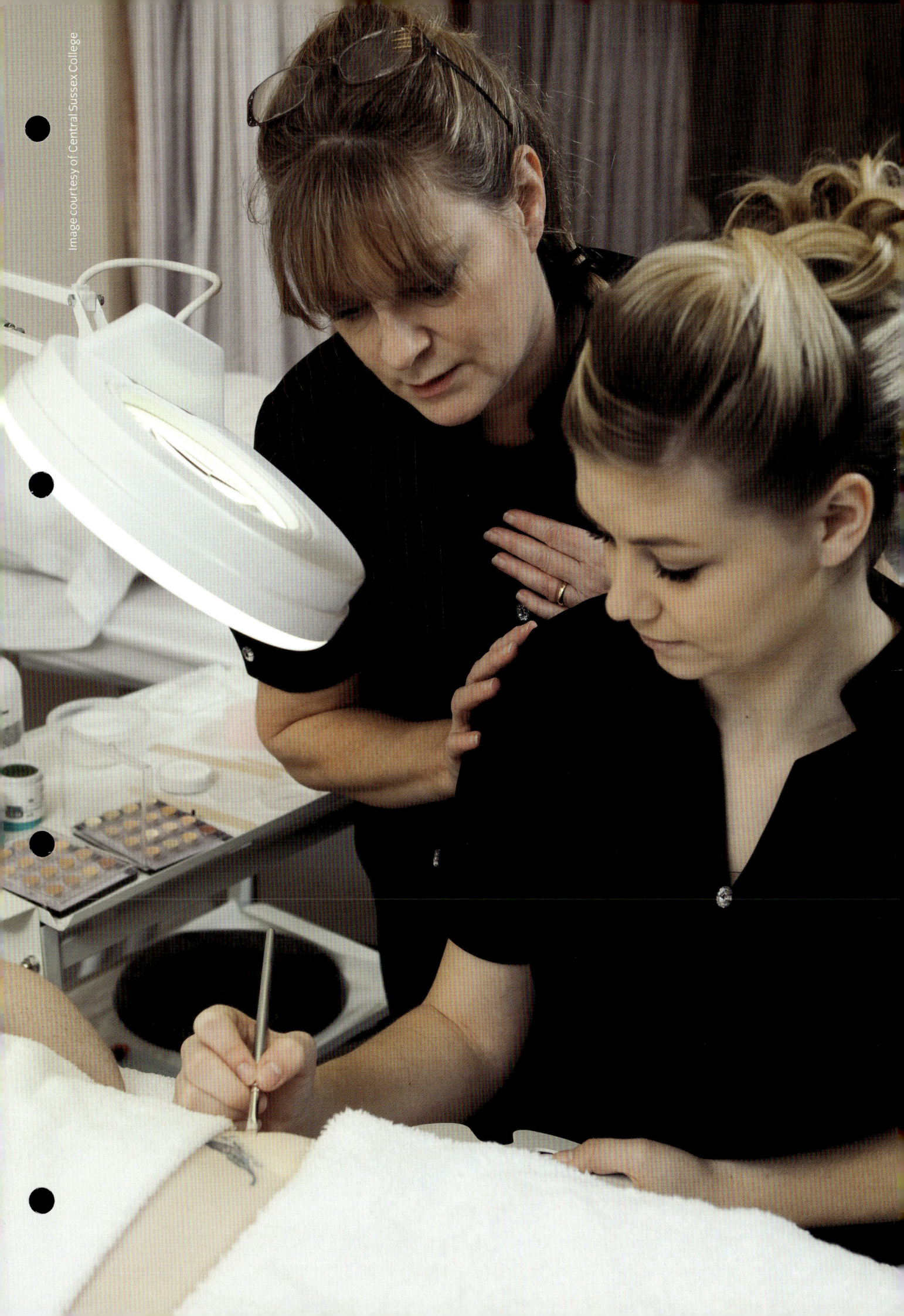

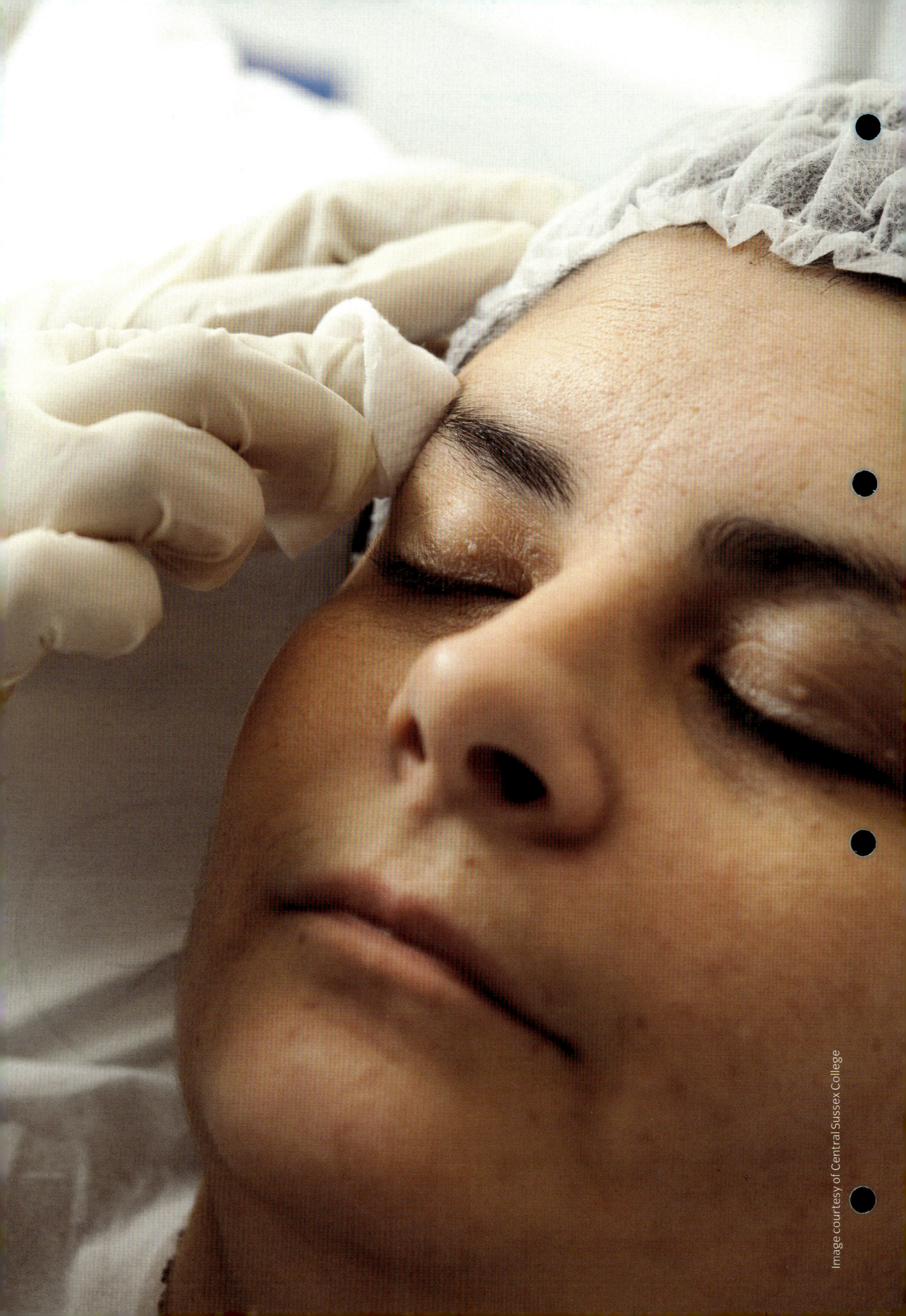

Image courtesy of Central Sussex College

302

Monitor and maintain health and safety practice in the salon

Whatever type of establishment you work in (beauty salon, spa or cruise liner, or on set), you need to know how to maintain a safe environment for the staff and clients or models. In this unit you'll learn when and how to carry out risk assessments and what to look out for. You'll get guidance on the types of insurance that are needed in the salon to make sure you are protected financially. Finally, you will look at how to induct new staff and the type of training and support they may need.

Assignment mark sheet
Unit 302 Monitor and maintain health and safety practice in the salon

This page is used to work out your overall grade for the unit. You must pass **all** parts of the tasks to be able to achieve a grade. There are no practical tasks in this unit.

What you must know	Tick when complete
Task 1a: produce an information sheet	
Task 1b: carry out a risk assessment and produce a report	
Or tick if covered by an online test	

Overall grade

Candidate name:

Candidate signature: Date:

Assessor signature: Date:

Quality assurance co-ordinator signature (where applicable):   Date:

External Verifier signature (where applicable):   Date:

If you need to know more about a potentially dangerous chemical you come across in the salon, ask for the safety data sheet.

What does it mean?
Some useful words are explained below

COSHH (control of substances hazardous to health)
The legislation that requires employers to control substances hazardous to the health of their employees and clients.

Employer's liability
Compulsory insurance that businesses must pay to meet the cost of compensation for any employee injuries or illnesses that occur as a result of their work.

Hazard
Anything with the potential to cause harm, eg electricity and chemicals.

Hazardous substance
Substances that are classified as either toxic, very toxic, corrosive, harmful or irritant.

   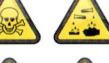

Hazard symbols
You might see one or more of these symbols on a single product. They tell us if the product is toxic, corrosive, harmful, explosive, oxidising or flammable.

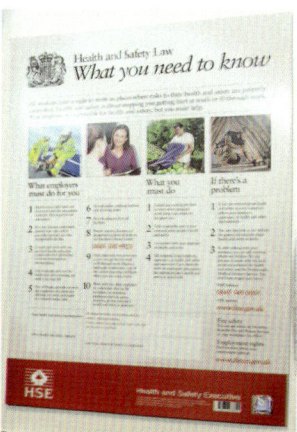

Health and Safety at Work Act
The 'umbrella' act under which all other health and safety legislation falls. It places a duty on all employers to ensure the health, safety and welfare at work of all their employees.

Legislation
Laws, in this case relating to health and safety practice, that you will need to be aware of.

Personal Protective Equipment (PPE)
Equipment in the workplace that protects you against risks to your health and safety, eg gloves, aprons, uniforms or respiratory protection.

Product and Treatment Liability
Insurance that protects salons against claims for injury or damage caused by treatments, services or products.

Public Liability Insurance
Protects the business financially from accidental injury to a client or member of the public, or from damage to their property.

Risk
The likelihood that damage, loss or injury will be caused by a hazard and how severe the outcome may be, eg trailing wires.

Risk assessment
A systematic process for looking at work activities, considering what could go wrong and the risks that exist, and deciding on suitable control measures to prevent damage or injury in the workplace.

Safety Data Sheet
Provides information on chemical products that helps users of those chemicals to make a risk assessment. It describes the hazards the chemical presents and gives information on handling, storage and emergency measures in case of an accident.

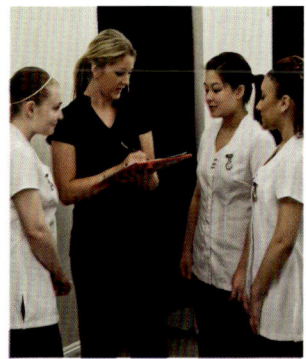

Staff induction
A process to introduce new employees to their jobs and working environment.

Revision tip

Carrying out a risk assessment is just the first step. Once it has been carried out, take steps to reduce any risks found. Also make sure that everyone involved in the activity or exposed to the risk is made aware of the findings.

What you must know
You must be able to:

1. State the reason for carrying out risk assessments
2. Describe the procedures for carrying out a risk assessment
3. Describe when risk assessments should be carried out
4. Outline necessary actions to take following a risk assessment
5. Outline the health and safety support that should be provided to staff
6. Outline procedures for dealing with different types of security breaches
7. Explain the need for insurance

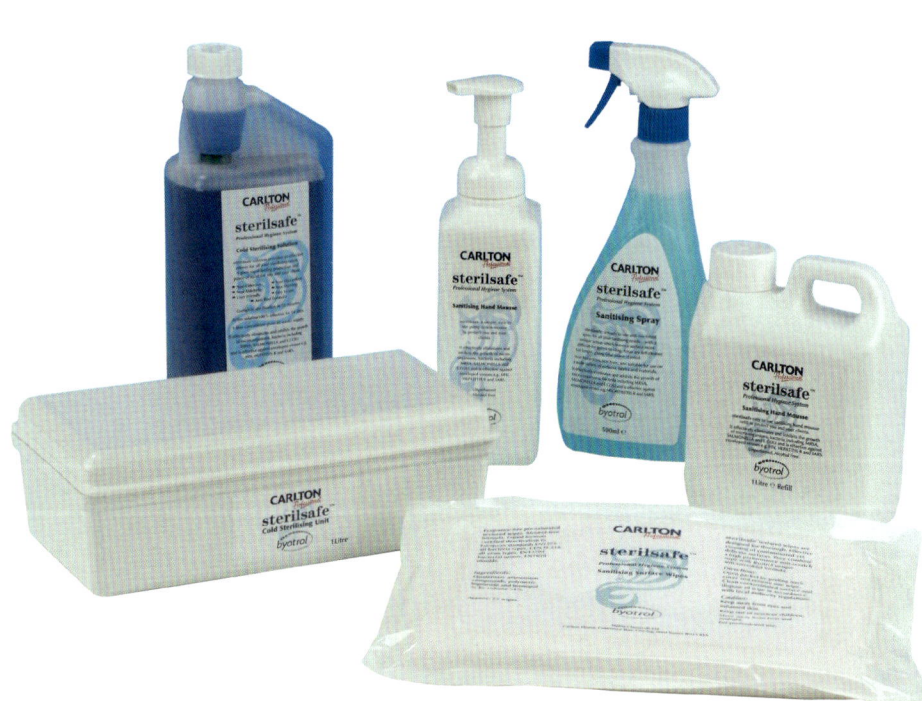

Image courtesy of Carlton Group

Revision tip

Everyone who is involved with the use of hazardous substances should be provided with the training, instruction and information required to ensure their safety.

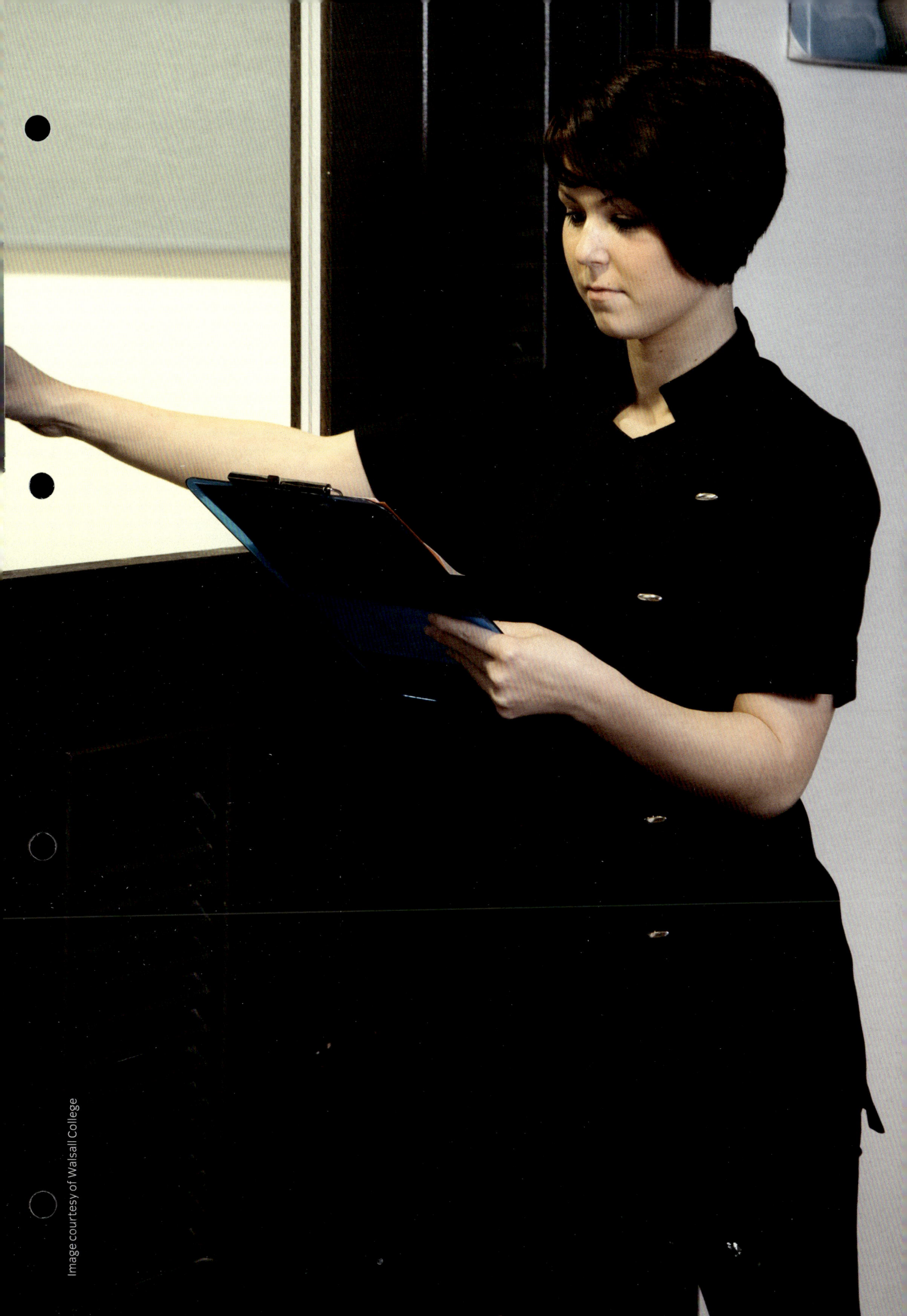

Image courtesy of Walsall College

Check accident reports and inspection and maintenance records to see if you can learn anything from existing records.

Health a

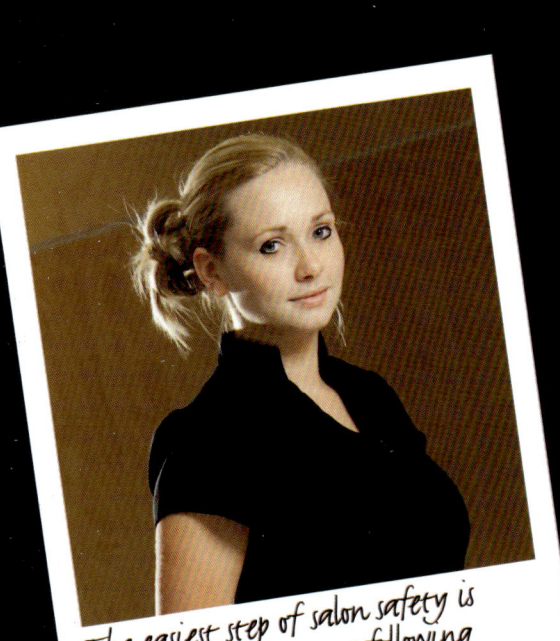

The easiest step of salon safety is ensuring that you are following the correct dress code.

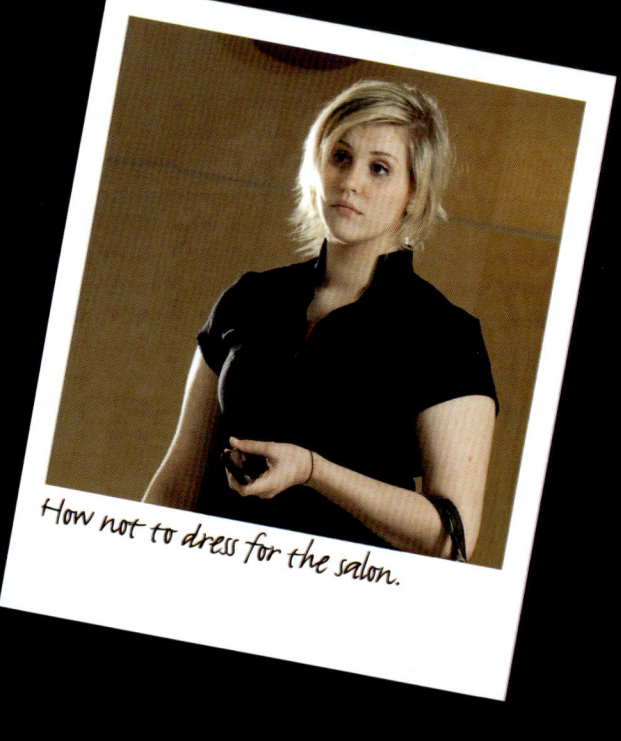

How not to dress for the salon.

Images courtesy of Hertford Regional College

Image courtesy of Walsall College

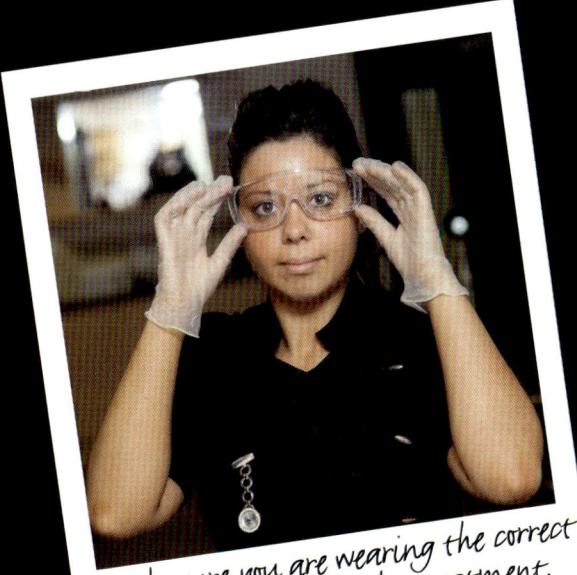

Make sure you are wearing the correct PPE before you start the treatment.

nd safety

Claims against therapists have risen in recent years. Compensation claims are made for damages and considerable legal fees are also added. Make sure you are covered by insurance!

Comment form
Unit 302 Monitor and maintain health and safety practice in the salon

This form can be used to record comments by you, your client, or your assessor.

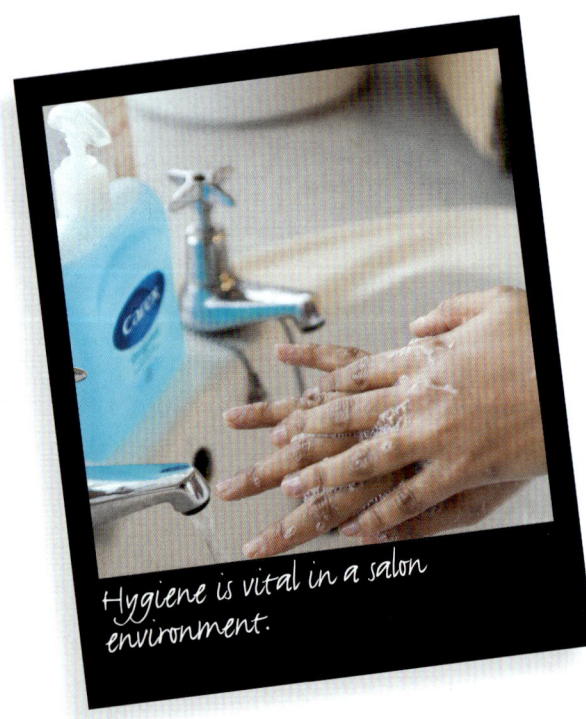
Hygiene is vital in a salon environment.

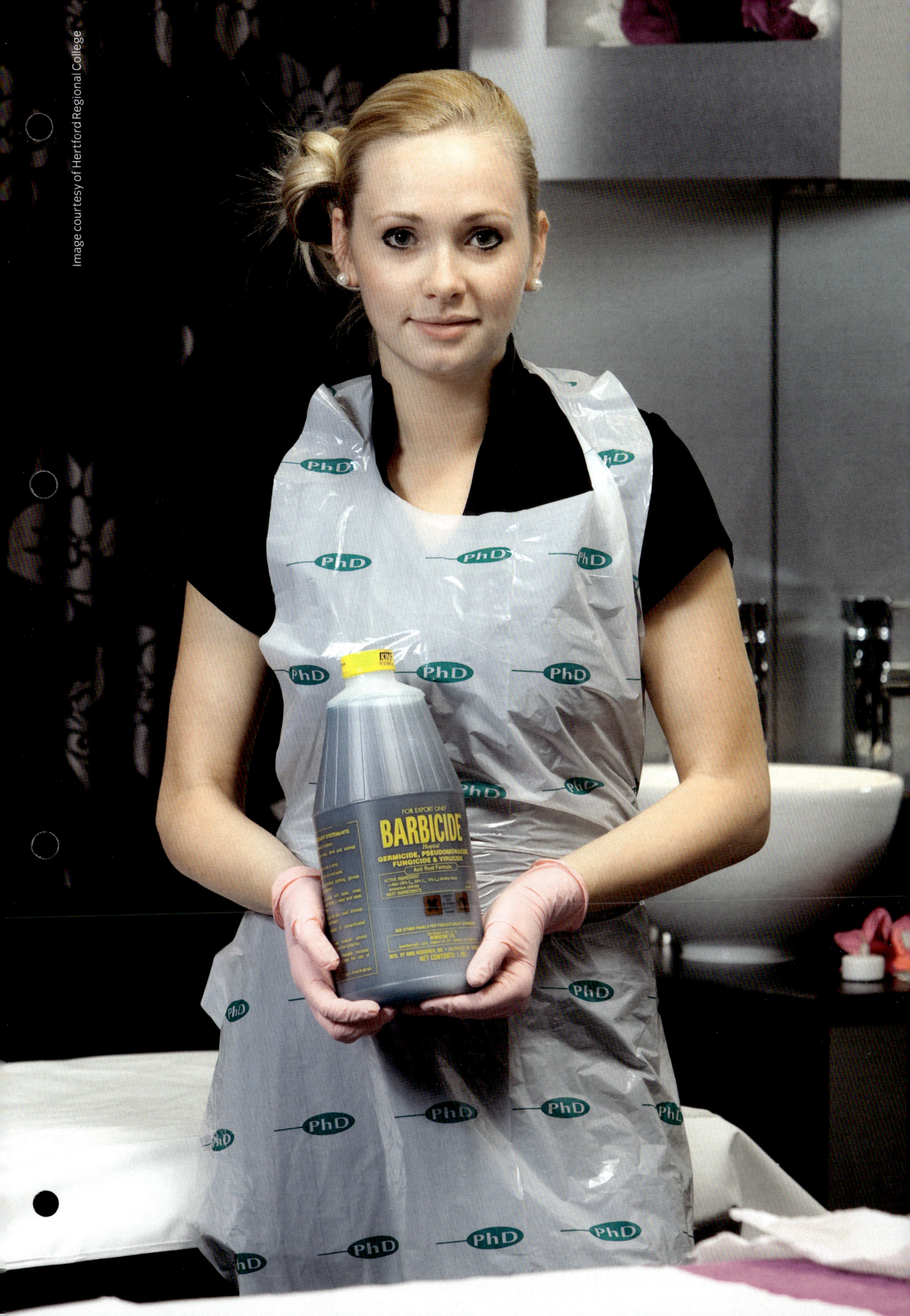

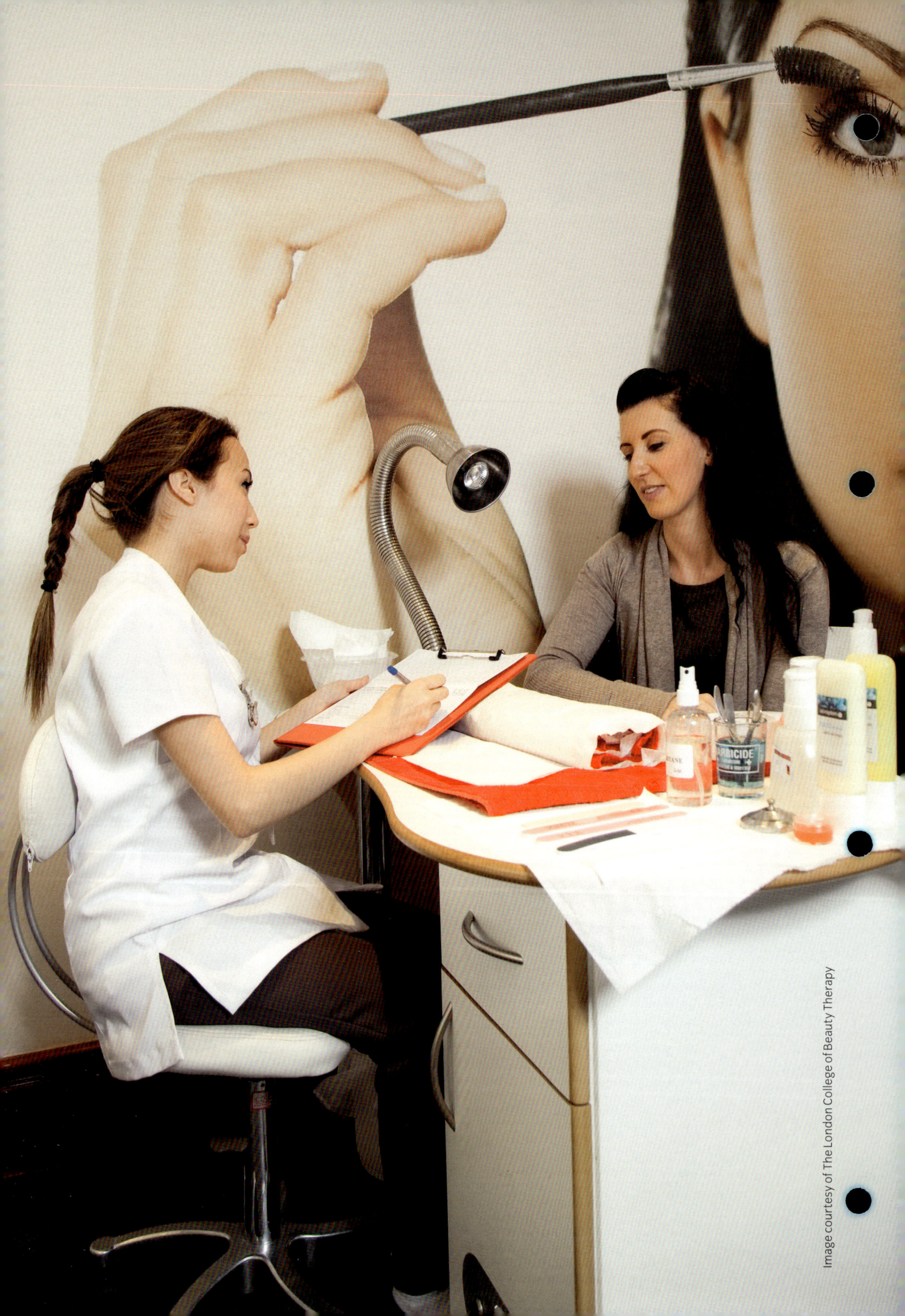

Image courtesy of The London College of Beauty Therapy

303

Client care and communication in beauty-related industries

Good communication skills are vital in this industry. Not only do you have to find out what the client wants, but also be able to deal with any unreasonable demands they may have. You will need excellent verbal skills, including knowing how and when to use different questioning techniques. Adjusting how you speak to suit each client will really make a difference to how they view you, as will your use of body language and eye contact. This unit covers how to behave in a salon situation with clients and colleagues, as well as the legal requirements you need to be aware of.

Assignment mark sheet
Unit 303 Client care and communication in beauty-related industries

Your assessor will mark you on each of the practical tasks in this unit. This page is used to work out your overall grade for the unit. You must pass **all** parts of the tasks to be able to achieve a grade. For each completed practical task, a pass equals 1 point, a merit equals 2 points and a distinction equals 3 points.

What you must know	Tick when complete
Task 1a: produce a report	
Task 1b: produce an information sheet	
Or tick if covered by an online test	

What you must do	Grade	Points
Task 2: Consultation		

Overall grade

Candidate name:

Candidate signature: Date:

Assessor signature: Date:

Quality assurance co-ordinator signature   Date:
(where applicable):

External Verifier signature   Date:
(where applicable):

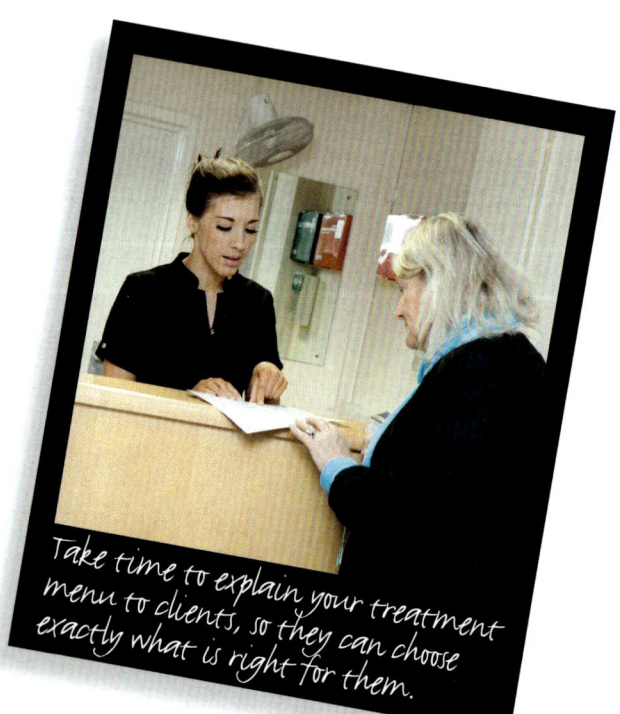

Take time to explain your treatment menu to clients, so they can choose exactly what is right for them.

Image courtesy of Central Sussex College

What does it mean?
Some useful words are explained below

Active listening
Using techniques to show that you are paying close attention to what is being said by a client or colleague. For example, using eye contact, or repeating back what the person has said, to confirm understanding.

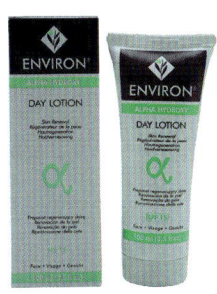

Benefits
These describe why the client would want to buy your products or services. For example, a product's benefit may be that it improves skin condition.

Body language
Non-verbal communication using gestures, facial expressions, eye contact and posture.

Closed questions
Questions that will result in an answer of 'yes' or 'no'. These are useful when specific factual information is needed.

Communication
Giving, receiving and responding to information, either verbally or non-verbally.

Confidential information
Data that must be handled properly and not shared with unauthorised persons.

Data Protection Act
The law that states how an individual's information should be processed and stored, and who is allowed access to it.

Features
A sales term meaning the characteristics of what you are selling. For example, a product's features are its size, colour, fragrance, and ingredients.

Open questions
These usually begin with 'who', 'when', 'where', 'why' or 'what'. These are useful when feelings or opinions are being sought.

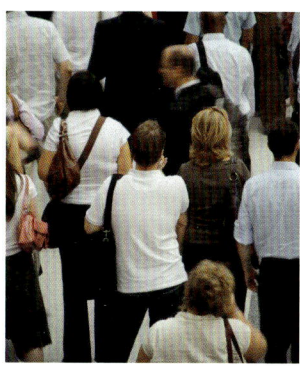

Personal space
The area surrounding a person. It varies between individuals, but invading it can lead to feelings of discomfort or anxiety.

Professionalism
The codes of conduct and behaviour that you must follow within a job role, and the behaviour expected by clients and colleagues.

Rapport
A relationship of understanding, trust and agreement between two or more people.

Sales techniques
Ways in which you will help the client to decide the product or service that will suit their needs.

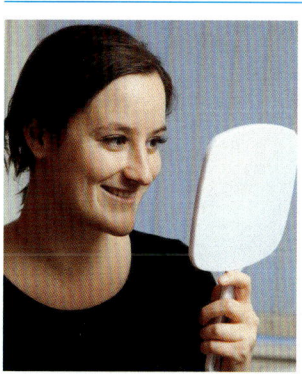

Treatment objectives
The aim or desired end result of the treatment.

> **Revision tip**
>
> Do you know your salon's policy for dealing with client complaints? Find out what it is now – not when you have an angry client to deal with!

What you must know
You must be able to:

1. Describe how to adapt methods of communication to suit the client and their needs
2. Explain what is meant by the term 'professionalism' within beauty-related industries
3. Explain the importance of respecting a client's 'personal space'
4. Describe how to use suitable consultation techniques to identify treatment objectives
5. Explain the importance of providing clear recommendations to the client
6. Evaluate measures used to maintain client confidentiality
7. Explain the importance of adapting retail sales techniques to meet client requirements
8. Identify methods of improving own working practices
9. Describe how to resolve client complaints

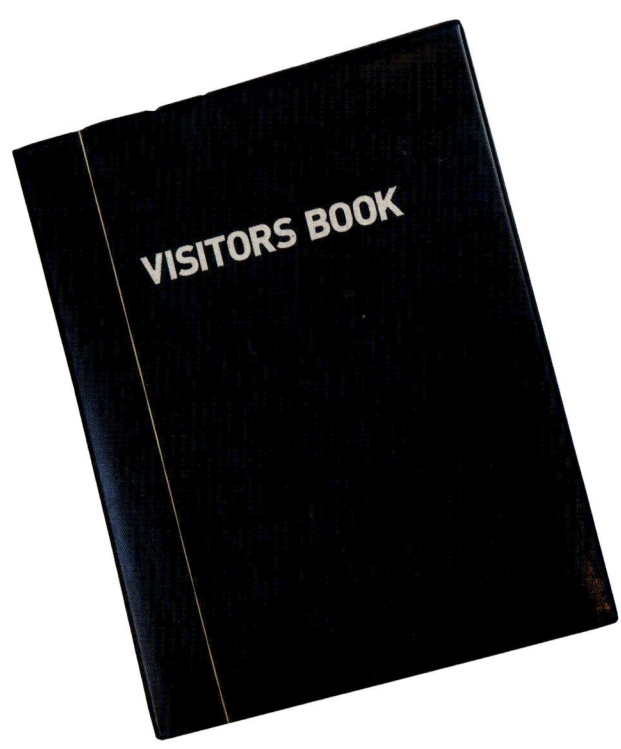

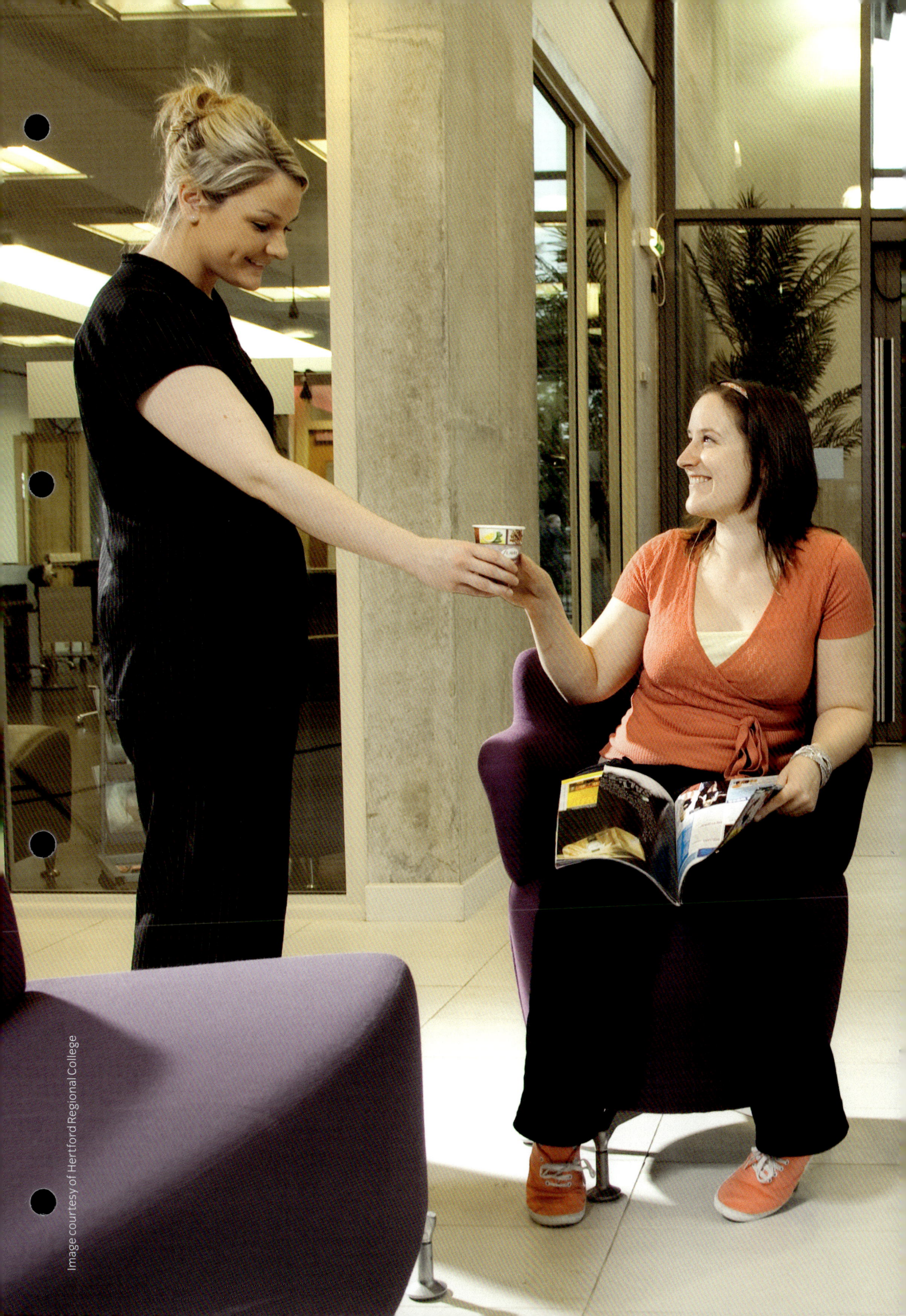
Image courtesy of Hertford Regional College

Clien

Always discuss the features and benefits of retail products with the client. They won't buy something unless they know why they need it and what it will do for them!

A detailed consultation allows you to tailor the treatment to the client.

Show your client that you're listening to them. Lean forward, nod and maintain appropriate eye contact. Summarise and confirm what they have said.

Image courtesy of Champneys Health Resorts (www.champneys.com)

t care

A friendly greeting is an excellent start to top class treatments!

Image courtesy of Champneys Health Resorts (www.champneys.com)

People vary in the amount of personal space they need. Read your client's body language and step back if he or she seems uneasy.

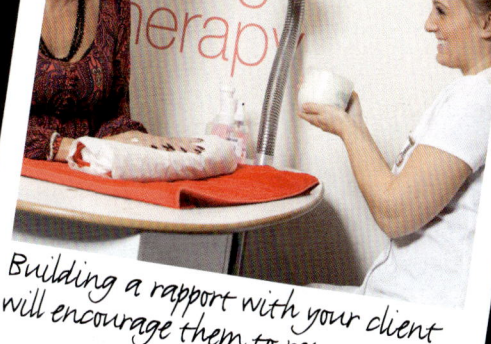

Building a rapport with your client will encourage them to return.

Image courtesy of The London College of Beauty Therapy

What you must do
Practical observations

This page shows what you need to do during your practical task. You can look at it beforehand, but you're **not** allowed to have it with you while carrying out your practical task. You must achieve **all** the criteria; you can achieve 1 mark, 2 marks or 3 marks for the criteria indicated with *.

Conversion chart

Grade	Marks
Pass	7–8
Merit	9–11
Distinction	12–13

	Consultation		
1 Behave in a professional manner	1		
2 Use and adapt effective communication techniques when dealing with clients *	1	2	3
3 Identify client treatment needs correctly	1		
4 Provide clear recommendations to the client *	1	2	3
5 Maintain client confidentiality in line with legislation	1		
6 Identify and recommend further treatments and/or products to meet the client's needs and requirements *	1	2	3
7 Evaluate client feedback	1		
Total			
Grade			
Candidate signature and date			
Assessor signature and date			

What you must do
Practical observations descriptors table

This table shows what you need to do to achieve 1, 2 or 3 marks for the criteria indicated with * on the previous page.

	1 mark	2 marks	3 marks
2 Use and adapt effective communication techniques when dealing with clients	Uses suitable questioning (open and/or closed questions) and listening techniques.	Uses suitable questioning (open and/or closed questions) and listening techniques, positive body language (eye contact and facial expression) and is friendly and polite to the client.	Uses suitable questioning (open and/or closed questions) and listening techniques, positive body language (eye contact and facial expression), is friendly and polite to the client, uses visual aids and client records (where applicable), adapts the terminology to client's level of understanding and tone of voice to match the setting/client/treatment, presents a confident manner.
4 Provide clear recommendations to the client	A basic treatment plan is recommended Example: explains treatment procedure and any adaptations to meet client treatment needs.	A good treatment plan is recommended Examples: explains treatment procedure and any adaptations to meet client treatment needs and expectations based on factors identified during consultation, explains the choice of products to be used.	A thorough treatment plan is recommended Examples: explains treatment procedure and any adaptations to meet client treatment needs and expectations based on factors identified during consultation, explains the choice of products to be used, invites the client to ask questions about the treatment plan and provides suitable answers.

Continues on next page

What you must do
Practical observations descriptors table (continued)

This table shows what you need to do to achieve 1, 2 or 3 marks for the criteria indicated with * on page 38.

	1 mark	2 marks	3 marks
6 Identify and recommend further treatments and/or products to meet the client's needs and requirements	Recommends basic suitable future treatment(s) and/or product(s) based on consultation and treatment.	Recommends suitable future treatment(s) and/or product(s) based on the factors identified during consultation and treatment to meet client's needs, including the frequency of treatment(s) (where applicable) and the main feature and benefit of the treatment(s) and/or product(s).	Recommends suitable future treatment(s) and/or product(s) based on the factors identified during consultation and treatment to meet client's needs, including the frequency of treatment(s) (where applicable), features and benefits of the treatment(s) and/or product(s) and relates these directly to the client's own needs and requirements.

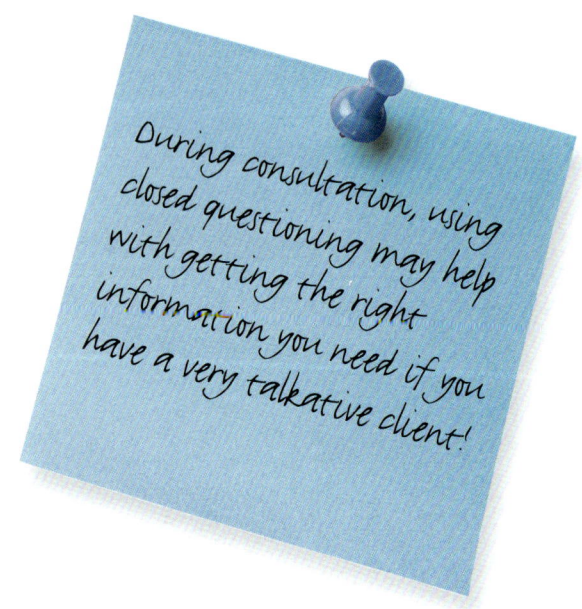

During consultation, using closed questioning may help with getting the right information you need if you have a very talkative client!

Comment form
Unit 303 Client care and communication in beauty-related industries

This form can be used to record comments by you, your client, or your assessor.

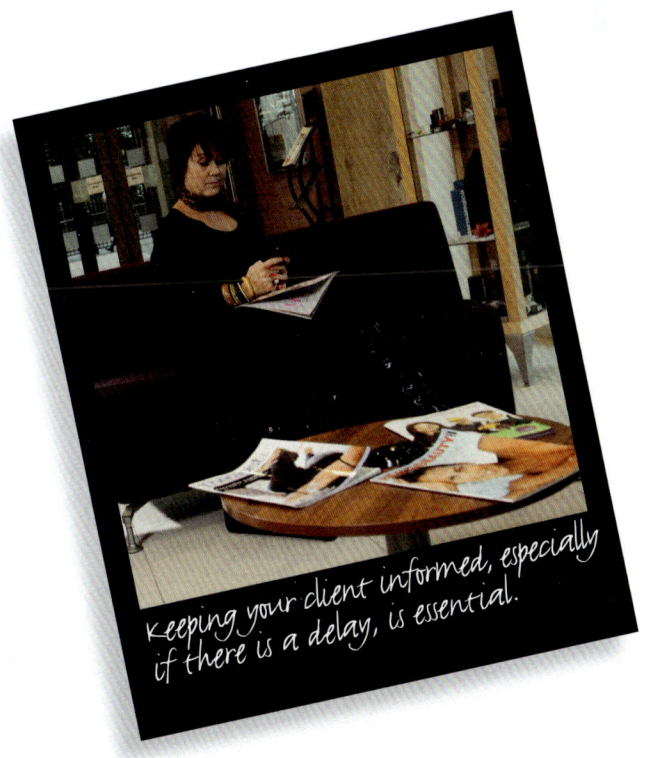

Keeping your client informed, especially if there is a delay, is essential.

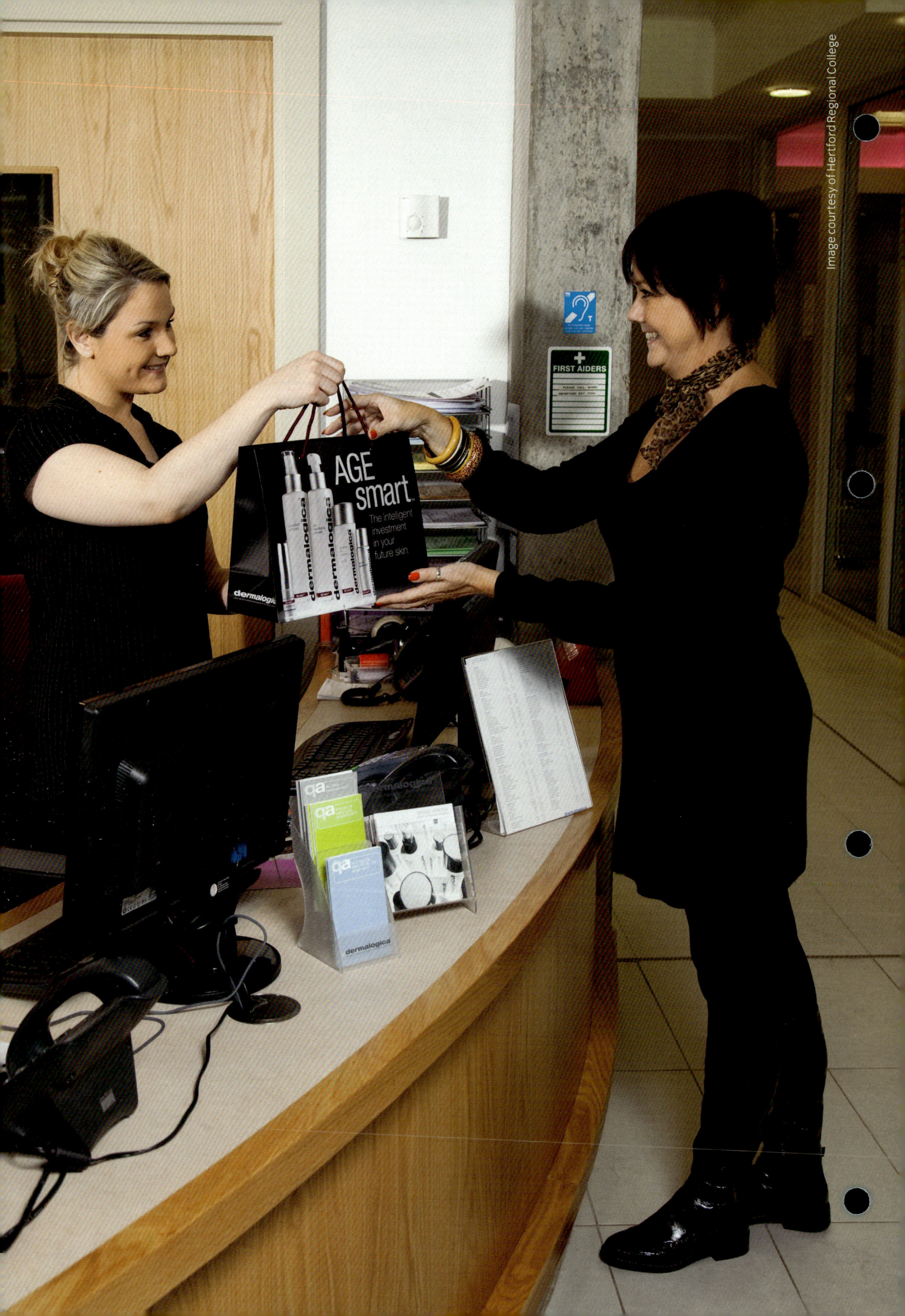

304

Promote and sell products and services to clients

Lots of people are frightened of selling, usually because they see it as being 'pushy'. This unit will help you to gain confidence by looking differently at the art of selling. You will be taken through the stages of the sales process, and how client objections can be viewed as buying signals. The ability to sell is a real asset and will increase your income and skill set. If done properly, the products and treatments you sell to clients will improve their experience, making them view you as a trusted and professional expert!

Assignment mark sheet
Unit 304 Promote and sell products and services to clients

Your assessor will mark you on each of the practical tasks in this unit. This page is used to work out your overall grade for the unit. You must pass **all** parts of the tasks to be able to achieve a grade. For each completed practical task, a pass equals 1 point, a merit equals 2 points and a distinction equals 3 points.

What you must know	Tick when complete
Task 1a: produce a report	
Task 1b: produce an information sheet	
Or tick if covered by an online test	

What you must do	Grade	Points
Task 2a: New products/services		
Task 2b: Products/services already used by client		

Conversion chart

Grade	Points
Pass	1–1.5
Merit	1.6–2.5
Distinction	2.6–3

	Points
Total points for graded tasks	
Divided by	÷ 2
= Average grade for tasks	
Overall grade (see conversion chart)	

Candidate name:

Candidate signature: Date:

Assessor signature: Date:

Quality assurance co-ordinator signature (where applicable): Date:

External Verifier signature (where applicable): Date:

What does it mean?
Some useful words are explained below

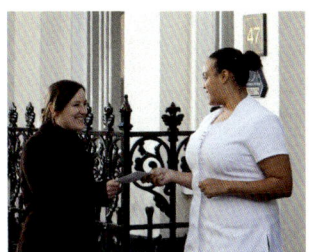

Advertising
Forms of communication with the purpose of persuading the client to buy.

Body language
Non-verbal communication, for example gestures, facial expressions, eye contact and postures. This is useful to use when selling, to inspire trust in the client. Also be aware of the client's body language, to gauge what they are thinking.

Buying signal
A comment from a client, which indicates that they are thinking about buying your product or service. The most common buying signal is the question: 'How much is it?'. Others are questions or comments such as: 'What sizes does it come in?'. Surprisingly, 'It's too expensive' or 'I already have a similar product at home' are also buying signals!

Closed question
A question that generally prompts an answer of either 'yes' or 'no'.

Closing the sale
Gaining agreement from the client to buy.

Communication
The giving and receiving of, and responding to, information.

Consumer
The client buying the treatment, service or product.

Data Protection Act
The law that states how an individual's information should be processed and stored, and who is allowed access to it.

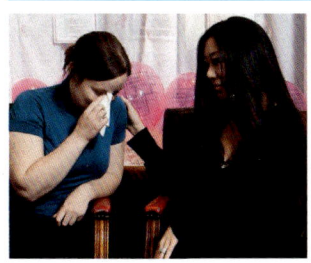

Empathy
Understanding how another person feels, and reflecting this back to the other person.

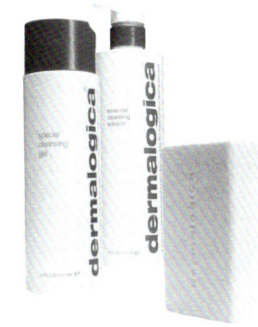

FABs
This stands for Features, Advantages, and Benefits and relates to the links between a product's description, its advantages over others, and the benefit the customer will get from using it.

Feedback
Information and evaluation of a process, activity or performance.

Objection/overcoming objections
An objection can be seen as the client putting up resistance to buying the product. A good sales person will be able to recognise if the objection is valid, and so close the discussion, or if the client just needs reassurance, in which case they will convince the client that they are doing the right thing by buying it.

Open question
A question that gains information, usually beginning with 'who', 'what', 'why', 'where', 'when', or 'how'.

Presentation/sales presentation
The process of explaining the product or service to the client, ideally including the product's features, advantages and benefits.

Prices Act
The law that deals with how goods are priced and marked.

Rapport
A relationship of understanding, trust and agreement between two or more people.

Target/sales target
The agreed level of sales to be made over a given period.

Trade Descriptions Act
The law that states that what is being sold must have an accurate description.

USP
This stands for Unique Selling Point. A USP is what makes the product better than others.

> **Revision tip**
> Know your products! Clients won't be convinced that something is right for them if you have to go and check the details.

What you must know
You must be able to:

1. Explain the benefits to the salon of promoting services and products to the client
2. Explain the importance of product and service knowledge when selling
3. Explain communication techniques used to promote products and services
4. Explain the differences between the terms 'features' and 'benefits'
5. Describe the stages of the sale process
6. Describe how to manage client expectations
7. Explain how to interpret buying signals
8. Explain the legislation that affects the selling of services or products
9. Explain the importance of reviewing selling techniques
10. Explain different methods of evaluating selling techniques
11. Describe how to implement improvements in your own selling techniques
12. Evaluate the effectiveness of advertising services and products to a target audience
13. Explain the importance of how to set and agree sales target/objectives

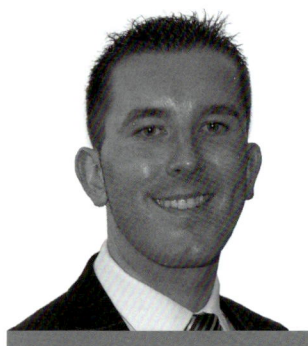

Follow in the footsteps of… *Matt Taylor*

Matt owns the Matthew Taylor Skin, Health & Body Therapy treatment rooms in Barnsley, South Yorkshire. He studied Beauty Therapy to Level 3 at Dearne Valley College, winning both the college's and the Dermalogica Student of the Year awards. Matt is a results-driven therapist who wants his clients to be happy every single time they visit his salon. He also wants men considering a career in the beauty industry to be inspired by his success. He believes that with passion and positivity, you can achieve your goals. Read on for Matt's top tips!

> **Revision tip**
> Make sure you understand the legislation involved in the selling process. These are legal requirements and ignoring them can result in heavy fines, or even imprisonment.

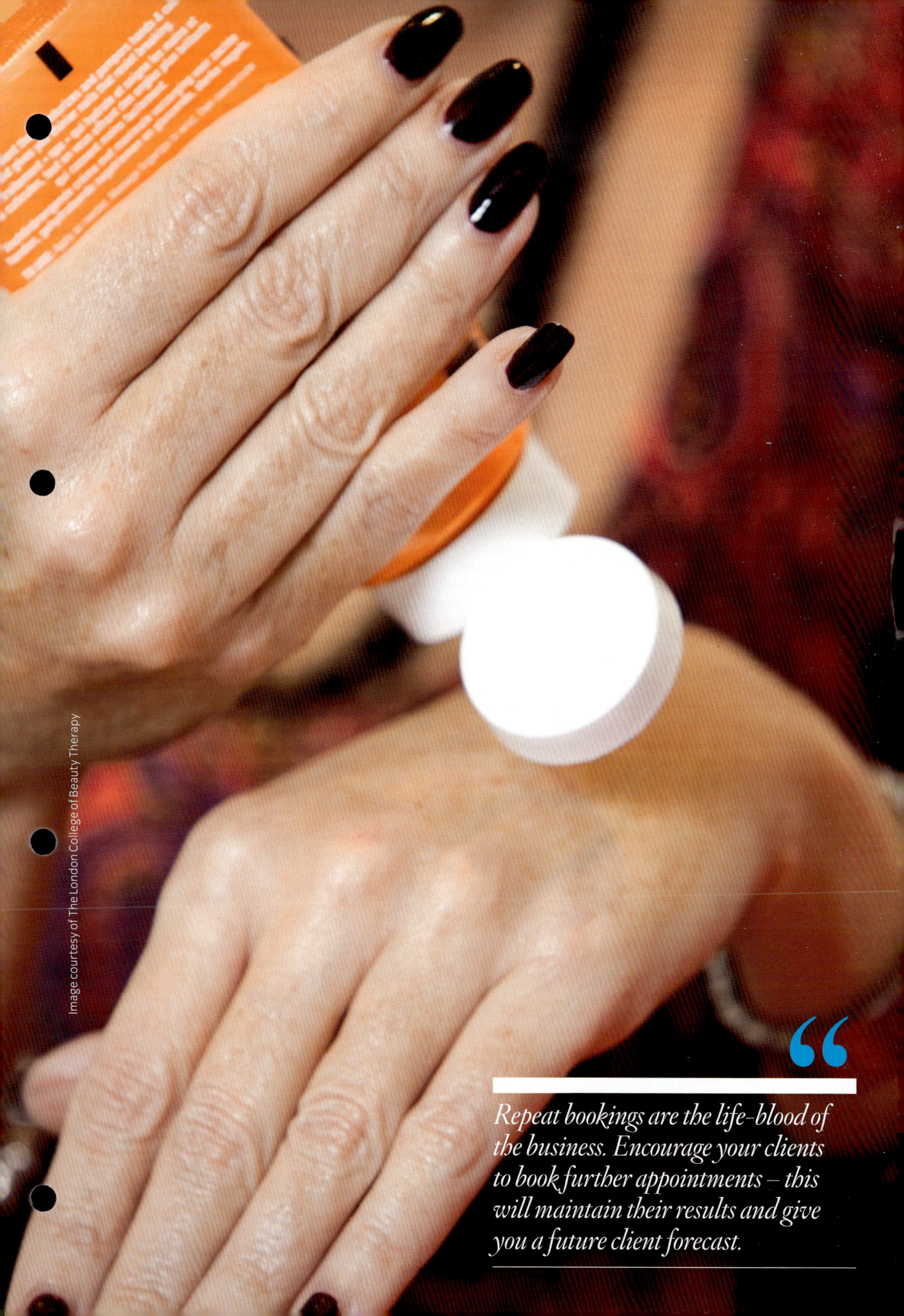

Image courtesy of The London College of Beauty Therapy

> "Repeat bookings are the life-blood of the business. Encourage your clients to book further appointments – this will maintain their results and give you a future client forecast.

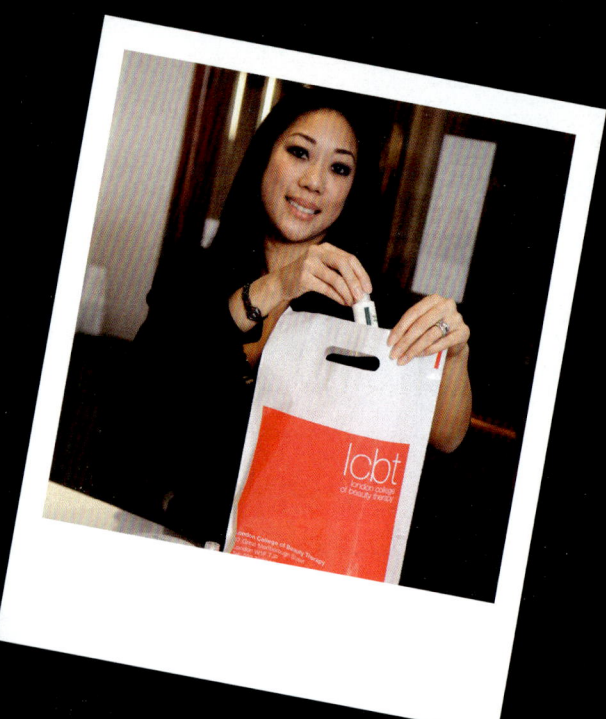

" Build up excellent rapport and trust with your clients. They will be more likely to book further treatments with you and purchase your product recommendations.

Promote

Believe in what you are selling! Whether it's a product or a treatment, why would your client want it, if you don't get excited about it?

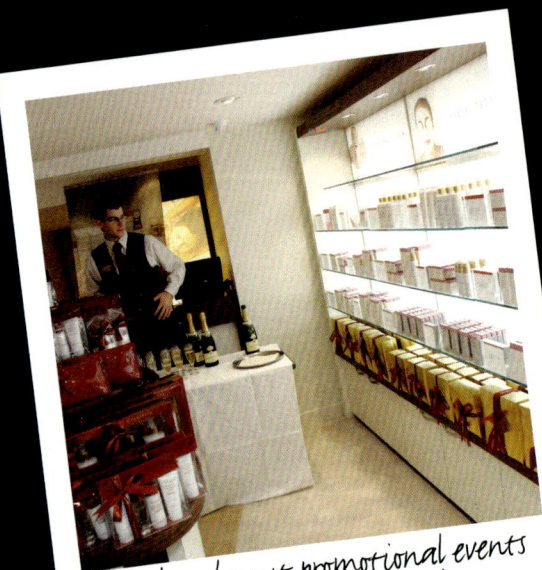

Well thought out promotional events increase sales, revenue and the client base.

The correct timing and use of questions is very important when gathering information, matching needs, and building rapport and empathy.

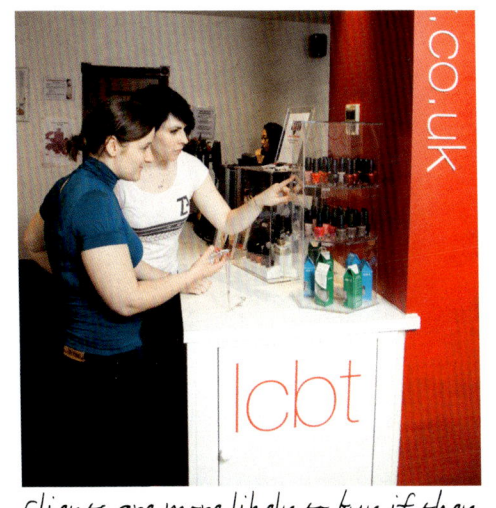

Clients are more likely to buy if they can see the product whilst you are talking about it.

and sell

" Clients don't just buy treatments, they buy time with you. Be sure to be the best therapist you can possibly be.

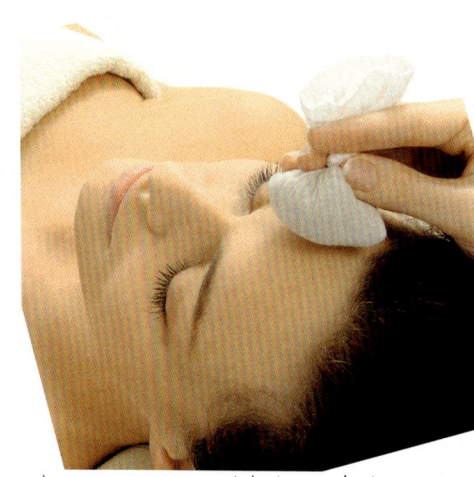

Clients are more likely to book in for unusual treatments if you explain their benefits.

What you must do
Practical observations

This page shows what you need to do during your practical task. You can look at it beforehand, but you're **not** allowed to have it with you while carrying out your practical task. You must achieve **all** the criteria; you can achieve 1 mark, 2 marks or 3 marks for the criteria indicated with *.

Conversion chart

Grade	Marks
Pass	7–8
Merit	9–12
Distinction	13–15

	Promote and sell					
	New products and/or services			Products and/or services already used by client		
1 Establish client's requirements	1			1		
2 Identify products and/or services to meet the requirements of the client *	1	2	3	1	2	3
3 Use effective communication techniques *	1	2	3	1	2	3
4 Introduce services and/or products to the client	1			1		
5 Give accurate and relevant information to ensure realistic client expectations *	1	2	3	1	2	3
6 Identify buying signals and interpret the client's intentions correctly *	1	2	3	1	2	3
7 Close the sale	1			1		
Total						
Grade						
Candidate signature and date						
Assessor signature and date						

> *Use the products and treatments you are selling. First-hand recommendations are the most convincing.*

What you must do
Practical observations descriptors table

This table shows what you need to do to achieve 1, 2 or 3 marks for the criteria indicated with * on the previous page.

	1 mark	2 marks	3 marks
2 Identify products and/or services to meet the requirements of the client	Correctly identified the main feature and benefit of the product(s) or service(s).	Correctly identified two main features and benefits of the product(s) or service(s).	Correctly identified all features and benefits of the product(s) or service(s).
3 Use effective communication techniques	Uses suitable open and/or closed questions and listening techniques.	Uses suitable open and/or closed questions and listening techniques, positive body language (eye contact and facial expression) and is polite to the client.	Uses suitable open and/or closed questions and listening techniques, positive body language (eye contact and facial expression), is polite to the client, uses visual aids and client records (where applicable), adapts the terminology to client's level of understanding and tone of voice to encourage the client to buy, presents a confident manner.
5 Give accurate and relevant information to ensure realistic client expectations	Gives basic information and advice Example: describes the main feature or use of the suitable product or service and how it can benefit the client.	Gives good information and advice Example: describes two main features or uses of suitable product or service and how each can benefit the client.	Detailed information and advice given Example: describes two main features and uses of suitable product or service with clear relevant links made to the client's own needs and requirements, ensure client understanding by inviting questions.

Continues on next page

What you must do
Practical observations descriptors table (continued)

This table shows what you need to do to achieve 1, 2 or 3 marks for the criteria indicated with * on page 50.

	1 mark	2 marks	3 marks
6 Identify buying signals and interpret the client's intentions correctly	Main buying signal and client's intentions are identified correctly. Example: verbal clue (eg the client asks about/comments on the product/service).	Two buying signals and client's intentions are identified correctly. Example: two clues (eg the client asks about/comments on the product/service, body language, handling the product).	Four or more buying signals and client's intentions are identified correctly. Example: clues (eg the client asks about/comments on the product/service, body language, handling the product, client talking as though product is already theirs, or about future treatments).

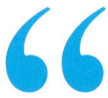

Selling home care products isn't all about making money – it's also about your client maintaining the great treatment results you've just achieved.

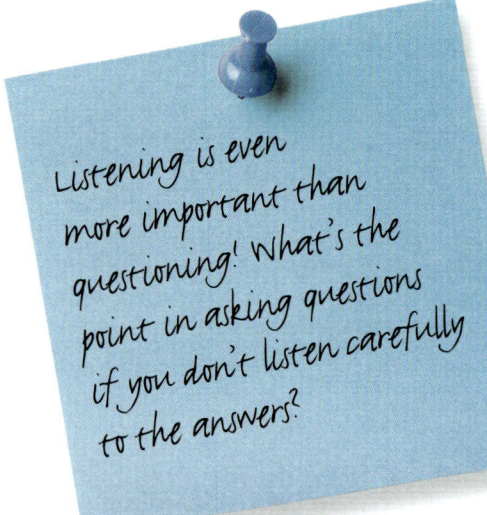

Listening is even more important than questioning! What's the point in asking questions if you don't listen carefully to the answers?

Comment form
Unit 304 Promote and sell products and services to clients

This form can be used to record comments by you, your client, or your assessor.

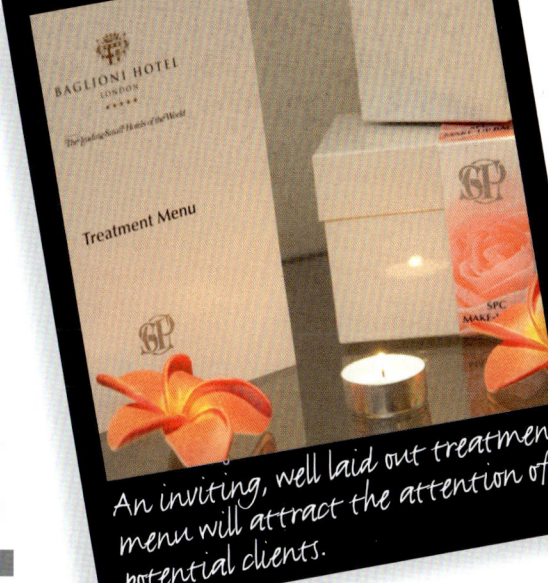

An inviting, well laid out treatment menu will attract the attention of potential clients.

> " *If a client decides not to buy a product you've recommended, give them a sample to try at home. They often return to buy once they've tried it for themselves and discovered how good it is.*

Image courtesy of Baglioni Spa by SPC (www.baglionispa.co.uk)

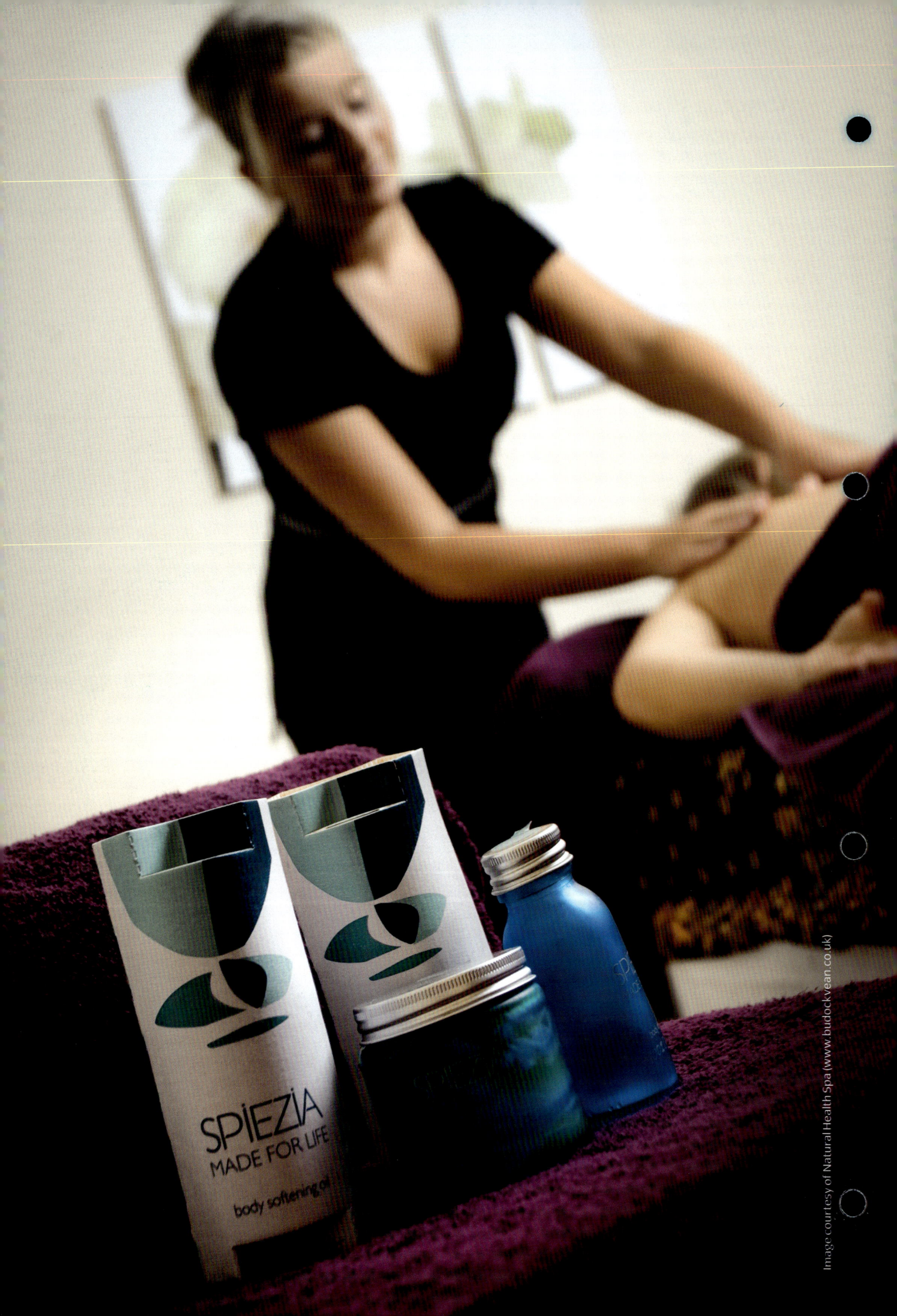

305

Provide body massage

Body massage is an ancient method of maintaining and promoting health and wellbeing. It can be physically demanding to carry out, but it can be extremely rewarding to feel your client relaxing as the massage progresses. In this unit, you will learn how to choose the correct products to suit the client, and which techniques will best meet their needs. You will also learn about the body and how its systems work. The use of infra-red and mechanical massage are also covered to give you a really broad knowledge base from which you can tailor the best possible treatment.

Assignment mark sheet
Unit 305 Provide body massage

Your assessor will mark you on each of the practical tasks in this unit. This page is used to work out your overall grade for the unit. You must pass **all** parts of the tasks to be able to achieve a grade. For each completed practical task, a pass equals 1 point, a merit equals 2 points and a distinction equals 3 points.

What you must know	Tick when complete
Task 1a: produce an information sheet	
Task 1b: produce a chart	
Task 1c: produce a fact sheet	
Task 1d: produce a fact sheet	
Task 1e: anatomy and physiology	
Or tick if covered by an online test	

What you must do	Grade	Points
Task 2: Provide body massage		

Overall grade

Candidate name:

Candidate signature: Date:

Assessor signature: Date:

Quality assurance co-ordinator signature   Date:
(where applicable):

External Verifier signature   Date:
(where applicable):

Don't work too deeply on knotted muscles at first. It's more relaxing for the client if you warm the muscles by using gentle movements and then slowly increase the pressure on tense muscles.

What does it mean?
Some useful words are explained below

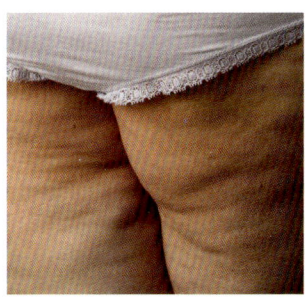

Cellulite
Congested tissue with a dimply 'orange peel' appearance. It is usually cold to the touch and commonly found on the thighs and buttocks.

Ectomorph
A long slender body type, this frame finds it hard to put on weight or muscle.

Effleurage
A stroking technique used to begin the massage and complete an area. It is also useful to link movements to provide flow and rhythm in the massage.

Endomorph
With this body type, the limbs tend to be short, and the hips wider than the shoulders. Weight gain may be a problem.

Infra-red lamp
A lamp producing infra-red light waves, which penetrate beyond the epidermis, used during the massage to warm and relax the client's skin and muscles.

Kyphosis
A postural condition where the upper thoracic area of the spine curves forward, rounding the shoulders and causing the head to 'poke' forward.

Lethargy
A feeling of tiredness and indifference.

Lordosis
A postural condition where the lower lumbar region of the spine curves in causing a 'hollow' back and the buttocks and abdomen to protrude.

Mechanical massage
A method of massage using a machine with interchangeable heads, giving a deeper effect than that which can be given manually.

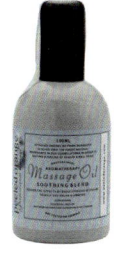

Medium
The product that is used to carry out a massage in order to provide slip and glide, eg oil/cream.

Mesomorph
With this body type, the client has narrow hips compared to their shoulders and muscle tone is usually well developed.

Petrissage
A technique that compresses the tissues of the body and lifts them away from the underlying structures.

Scoliosis
A sideways curvature to the spine, which can result in uneven hip and shoulder height.

Tapotement/percussion
A rhythmic movement performed to stimulate the skin and muscle tissues.

Treatment objective
The desired outcome of the massage, eg relaxation.

Vibrations
Fine trembling movements that can stimulate or relax nerves depending on how they are applied.

Revision tip

If you remember what each of the massage movements does, it will make it easier for you to decide which ones will be the best to meet your client's needs.

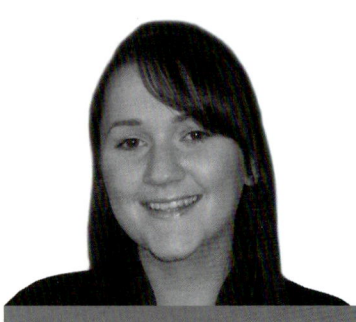

Follow in the footsteps of...
Stephanie Pedrini

I am currently studying VRQ Level 3 Beauty Therapy at Bournemouth and Poole College. I have always had an interest in beauty therapy, enjoying the practical element as well as the opportunity to meet, treat and help new people on a daily basis. Last year I completed four weeks of work experience in two top UK spas, 'Senspa' and 'Chewton Glen Spa'.

In the future I hope to work within the spa environment or travel whilst working on cruise ships, eventually leading to setting up my own business within the industry. Read the blue quotes for Stephanie's handy hints!

What you must know
You must be able to:

1. Describe salon requirements for preparing yourself, the client and work area
2. Describe the environmental conditions suitable for body massage treatments
3. Describe the different consultation techniques used to identify treatment objectives
4. Describe how to select products and tools to suit client treatment needs, skin types and conditions
5. Describe the different skin types and conditions
6. Explain the contra-indications that prevent or restrict body massage treatments
7. State the objectives of massage treatments
8. State the benefits derived from massage treatments
9. Identify general body types
10. Describe the different types of body fat
11. Outline common postural faults
12. Explain how to communicate and behave in a professional manner
13. Describe health and safety working practices
14. Explain the importance of positioning yourself and the client correctly throughout the treatment
15. Explain the importance of using products, tools and techniques to suit client's treatment needs, skin types and conditions

Continues on next page

16 Describe the benefits and uses of mechanical massage and pre-heat treatments

17 Describe how treatments can be adapted to suit client treatment needs, skin types and conditions

18 State the contra-actions that may occur during and following treatments and how to respond

19 Explain the importance of completing the treatment to the satisfaction of the client

20 Explain the importance of completing treatment records

21 Describe the methods of evaluating the effectiveness of the treatment

22 Describe the aftercare advice that should be provided

23 Describe the structure and the main functions of the following body systems in relation to massage:
- skin
- skeletal
- muscular
- cardio-vascular
- lymphatic
- nervous
- digestive
- urinary
- endocrine

24 Describe the main diseases and disorders of body systems

25 Describe the effects of massage on the body

26 Describe the uses of the five classical massage movements

27 Describe the uses of different massage mediums

28 Describe the legislation relating to the provision of massage treatments

> The infra-red lamp is really useful to use when a client has tight, tense muscles which need warming up in order to fully benefit from the massage.

> *The client's modesty should be respected at all times and every effort should be made to ensure the client is at ease and relaxed in the therapist's presence. This can easily be achieved by small gestures such as a smile, eye contact, care and understanding.*

Revision tip

Remember the uses of the different types of medium, so you can select what is most suitable for your client's needs.

> *Before giving a body massage and throughout the treatment, stay 'grounded' to prevent dizziness.*

Mas

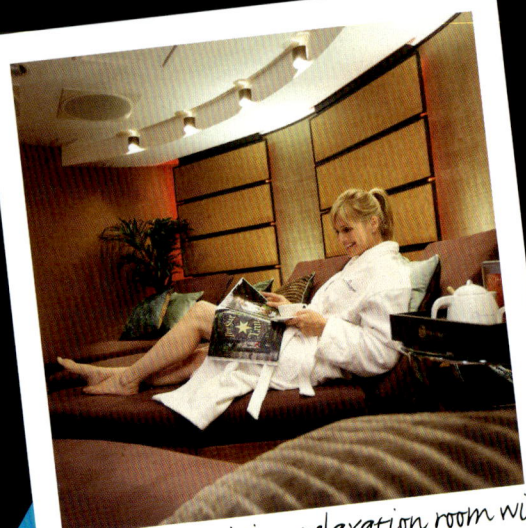

A warm, inviting relaxation room will help the client stay relaxed even after their treatment.

Concentrate on your client during the massage. It helps you to provide a better massage if you can focus on the way the client's muscle, fat and skin tissue react to the movements.

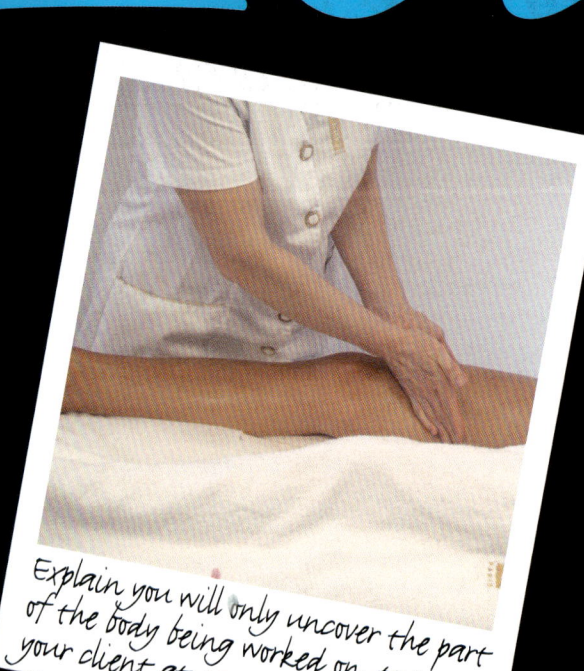

Explain you will only uncover the part of the body being worked on, to put your client at ease.

You may wish to add specialised techniques to your training.

> To make a body massage more personal, make sure you ask the client if they are warm enough and comfortable. Once started, ask if the pressure is to their liking and adapt the treatment if not.

ssage

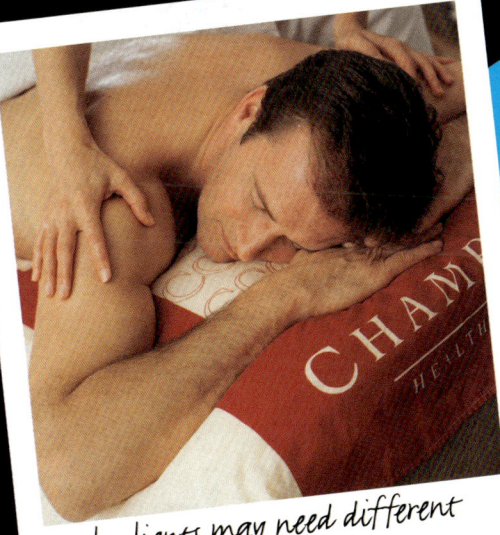

Male clients may need different pressures and mediums from female clients.

What you must do
Practical observations

This page shows what you need to do during your practical task. You can look at it beforehand, but you're **not** allowed to have it with you while carrying out your practical task. You must achieve **all** the criteria; you can achieve 1 mark, 2 marks or 3 marks for the criteria indicated with *.

Conversion chart

Grade	Marks
Pass	13–15
Merit	16–21
Distinction	22–25

○ Please tick when all pre-observation requirements have been met

	Provide body massage		
1 Prepare yourself, client and work area for body massage treatment	1		
2 Use suitable consultation techniques to identify treatment objectives *	1	2	3
3 Carry out a body analysis *	1	2	3
4 Advise the client how to prepare for the treatment	1		
5 Provide clear recommendations to the client *	1	2	3
6 Position yourself and the client correctly throughout the treatment	1		
7 Follow health and safety working practices	1		
8 Communicate and behave in a professional manner	1		
9 Apply and use massage medium to suit client's skin type and conditions	1		
10 Use and adapt massage techniques correctly to suit client treatment needs *	1	2	3
11 Complete the treatment to the satisfaction of the client *	1	2	3
12 Record and evaluate the results of the treatment	1		
13 Provide suitable aftercare advice *	1	2	3

Total

Grade

Candidate signature and date

Assessor signature and date

Unit 305 Level 3 VRQ Beauty Therapy

What you must do
Practical observations descriptors table

This table shows what you need to do to achieve 1, 2 or 3 marks for the criteria indicated with * on the previous page.

	1 mark	2 marks	3 marks
2 Use suitable consultation techniques to identify treatment objectives	Basic consultation Examples: uses open and closed questions, checks for contra-indications, identifies the treatment objectives correctly.	Good consultation Examples: positive body language, uses open and closed questions to identify contra-indications, general health, lifestyle and expectations; identifies the treatment objectives and any factors that may limit or restrict the treatment.	Thorough consultation Examples: positive body language, uses open and closed questions to identify contra-indications, general health, lifestyle and expectations, how client feels about their body and what improvement they would like to achieve; identifies the treatment objectives and any factors that may limit or restrict the treatment, allows the client to ask any questions to confirm understanding.
3 Carry out a body analysis	Carries out a basic analysis, identifies client's posture, records findings.	Carries out a good analysis, identifies client's posture and any figure faults, body and skin type, records findings.	Carries out a detailed analysis, identifies client's posture and any figure faults, body type, and skin type and condition (ie soft fat, hard fat, cellulite), records findings.

Continues on next page

Provide body massage Unit 305

What you must do
Practical observations descriptors table (continued)

This table shows what you need to do to achieve 1, 2 or 3 marks for the criteria indicated with * on page 62.

	1 mark	2 marks	3 marks
5 Provide clear recommendations to the client	A basic treatment plan is recommended. Example: explains treatment procedure and any adaptations to meet client treatment needs.	A good treatment plan is recommended. Example: explains treatment procedure and any adaptations to meet client treatment needs based on factors identified during consultation (lifestyle, medication (if any), contra-indications, results of postural diagnosis), a choice of products to be used.	A thorough treatment plan is recommended. Example: explains treatment procedure and any adaptations to meet client treatment needs based on factors identified during consultation (lifestyle, medication (if any), contra-indications, results of postural diagnosis), a choice of products to be used, adaptation of massage movements to suit client treatment needs, allows the client to ask questions about the treatment plan.
10 Use and adapt massage techniques correctly to suit client treatment needs	Adapts the massage routine to suit client treatment objectives. Uses a variety of movements, movements are even and flowing, uses appropriate pressure for the client.	Adapts the massage routine to suit client treatment objectives, muscle and fat type. Carries out massage movements correctly and fully with even flow showing variations in rate and rhythm according to treatment objectives, uses appropriate pressure for the client.	Adapts the massage routine to suit client treatment objectives, muscle and fat type, taking into account findings of the postural diagnosis. The whole routine flows throughout, uses appropriate pressure for the client, checks the client's comfort and wellbeing at appropriate times.

Continues on next page

	1 mark	2 marks	3 marks
11 Complete the treatment to the satisfaction of the client	The treatment is completed within the agreed time and brought to a satisfactory close.	The treatment is completed within the agreed time, brought to a satisfactory close, excess massage medium is removed from the skin correctly.	The treatment is completed within the agreed time, brought to a satisfactory close, excess massage medium is removed from the skin correctly, the client is asked for feedback and is allowed sufficient time to get dressed.
13 Provide suitable aftercare advice	Basic aftercare advice Examples: how to deal with possible contra-actions, product(s) to use, importance of rest and relaxation, future treatment needs.	Good level of aftercare advice Examples: how to deal with possible contra-actions, product(s) to use, importance of rest and relaxation, specific lifestyle advice (ie dealing with stress, fluid intake, healthy eating), future treatment needs.	Excellent aftercare advice Examples: how to deal with possible contra-actions, product(s) to use, importance of rest and relaxation, specific lifestyle advice (ie dealing with stress, fluid intake, healthy eating), postural awareness, recommends future treatment programme (regular massage, introduction of new/alternative treatments).

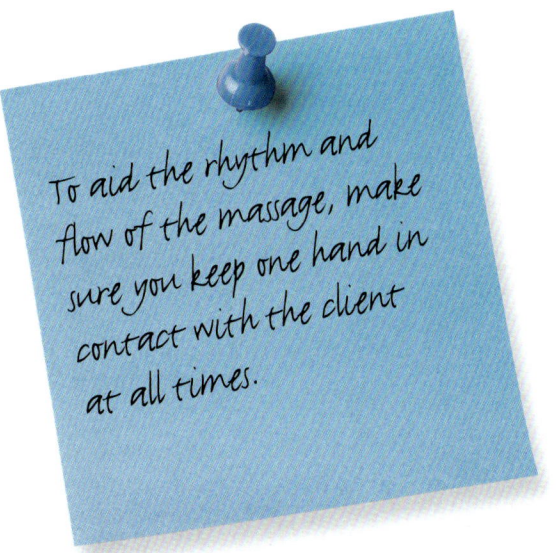

To aid the rhythm and flow of the massage, make sure you keep one hand in contact with the client at all times.

Comment form
Unit 305 Provide body massage

This form can be used to record comments by you, your client, or your assessor.

Clear and concise aftercare advice should be given to the client after a body massage so the full effects of the massage can be experienced. This will increase the chance of another treatment being booked.

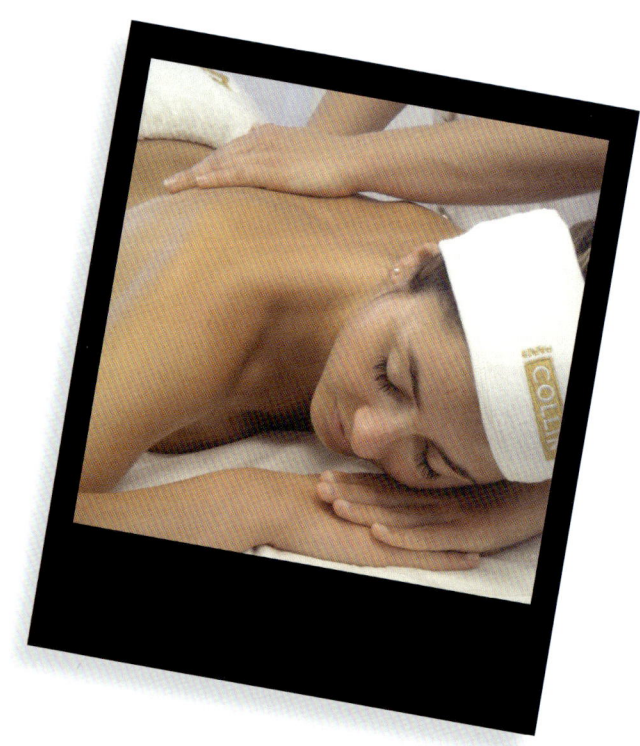

Image courtesy of Collin UK

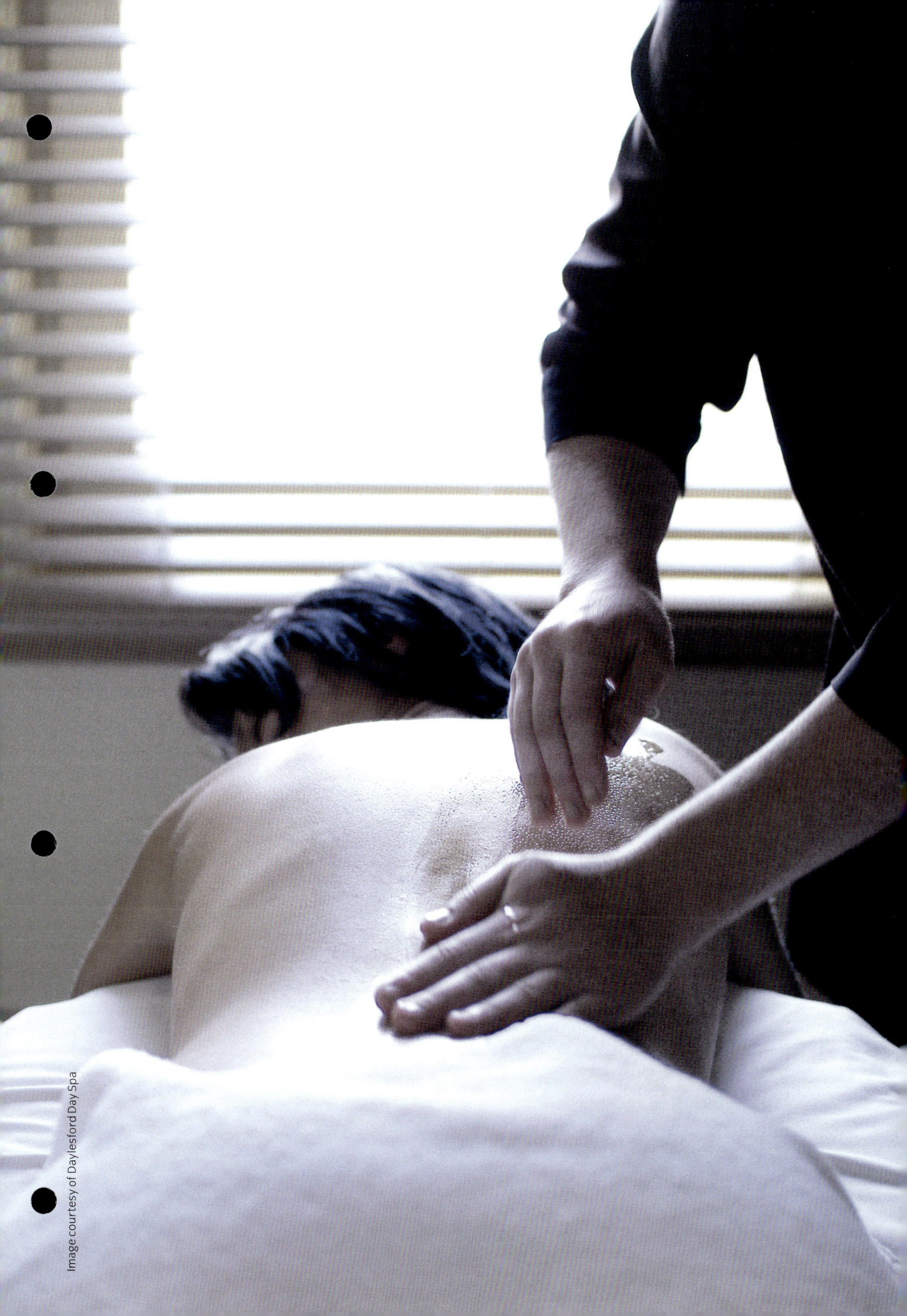

Image courtesy of Daylesford Day Spa

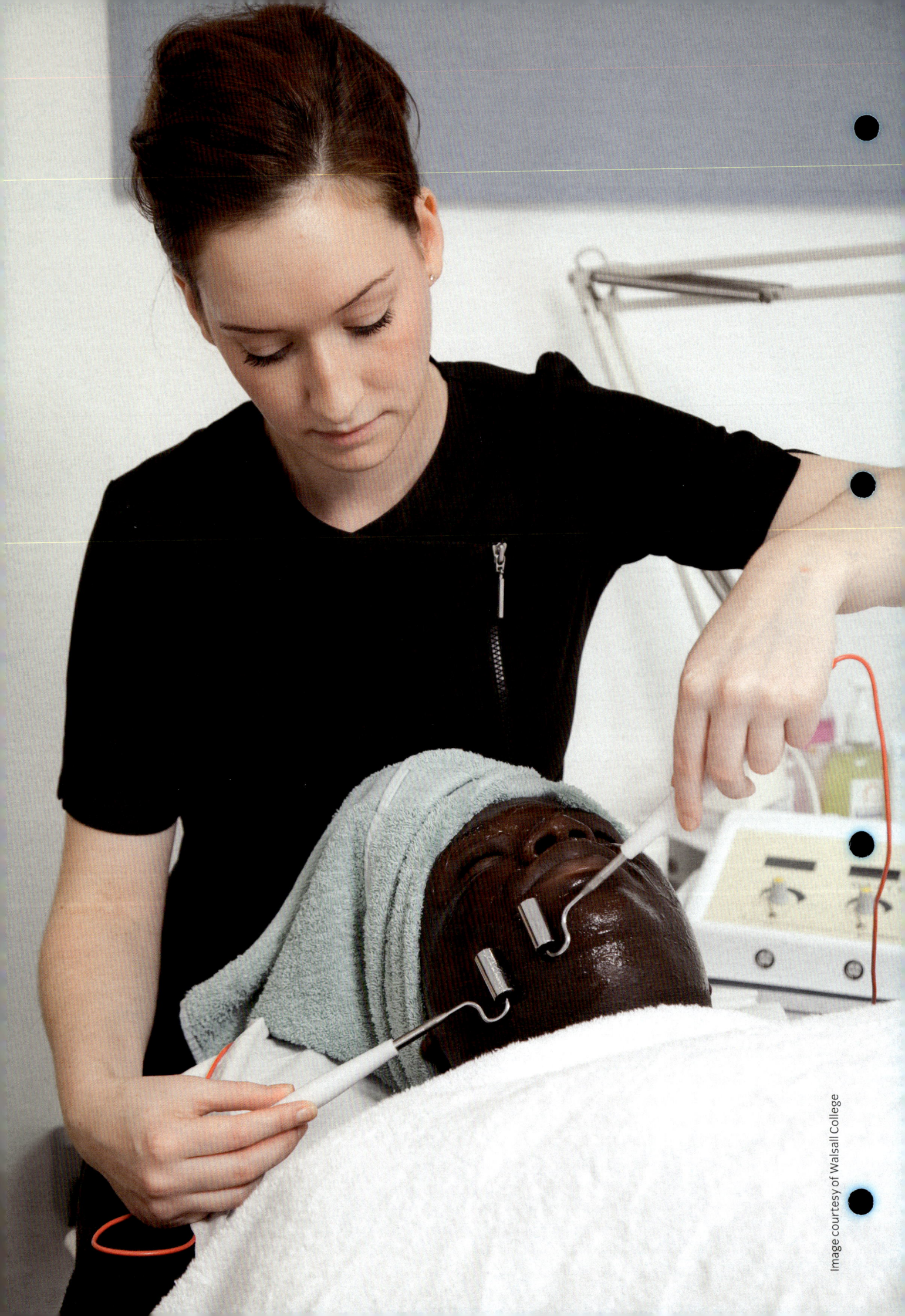

Image courtesy of Walsall College

306

Provide facial electrotherapy treatments

This is where skincare gets exciting! For those of you who are serious about improving your clients' skin, this unit will give you the knowledge, techniques and expertise to really make a difference. You will be able to provide a really deep cleanse for those with congestion and blackheads, and make dry, scaly skin dewy and soft. These treatments are a pleasure to receive, but as a bonus they are also very relaxing and therapeutic to give!

Assignment mark sheet
Unit 306 Provide facial electrotherapy treatments

Your assessor will mark you on each of the practical tasks in this unit. This page is used to work out your overall grade for the unit. You must pass **all** parts of the tasks to be able to achieve a grade. For each completed practical task, a pass equals 1 point, a merit equals 2 points and a distinction equals 3 points.

Conversion chart

Grade	Points
Pass	1–1.5
Merit	1.6–2.5
Distinction	2.6–3

What you must know	Tick when complete
Task 1a: produce an information sheet	
Task 1b: produce a chart	
Task 1c: produce a fact sheet	
Task 1d: anatomy and physiology	
Or tick if covered by an online test	

What you must do	Grade	Points
Task 2a: Treatment 1		
Task 2b: Treatment 2		
Task 2c: Treatment 3		
Task 2d: Treatment 4		

Total points for graded tasks	
Divided by	÷ 4
= Average grade for tasks	
Overall grade (see conversion chart)	

Candidate name:

Candidate signature: Date:

Assessor signature: Date:

Quality assurance co-ordinator signature (where applicable): Date:

External Verifier signature (where applicable): Date:

What does it mean?
Some useful words are explained below

Acid mantle
The layer of sebum and sweat on the skin's surface that provides lubrication and protects against bacteria.

Comedone
Commonly known as a blackhead, this is a plug of oxidised sebum in the opening of a pore or follicle.

Contra-indication
A condition that prevents treatment from taking place, or makes it necessary to modify the treatment.

Dehydrated skin
This is a lack of water or moisture within the skin as opposed to a lack of oil, and can occur on any skin type.

Desincrustation
A treatment using a negatively changed galvanic current to break down the acid mantle, soften keratin, dilate pores, and saponify sebum to make deep extraction work possible.

Direct high frequency
A treatment using ozone to control an oily, pustular or acnied skin.

EMS
This stands for electro muscle stimulator. It uses a faradic current to tighten and tone muscles, for a lifting, anti-ageing effect.

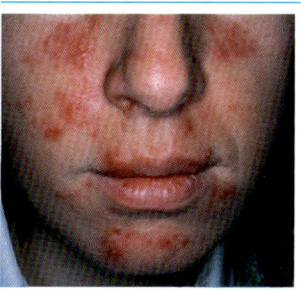

Erythema
Redness of the skin resulting from dilation of blood vessels, due to stimulation, irritation or allergy.

Faradic current
A direct, interrupted, surging current used in EMS to cause muscle contraction.

Galvanic current
A constant, direct current where the client forms part of the circuit, used in iontophoresis and desincrustation.

Impetigo
A bacterial skin infection where small blisters break open and then crust over to form honey-coloured scabs.

Indirect high frequency
This uses an alternating oscillating current, which flows through both the client and the therapist during facial massage to provide a warming and stimulating effect.

Iontophoresis
Uses a galvanic current to 'push' the selected product into the skin using a charged electrode.

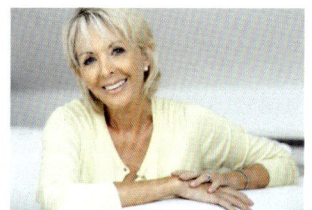

Mature skin
In beauty therapy terms, this is any skin over the age of 25. However, the skin is generally not classed as being mature until the signs of ageing are apparent.

Micro-current
Sometimes referred to as a non-surgical face lift. This treatment uses a low frequency current to re-educate the facial muscles and increase production of collagen and elastin.

Oxygenating cream/serum
A product used with direct high frequency (DHF) to improve and enhance its effects.

Ringworm
A contagious fungal infection where there are circles of red itchy skin, which heal from the centre.

Skin analysis
A careful assessment of the skin to determine its type and condition, taking into account contributory factors.

Skin type
A way of classifying the skin according to the amount of oil it produces. The skin types are: normal, dry, oily, and combination.

Sterilisation
The complete destruction of micro-organisms and their spores.

Vacuum suction
A treatment designed to stimulate lymphatic drainage, remove excess waste, reduce puffiness, and temporarily fill out fine lines and wrinkles.

> **Revision tip**
>
> A detailed skin analysis will allow you to choose the most appropriate treatment and products to improve and maintain the condition of the skin.

What you must know
You must be able to:

1. Describe salon requirements for preparing themselves, the client and work area
2. Describe the environmental conditions suitable for facial electrotherapy treatments
3. Describe the different consultation techniques used to identify treatment objectives
4. Explain the importance of carrying out a detailed skin analysis and relevant tests
5. Describe how to select products, tools and equipment to suit client treatment needs, skin types and conditions
6. Describe the different skin types, conditions and characteristics
7. Explain the contra-indications that prevent or restrict facial electrotherapy treatments
8. Explain how to communicate and behave in a professional manner
9. Describe health and safety working practices
10. Explain the importance of positioning themselves and the client correctly throughout the treatment
11. Explain the importance of using products, tools, equipment and techniques to suit client's treatment needs, skin type and conditions
12. Describe the effects and benefits of electrotherapy equipment and products on the skin and underlying structures

Continues on next page

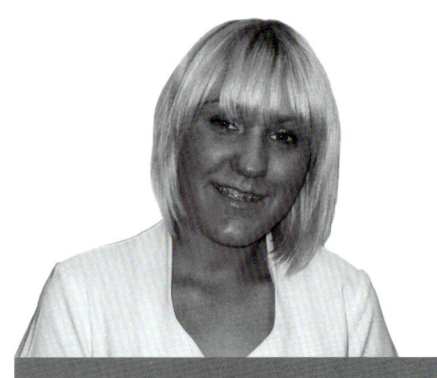

Follow in the footsteps of... *Alice O'Shea*

Alice is currently taking her Level 3 VRQ in Beauty Therapy at The London College of Beauty Therapy. Facial electrotherapy is her favourite treatment, because it gives such great results. As well as finishing her qualification, Alice loves working at the Caci Clinic. In the future Alice would like to do more training and one day open her very own Beauty salon. Read on for Alice's electrotherapy tips!

13. Explain the principles of electrical currents
14. Describe how treatments can be adapted to suit client treatment needs, skin types and conditions
15. State the contra-actions that may occur during and following treatments and how to respond
16. Explain the importance of completing the treatment to the satisfaction of the client
17. Explain the importance of completing treatment records
18. Describe the methods of evaluating the effectiveness of the treatment
19. Describe the aftercare advice that should be provided
20. Describe the structure, growth and repair of the skin
21. Describe skin types, conditions, diseases and disorders
22. Describe the structure, function, position and action of the head, neck and shoulder muscles
23. Describe the location, function and structure of the bones of the head, neck and shoulder
24. Describe the structure and function of the circulatory and lymphatic systems for the head, neck and shoulder
25. Explain how the ageing process, lifestyle and environmental factors affect the condition of skin and underlying structures

Revision tip

A dry skin will have small pores, with a matt appearance. It lacks sebum and so blemishes are rare, but the downside is that it is prone to ageing more than other skins.

Make sure you apply plenty of oil when using vacuum suction and that your vacuum is not set too high. This prevents bruising.

Facial

Modifying and adapting the treatment by altering the time, pressure, products and techniques to suit the client's skin on the day will show the best results and keep the client coming back.

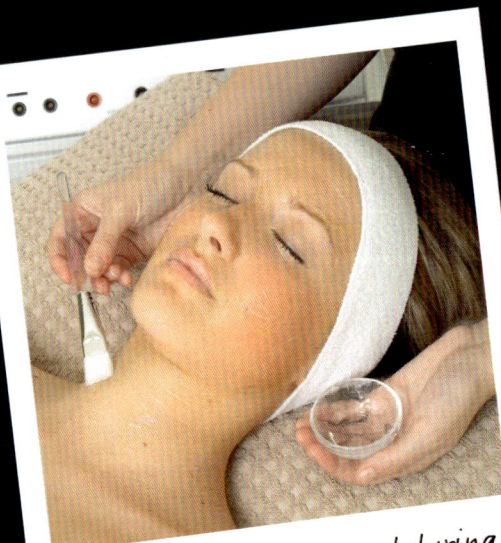

The specialised products used during electrotherapy support the action of the various currents.

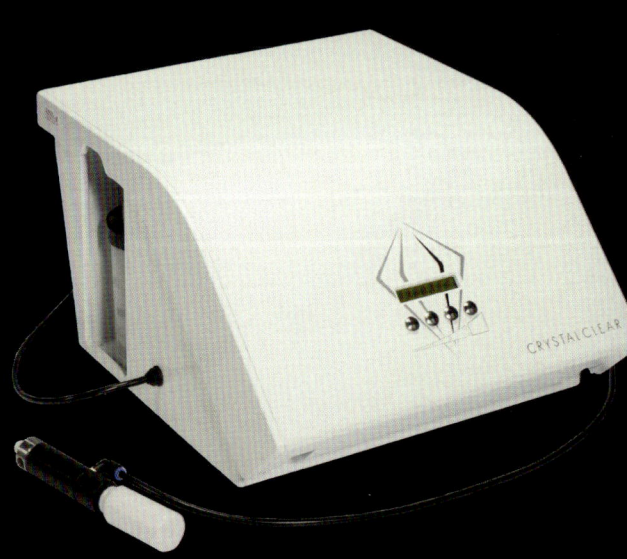

Include your client when planning the treatment. Finding out how the client feels about their skin, and what matters to them is as important as carrying out the visual skin analysis.

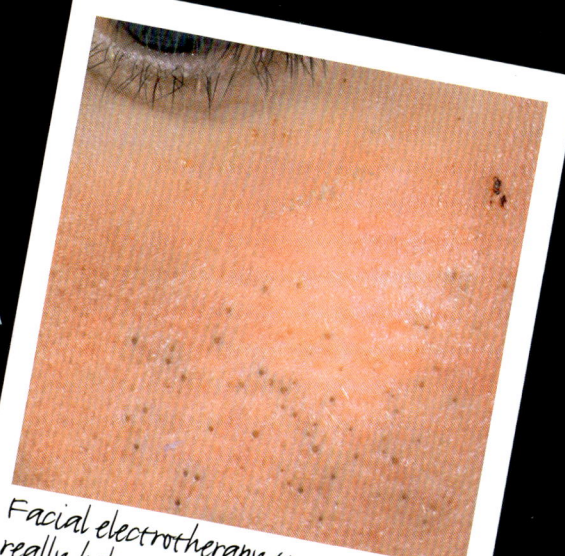

Facial electrotherapy treatments can really help treat comedones.

Electric

> " *Make sure you position yourself well and maintain a good posture throughout the treatment.*

Image courtesy of Science Photo Library

What you must do
Practical observations

This page shows what you need to do during your practical task. You can look at it beforehand, but you're **not** allowed to have it with you while carrying out your practical task. You must achieve **all** the criteria; you can achieve 1 mark, 2 marks or 3 marks for the criteria indicated with *.

Conversion chart

Grade	Marks
Pass	11–13
Merit	14–19
Distinction	20–23

○ Please tick when all pre-observation requirements have been met

	Provide a facial electrotherapy treatment											
	Treatment 1			Treatment 2			Treatment 3			Treatment 4		
State the electrotherapy chosen												
1 Prepare yourself, client and work area for facial electrotherapy treatment	1			1			1			1		
2 Use suitable consultation techniques to identify treatment objectives *	1	2	3	1	2	3	1	2	3	1	2	3
3 Carry out a skin analysis and relevant tests *	1	2	3	1	2	3	1	2	3	1	2	3
4 Provide clear recommendations to the client *	1	2	3	1	2	3	1	2	3	1	2	3
5 Position yourself and client correctly throughout the treatment	1			1			1			1		
6 Select and use products, tools, electrotherapy equipment and techniques to suit the client treatment needs, skin type and conditions *	1	2	3	1	2	3	1	2	3	1	2	3
7 Communicate and behave in a professional manner	1			1			1			1		
8 Follow health and safety working practices	1			1			1			1		
9 Complete the treatment to the satisfaction of the client *	1	2	3	1	2	3	1	2	3	1	2	3
10 Record and evaluate the results of the treatment	1			1			1			1		
11 Provide suitable aftercare advice *	1	2	3	1	2	3	1	2	3	1	2	3
Total												
Grade												
Candidate signature and date												
Assessor signature and date												

Unit 306 Level 3 VRQ Beauty Therapy

What you must do
Practical observations descriptors table

This table shows what you need to do to achieve 1, 2 or 3 marks for the criteria indicated with * on the previous page.

	1 mark	2 marks	3 marks
2 Use suitable consultation techniques to identify treatment objectives	Basic consultation Examples: uses open and closed questions, checks for contra-indications, identifies the treatment objectives correctly.	Good consultation Examples: positive body language, uses open and closed questions to identify contra-indications, general health, lifestyle and expectations; identifies the treatment objectives and any factors that may limit or restrict the treatment.	Thorough consultation Examples: positive body language, uses open and closed questions to identify contra-indications, general health, lifestyle and expectations, how client feels about their skin and what improvement they would like to achieve; identifies the treatment objectives and any factors that may limit or restrict the treatment, allows the client to ask any questions to confirm understanding.
3 Carry out a skin analysis and relevant tests	Skin cleansed, magnifier and light used. Some recording of skin characteristics.	Skin cleansed, magnifier and light used, good observations of skin characteristics recorded.	Skin is cleansed thoroughly, magnifier and light used, detailed observations of skin characteristics recorded.

Continues on next page

What you must do
Practical observations descriptors table (continued)

This table shows what you need to do to achieve 1, 2 or 3 marks for the criteria indicated with * on page 76.

	1 mark	2 marks	3 marks
4 Provide clear recommendations to the client	A basic treatment plan is recommended. Examples: explains treatment procedure and any adaptations to meet client treatment needs, equipment to be used.	A good treatment plan is recommended. Examples: explains treatment procedure and any adaptations to meet client treatment needs, equipment to be used based on factors identified during consultation (lifestyle, medication (if any), contra-indications, results of skin analysis), a choice of products to be used.	A thorough treatment plan is recommended. Examples: explains treatment procedure and any adaptations to meet client treatment needs, equipment to be used based on factors identified during consultation (lifestyle, medication (if any), contra-indications, results of skin analysis), a choice of products to be used, explains effects and benefits of the type of equipment used and the adaptation/modification to suit client treatment needs, allows the client to ask questions about the treatment plan.
6 Select and use products, tools, electrotherapy equipment and techniques to suit the client treatment needs, skin type and conditions	Selects and uses the correct equipment, tools, techniques and basic products based on factors identified in skin analysis.	Selects and uses the correct equipment, tools, techniques and a variety of products based on factors identified in skin analysis, explains effects and benefits of the products and equipment to the client as appropriate throughout.	Selects and uses the correct equipment, tools, techniques and a variety of products based on factors identified in skin analysis, explains effects and benefits of the products and equipment to the client as appropriate throughout, adapts and modifies the techniques used, explains the treatment to the client as appropriate throughout.

Continues on next page

	1 mark	2 marks	3 marks
9 Complete the treatment to the satisfaction of the client	The treatment is completed within the agreed time and brought to a satisfactory close.	The treatment is completed within the agreed time, brought to a satisfactory close and positive feedback is gained from the client.	The treatment is completed within the agreed time, brought to a satisfactory close and positive feedback is gained from the client, shows the client the results of the treatment and allows the client to ask questions.
11 Provide suitable aftercare advice	Basic aftercare advice Examples: how to deal with possible contra-actions, product(s) to use, future treatment needs.	Good level of aftercare advice Examples: how to deal with possible contra-actions, product(s) to use, specific advice (ie what to avoid immediately after the treatment, fluid intake, healthy eating), future treatment needs.	Excellent aftercare advice Examples: how to deal with possible contra-actions, product(s) to use, specific advice (ie what to avoid immediately after the treatment, fluid intake, healthy eating), recommends future treatment programme (regular treatments, introduction of new/alternative treatments).

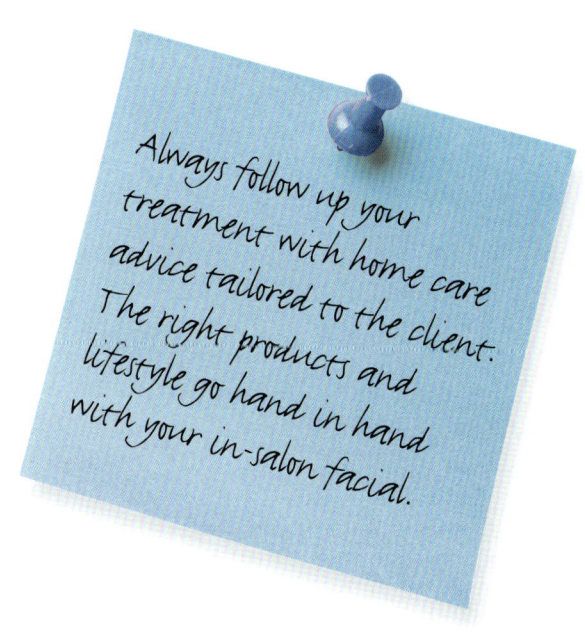

Always follow up your treatment with home care advice tailored to the client. The right products and lifestyle go hand in hand with your in-salon facial.

Comment form
Unit 306 Provide facial electrotherapy treatments

This form can be used to record comments by you, your client, or your assessor.

> *Apply enough gel during galvanic treatments and maintain contact with the client while turning the current up slowly.*

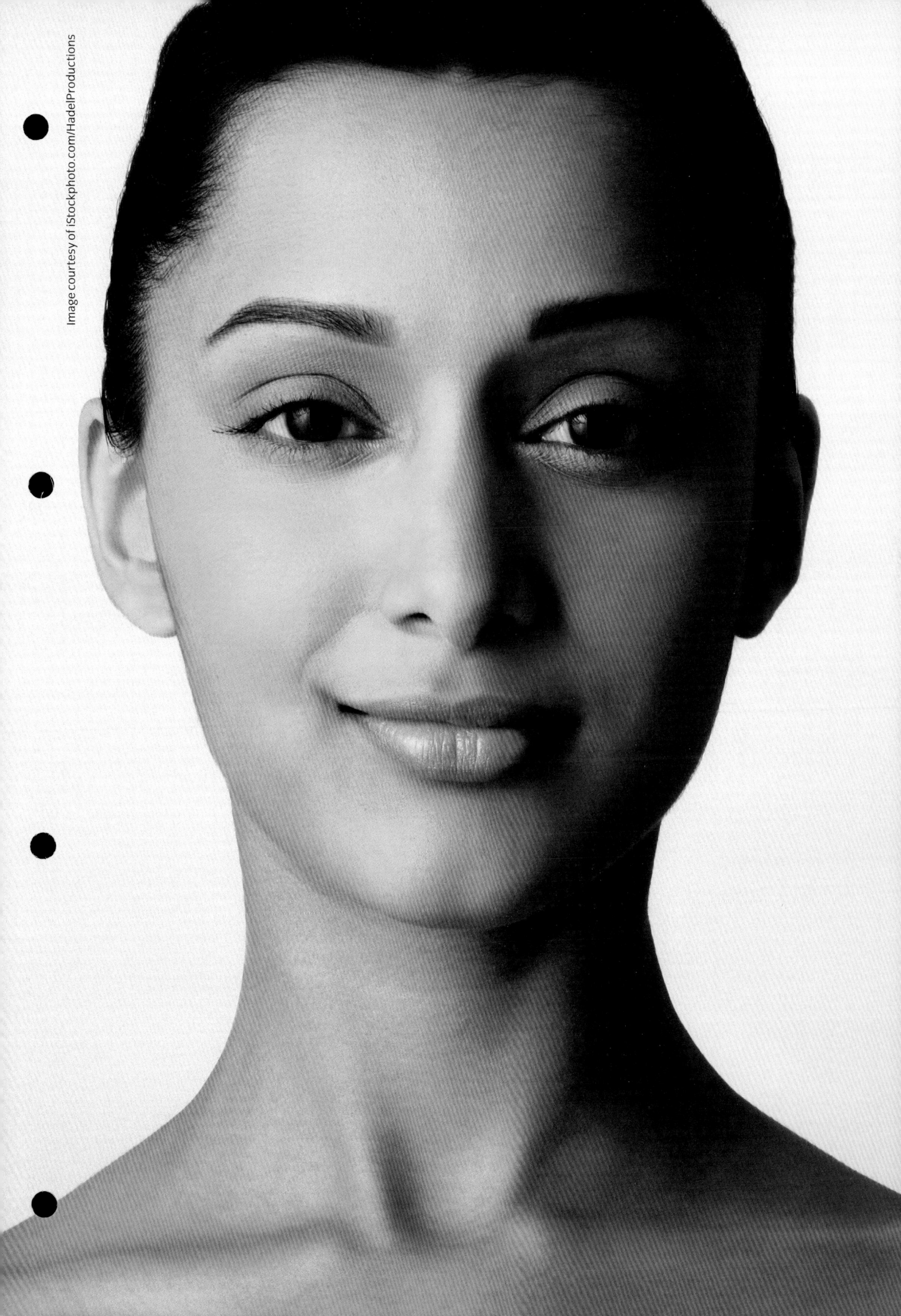

Image courtesy of iStockphoto.com/HadelProductions

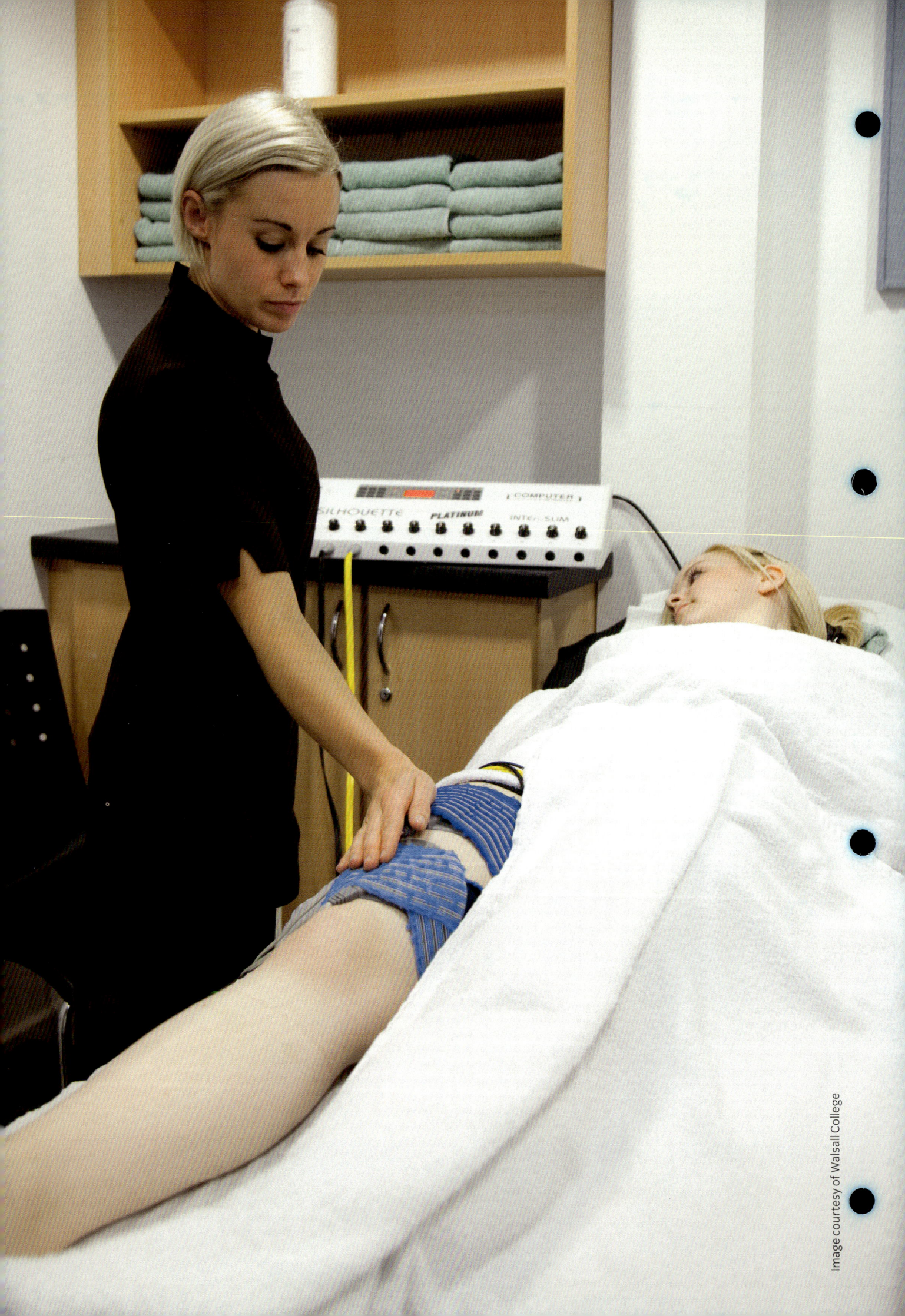

Image courtesy of Walsall College

307

Provide body electrotherapy treatments

As a beauty therapist, you will come across bodies of all shapes and sizes. Whether it's toning, firming, skin improvement, cellulite reduction or pure relaxation that your client wants, you will learn how to meet their needs in this unit. You'll find out how to diagnose their basic body type, in order to adapt how the treatment is carried out, but also to make sure a realistic outcome can be achieved. With your knowledge of the benefits and effects of body electrotherapy treatments, plus the home care and lifestyle advice that you will give them, your clients will be well on their way to getting the figure they want.

Assignment mark sheet
Unit 307 Provide body electrotherapy treatments

Your assessor will mark you on each of the practical tasks in this unit. This page is used to work out your overall grade for the unit. You must pass **all** parts of the tasks to be able to achieve a grade. For each completed practical task, a pass equals 1 point, a merit equals 2 points and a distinction equals 3 points.

Conversion chart

Grade	Points
Pass	1–1.5
Merit	1.6–2.5
Distinction	2.6–3

What you must know	Tick when complete
Task 1a: produce an information sheet	
Task 1b: produce a chart	
Task 1c: produce a fact sheet	
Task 1d: anatomy and physiology	
Or tick if covered by an online test	

What you must do	Grade	Points
Task 2a: Treatment 1		
Task 2b: Treatment 2		
Task 2c: Treatment 3		
Task 2d: Treatment 4		

Total points for graded tasks	
Divided by	÷ 4
= Average grade for tasks	
Overall grade (see conversion chart)	

Candidate name:

Candidate signature: Date:

Assessor signature: Date:

Quality assurance co-ordinator signature (where applicable):   Date:

External Verifier signature (where applicable):   Date:

What does it mean?
Some useful words are explained below

Adipose tissue
The layer of fat cells which lies beneath the dermis, otherwise known as the subcutaneous layer.

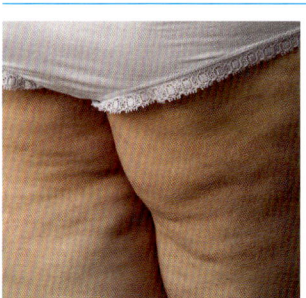

Cellulite
Congested tissue with a dimply 'orange peel' appearance. It is usually cold to the touch and found on the thighs and buttocks.

Contra-action
An undesirable outcome as a result of a treatment. Some of these cannot be helped and are a natural reaction, but others are the result of poor practice.

Deep vein thrombosis (DVT)
A blood clot in a deep vein. It commonly affects the leg veins such as the femoral or popliteal vein.

Direct high frequency
A treatment using ozone to control an oily, pustular or acnied back.

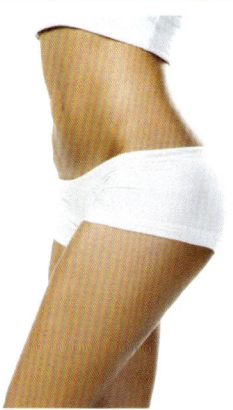

Ectomorph
A long slender body type, this frame finds it hard to put on weight or muscle.

EMS
This stands for electro muscle stimulator. It uses a faradic current to tighten and tone muscles, for a lifting, slimming effect.

Endomorph
With this body type, the limbs tend to be short, and the hips wider than the shoulders. Weight gain may be a problem.

Faradic current
A direct, interrupted, surging current used in EMS to cause muscle contraction.

Galvanic current
A constant, direct current where the client forms part of the circuit, used in iontophoresis and desincrustation.

Hard fat
Hard fat – feels solid to touch. Often found at the tops of thighs.

Lifestyle patterns
Habits such as smoking, alcohol intake, sleeping, relaxation, exercise patterns, diet and fluid intake, which have an effect on the body.

Mechanical massage
A method of massage using a machine with interchangeable heads, giving a deeper effect than that which can be given manually.

Mesomorph
With this body type, the client has narrow hips compared to their shoulders and muscle tone is usually well developed.

Micro-current
A treatment which tones, lifts, firms and re-educates muscles, improving collagen and elastin production to help improve body contours and shape.

Soft fat
Wobbly and spongy to touch. Often found on the abdomen.

Sterilisation
The complete destruction of micro-organisms and their spores.

Vacuum suction
A treatment designed to stimulate lymphatic drainage, remove excess waste, reduce puffiness, and cellulite.

Provide body electrotherapy treatments Unit 307

Revision tip

Learn where the muscles of the body are, and what they do. This will help you when carrying out EMS, as you will know where to place the pads when the client decides the areas they want toning.

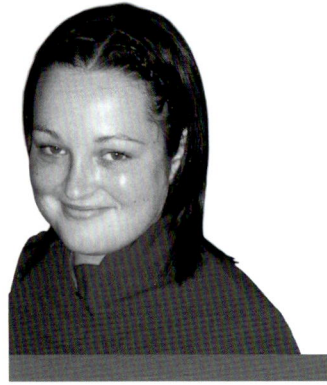

Follow in the footsteps of...
Charlotte Byrne

Charlotte is currently taking her Level 3 VRQ in Beauty Therapy at the Folkestone Academy. Body electrotherapy is her favourite treatment. Charlotte won the Academy's Student of the Year Award last year. She intends to continue with her training in Beauty Therapy to gain more qualifications, but eventually wants to work in a salon. Read on for Charlotte's electrotherapy tips!

What you must know
You must be able to:

1 Describe salon requirements for preparing yourself, the client and work area

2 Describe the environmental conditions suitable for body electrotherapy treatments

3 Describe the different consultation techniques used to identify treatment objectives

4 Explain the importance of carrying out a detailed body analysis and relevant tests

5 Describe how to select products, tools and equipment to suit client treatment needs, body types and conditions

6 Describe the different body types, conditions and characteristics

7 Explain the contra-indications that prevent or restrict body electrotherapy treatments

8 Explain how to communicate and behave in a professional manner

9 Describe health and safety working practices

10 Explain the importance of positioning yourself and the client correctly throughout the treatment

11 Describe different body types and conditions

12 Explain the importance of using products, tools, equipment and techniques to suit client's treatment needs, body type and conditions

13 Explain the effects and benefits of electrotherapy equipment and products on the skin and underlying structures

14 Explain the principles of electrical currents

15 Describe how treatments can be adapted to suit client treatment needs, body types and conditions

16 State the contra-actions that may occur during and following treatments and how to respond

Continues on next page

17 Explain the importance of completing the treatment to the satisfaction of the client

18 Explain the importance of completing treatment records

19 Describe the methods of evaluating the effectiveness of the treatment

20 Describe the aftercare advice that should be provided

21 Describe the structure, growth and repair of the skin

22 Describe body types, conditions, diseases and disorders

23 Describe the structure, function, position and action of the muscles of the body

24 Describe the location, function and structure of the bones of the body

25 Describe the structure and function of the circulatory and lymphatic systems for the body

26 Outline the structure and function of the digestive system

27 Outline the structure and function of the endocrine system

28 Describe the structure and function of the nervous system for the body

29 Explain how the ageing process, lifestyle and environmental factors affect the skin, body conditions and underlying structures

> *The G5 treatment is great for clients that are trying to lose weight or who have very tense muscles.*

Revision tip

Think of an **end**omorph as having a heavy rear **end**. A mesomorph begins with **m** and is **m**uscular. This may help you to remember which is which.

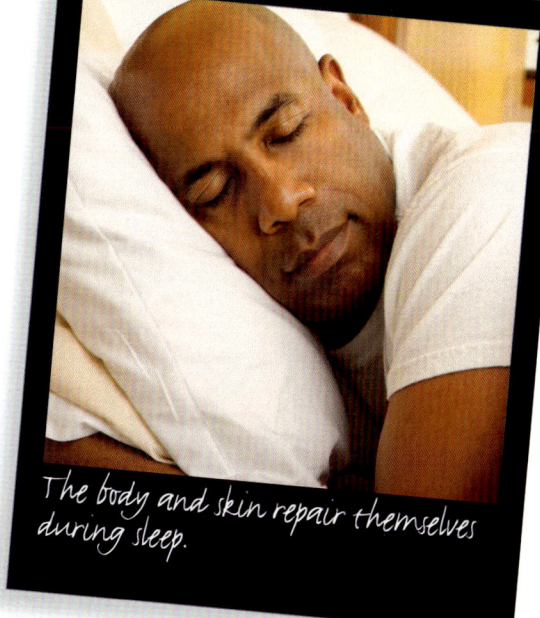

The body and skin repair themselves during sleep.

Make sure you know the maximum safe setting for body galvanic. This is worked out according to the size of pads used.

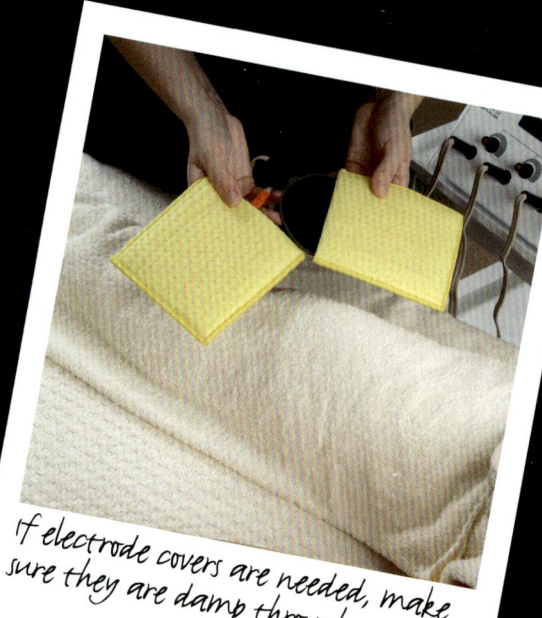

If electrode covers are needed, make sure they are damp throughout.

Body E

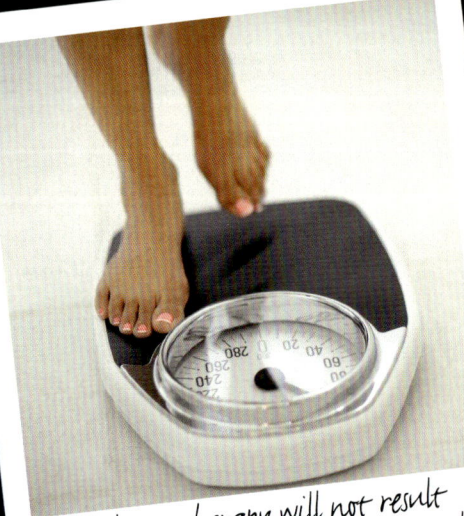

Body electrotherapy will not result in weight loss but toning the muscles make the body look more streamlined.

> During EMS check the contractions on both sides of the body are equal. Don't worry if the setting dials are different, as our muscle tone and strength differs on each side of the body.

> " The infra red lamp is very effective on cold, tense clients as it really helps them to relax and can relieve muscle pain.

Electric

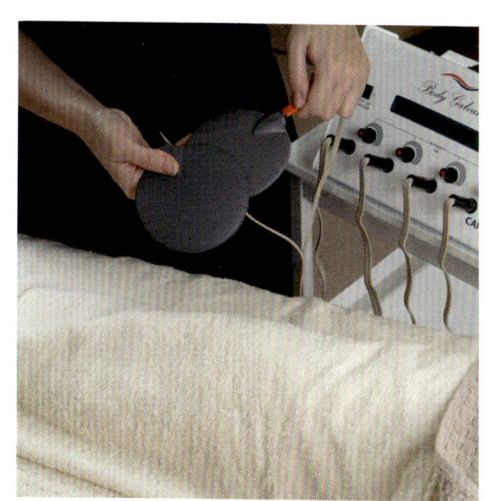

Health and safety should always be at the forefront of your mind when performing electrical treatments.

Image courtesy of Carlton Group

What you must do
Practical observations

This page shows what you need to do during your practical task. You can look at it beforehand, but you're **not** allowed to have it with you while carrying out your practical task. You must achieve **all** the criteria; you can achieve 1 mark, 2 marks or 3 marks for the criteria indicated with *.

Conversion chart

Grade	Marks
Pass	11–13
Merit	14–19
Distinction	20–23

○ Please tick when all pre-observation requirements have been met

	Provide a body electrotherapy treatment			
	Treatment 1	Treatment 2	Treatment 3	Treatment 4
State the electrotherapy chosen				
1 Prepare yourself, client and work area for body electrotherapy treatment	1	1	1	1
2 Use suitable consultation techniques to identify treatment objectives *	1 2 3	1 2 3	1 2 3	1 2 3
3 Carry out a body analysis and relevant tests *	1 2 3	1 2 3	1 2 3	1 2 3
4 Provide clear recommendations to the client *	1 2 3	1 2 3	1 2 3	1 2 3
5 Position yourself and client correctly throughout the treatment	1	1	1	1
6 Select and use products, tools, electrotherapy equipment and techniques to suit the client treatment needs, body type and conditions *	1 2 3	1 2 3	1 2 3	1 2 3
7 Communicate and behave in a professional manner	1	1	1	1
8 Follow health and safety working practices	1	1	1	1
9 Complete the treatment to the satisfaction of the client *	1 2 3	1 2 3	1 2 3	1 2 3
10 Record and evaluate the results of the treatment	1	1	1	1
11 Provide suitable aftercare advice *	1 2 3	1 2 3	1 2 3	1 2 3
Total				
Grade				
Candidate signature and date				
Assessor signature and date				

What you must do
Practical observations descriptors table

This table shows what you need to do to achieve 1, 2 or 3 marks for the criteria indicated with * on the previous page.

	1 mark	2 marks	3 marks
2 Use suitable consultation techniques to identify treatment objectives	Basic consultation Examples: uses open and closed questions, checks for contra-indications, identifies the treatment objectives correctly.	Good consultation Examples: positive body language, uses open and closed questions to identify contra-indications, general health, lifestyle and expectations; identifies the treatment objectives and any factors that may limit or restrict the treatment.	Thorough consultation Examples: positive body language, uses open and closed questions to identify contra-indications, general health, lifestyle and expectations, how client feels about their body and what improvement they would like to achieve; identifies the treatment objectives and any factors that may limit or restrict the treatment, allows the client to ask any questions to confirm understanding.
3 Carry out a body analysis and relevant tests	Carries out a basic analysis, identifies client's body type, carries out heat sensitivity and tactile sensation tests, records findings.	Carries out a good analysis, identifies client's body type and conditions, carries out heat sensitivity and tactile sensation tests, records findings.	Carries out a detailed analysis, identifies client's posture, body type and conditions (ie soft fat, hard fat, cellulite) and skin type and characteristics, records findings.

Continues on next page

Provide body electrotherapy treatments **Unit 307**

What you must do
Practical observations descriptors table (continued)

This table shows what you need to do to achieve 1, 2 or 3 marks for the criteria indicated with * on page 90.

	1 mark	2 marks	3 marks
4 Provide clear recommendations to the client	A basic treatment plan is recommended Examples: explains treatment procedure and any adaptations to meet client treatment needs, equipment to be used.	A good treatment plan is recommended Examples: explains treatment procedure and any adaptations to meet client treatment needs, equipment to be used based on factors identified during consultation (lifestyle, medication (if any), contra-indications, results of body analysis), a choice of products to be used.	A thorough treatment plan is recommended Examples: explains treatment procedure and any adaptations to meet client treatment needs, equipment to be used based on factors identified during consultation (lifestyle, medication (if any), contra-indications, results of body analysis), a choice of products to be used, explains effects and benefits of the type of equipment used and the adaptation/modification to suit client treatment needs, allows the client to ask questions about the treatment plan.

Continues on next page

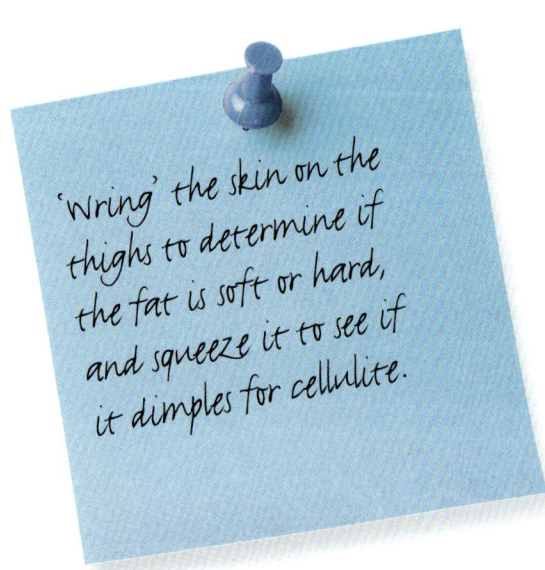

'Wring' the skin on the thighs to determine if the fat is soft or hard, and squeeze it to see if it dimples for cellulite.

	1 mark	2 marks	3 marks
6 Select and use products, tools, electrotherapy equipment and techniques to suit the client treatment needs, body type and conditions	Selects and uses the correct equipment, tools, techniques and basic products based on factors identified in body analysis.	Selects and uses the correct equipment, tools, techniques and a variety of products based on factors identified in body analysis, explains effects and benefits of the products and equipment to the client as appropriate throughout.	Selects and uses the correct equipment, tools, techniques and a variety of products based on factors identified in body analysis, explains effects and benefits of the products and equipment to the client as appropriate throughout, adapts and modifies the techniques used, explains the treatment to the client as appropriate throughout.
9 Complete the treatment to the satisfaction of the client	The treatment is completed within the agreed time and brought to a satisfactory close.	The treatment is completed within the agreed time, brought to a satisfactory close and positive feedback is gained from the client.	The treatment is completed within the agreed time, brought to a satisfactory close and positive feedback is gained from the client, shows the client the results of the treatment and allows the client to ask questions.
11 Provide suitable aftercare advice	Basic aftercare advice Examples: how to deal with possible contra-actions, product(s) to use, future treatment needs.	Good level of aftercare advice Examples: how to deal with possible contra-actions, product(s) to use, specific advice (ie what to avoid immediately after the treatment, fluid intake, healthy eating), future treatment needs.	Excellent aftercare advice Examples: how to deal with possible contra-actions, product(s) to use, specific advice (ie what to avoid immediately after the treatment, fluid intake, healthy eating), recommends future treatment programme (regular treatments, introduction of new/alternative treatments).

Comment form
Unit 307 Provide body electrotherapy treatments

This form can be used to record comments by you, your client, or your assessor.

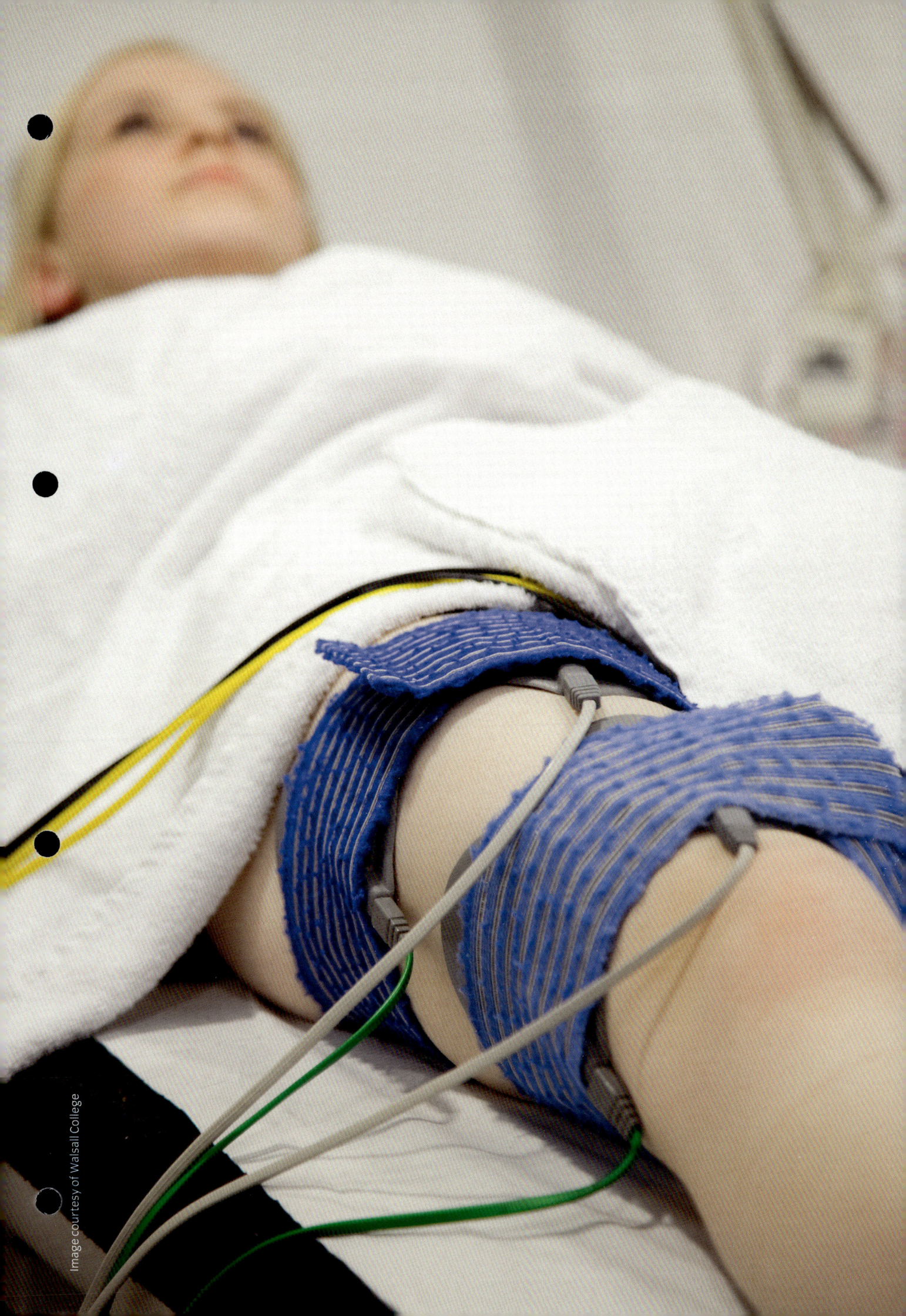

Image courtesy of Walsall College

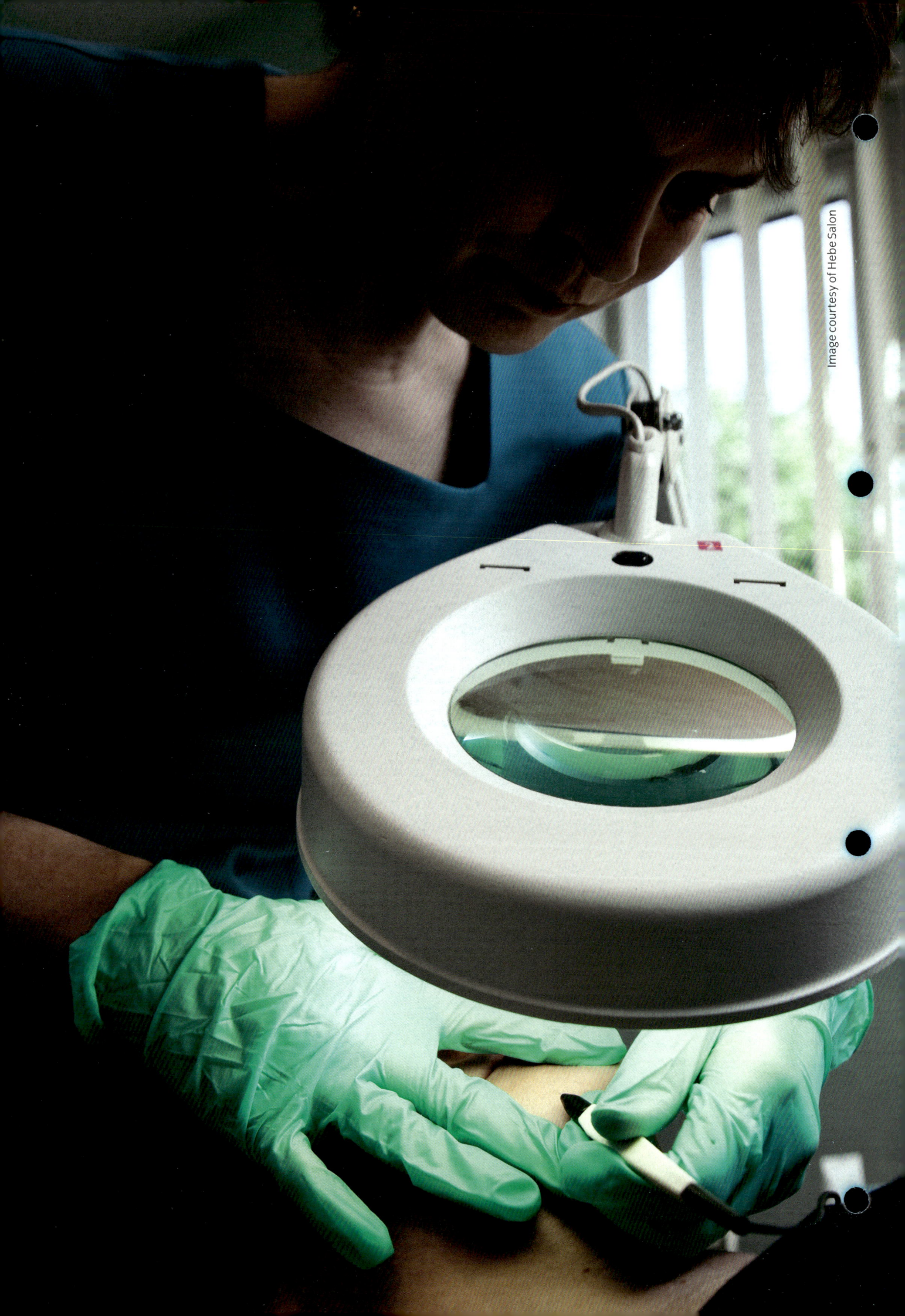

Image courtesy of Hebe Salon

308

Provide electrical epilation

Excess hair can be a huge embarrassment, whatever the age of the client. Plucking might make the hair grow back thicker, and shaving makes the skin sore, irritated and stubbly. So, the removal by an electrical current, known as either electrolysis or electrical epilation (sometimes shortened to epilation), may be the answer. This unit covers the causes of excess hair, the tact and sensitivity you will need to use when dealing with the client, as well as how to carry out removal professionally and successfully. It's very rewarding for the therapist, involving a high level of skill, and can make a vast difference to the confidence of the client.

Assignment mark sheet
Unit 308 Provide electrical epilation

Your assessor will mark you on each of the practical tasks in this unit. This page is used to work out your overall grade for the unit. You must pass **all** parts of the tasks to be able to achieve a grade. For each completed practical task, a pass equals 1 point, a merit equals 2 points and a distinction equals 3 points.

What you must know	Tick when complete
Task 1a: produce a report	
Task 1b: produce an information sheet	
Task 1c: produce a fact sheet	
Task 1d: anatomy and physiology	
Or tick if covered by an online test	

What you must do	Grade	Points
Task 2a: Short wave diathermy		
Task 2b: Blend		

Conversion chart

Grade	Points
Pass	1–1.5
Merit	1.6–2.5
Distinction	2.6–3

Total points for graded tasks

Divided by ÷ 2

= Average grade for tasks

Overall grade
(see conversion chart)

Candidate name:

Candidate signature: Date:

Assessor signature: Date:

Quality assurance co-ordinator signature   Date:
(where applicable):

External Verifier signature   Date:
(where applicable):

What does it mean?
Some useful words are explained below

Anagen hair
The active stage of hair growth, where the hair is still attached to its blood supply. This is the best stage for successful epilation.

Anaphoresis
The use of a negative galvanic current to help dilate small, tight follicles before treatment, making insertion easier.

Blend method
A combination of direct galvanic current and alternating high frequency current (diathermy) passing down the same needle. This has the efficiency of galvanic electrolysis, with a faster speed. It can result in a more effective, less painful treatment.

Cataphoresis
A technique used after epilation to help constrict follicles, reduce redness and rebalance the acid mantle, making bacterial infection less likely.

Compound hair
A single follicle, which produces two or more hairs.

Diathermy
The fastest method of epilation. Uses an alternating oscillating current to produce heat.

Electrolysis
A permanent method of hair removal. Uses a galvanic current, which reacts with the skin's moisture resulting in chemical destruction of the hair follicle. It is very effective but the slowest to perform.

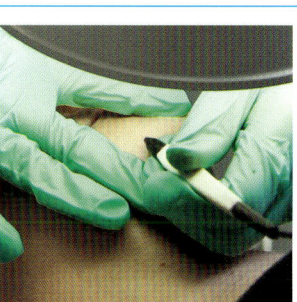

Endocrine system
A system of glands which secrete hormones. These have an effect on particular organs and body systems, and help to regulate the body.

Hirsutism
A male hair growth pattern on women, as a result of hormonal imbalance.

Hormone
A chemical messenger that travels around the body via the blood circulation where it will affect its target organ.

Insulated needle
A needle with a coating along its length, leaving only the tip exposed.

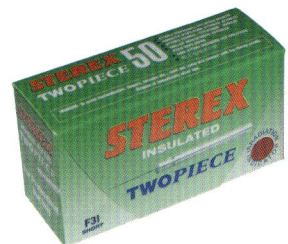

Moisture gradient
The levels of moisture in the skin (needed for successful epilation) are higher in the deeper levels of the dermis, becoming drier towards the surface.

Repetitive strain injury (RSI)
Soft tissue injury, usually in the wrists, as a result of overuse.

Superfluous hair
A term used to describe any unwanted hair.

Terminal hair
Thick, coarse hair with a deep root and rich blood supply.

Topical hair growth
This is caused by an increase in blood to the area, and may be the result of waxing or plucking.

Vellus hair
Fine, soft hair, which does not always contain a medulla. Can be stimulated into terminal hair.

Revision tip

It's important to know why some conditions contra-indicate epilation. For example, with haemophilia the blood does not clot properly so damage to the skin would be dangerous for the client.

What you must know
You must be able to:

1. Describe the different consultation techniques used to identify treatment objectives
2. Explain the contra-indications that prevent or restrict electrical epilation treatment
3. Describe health and safety working practices
4. Explain the importance of carrying out a detailed hair and skin analysis
5. Describe how to select products, tools and equipment to suit client needs
6. Describe the environmental conditions suitable for electrical epilation treatments
7. Describe how to select the needle type and size to suit hair and skin types
8. Describe how to work on different hair growth patterns and treatment areas
9. Explain the consequences of inaccurate probing
10. Explain the principles, uses and benefits of galvanic, short wave diathermy and blend

Continues on next page

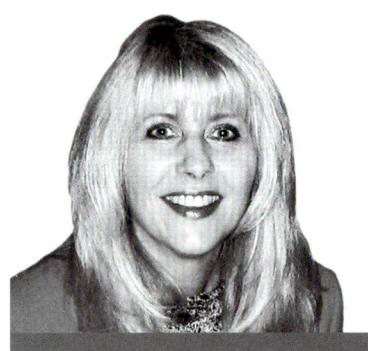

Follow in the footsteps of... *Elaine Stoddart*

Elaine Stoddart is Director of Education & PR for brand leader Sterex Electrolysis International and runs two specialist electrolysis clinics in Harley Street and Buckinghamshire. Elaine is the most prolific trainer in the UK in advanced techniques using electrolysis and has trained surgeons, GPs, nurses, other medical practitioners and therapists in these procedures. She is also a published author and international speaker in Electrolysis and Advanced Electrolysis/Cosmetic Procedures. **Read on for Elaine's fab epilation tips!**

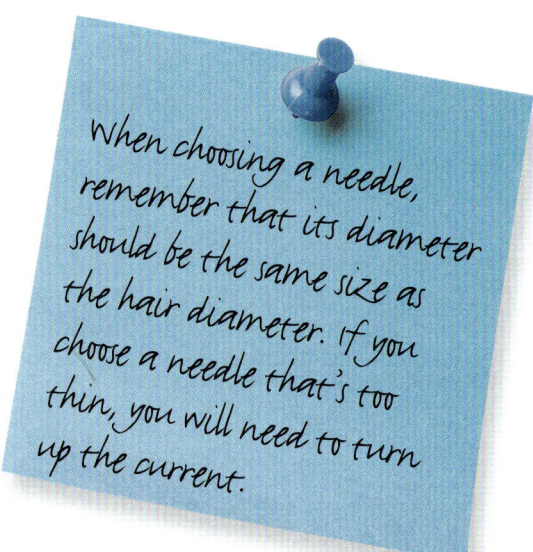

When choosing a needle, remember that its diameter should be the same size as the hair diameter. If you choose a needle that's too thin, you will need to turn up the current.

11 Describe how treatments can be adapted to suit client treatment needs, skin, hair types and conditions

12 Describe how moisture gradient in the skin affects the electrical epilation treatment

13 State the contra-actions that may occur during and following treatments

14 Describe the methods of evaluating the effectiveness of the treatment

15 Describe the aftercare advice that should be provided

16 Describe the suitable methods of dealing with regrowth between treatments

17 Describe different skin types, conditions, diseases and disorders

18 Describe the structure, growth and repair of the skin

19 Describe the structure and function of the hair

20 Describe the hair types, growth patterns and causes of hair growth

21 Describe the structure and function of the endocrine system and its effect on hair growth

22 Describe the structure and function of circulatory and lymphatic systems

Revision tip

Epilation is most successful on hairs in the anagen phase – therefore a hair is best treated while it is still actively growing.

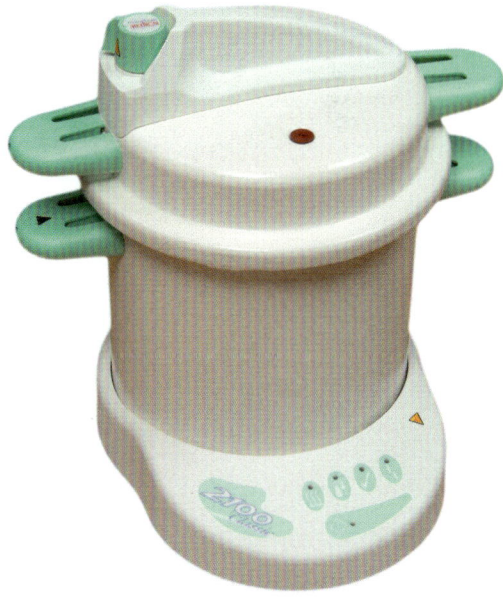

Image courtesy of Ellisons

Gloves used for the treatment are not sterile. After putting on gloves just before the treatment wash your gloved hands with an antibacterial dry handwash.

Epil...

> "The needle should slide down the follicle easily. If there is any resistance at all then retract the needle, realign the insertion approach and try again.

The needle should be inserted into the hair follicle at the same angle as the hair. Stop as soon as the bottom of the follicle is felt and/or dimpling on the surface of the skin is seen.

Image courtesy of Sterex

ation

When treating dense hair growth where the hairs are growing closely together, the 'checkerboard method' should be used, ie treat one, miss one.

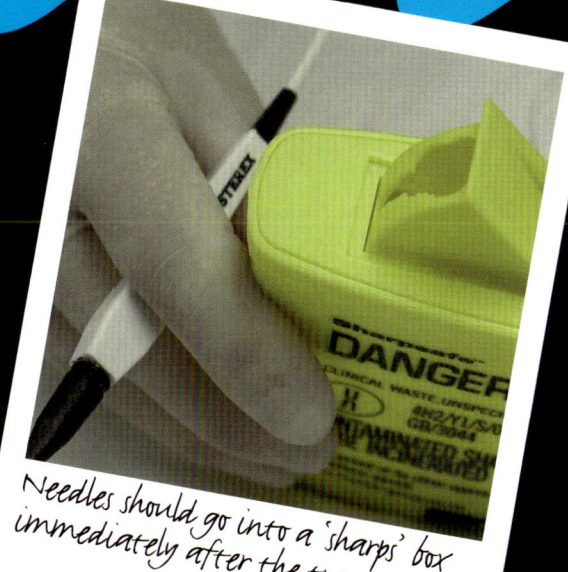

Needles should go into a 'sharps' box immediately after the treatment.

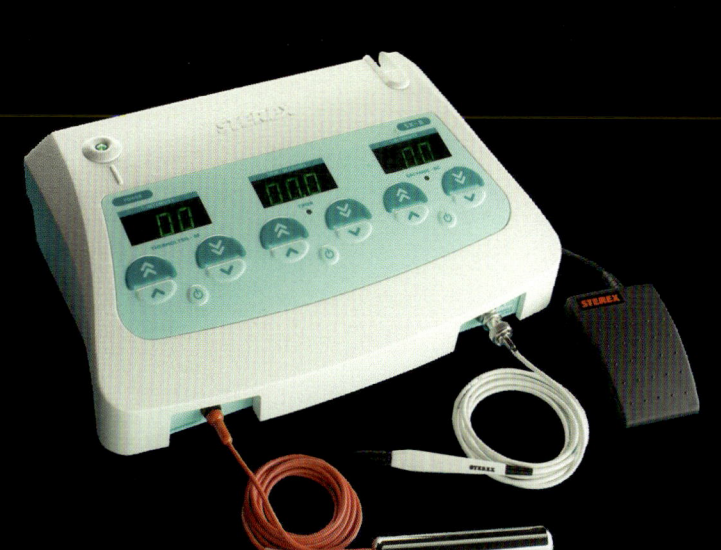

Images courtesy of Sterex

What you must do
Practical observations

This page shows what you need to do during your practical task. You can look at it beforehand, but you're **not** allowed to have it with you while carrying out your practical task. You must achieve **all** the criteria; you can achieve 1 mark, 2 marks or 3 marks for the criteria indicated with *.

Conversion chart

Grade	Marks
Pass	14–16
Merit	17–22
Distinction	23–26

○ Please tick when all pre-observation requirements have been met

	Electrical epilation					
	Short wave diathermy			Blend		
1 Prepare yourself, client and work area for electrical epilation	1			1		
2 Use suitable consultation techniques to identify treatment objectives *	1	2	3	1	2	3
3 Carry out skin and hair analysis	1			1		
4 Provide clear recommendations to the client *	1	2	3	1	2	3
5 Position yourself and client correctly throughout the treatment	1			1		
6 Follow health and safety working practices	1			1		
7 Communicate and behave in a professional manner	1			1		
8 Select and use products, tools, equipment and techniques to suit client treatment needs, skin type and conditions *	1	2	3	1	2	3
9 Stretch and support skin tissues effectively for safe and accurate insertion of needle	1			1		

Continues on next page

| | Electrical epilation ||||||
| | Short wave diathermy ||| Blend |||
	1	2	3	1	2	3
10 Correctly insert the needle into the hair follicle with regards to depth and angle *	1	2	3	1	2	3
11 Remove hair from follicles without traction	1			1		
12 Complete the treatment to the satisfaction of the client *	1	2	3	1	2	3
13 Record and evaluate the results of the treatment	1			1		
14 Provide suitable aftercare advice *	1	2	3	1	2	3
Total						
Grade						
Candidate signature and date						
Assessor signature and date						

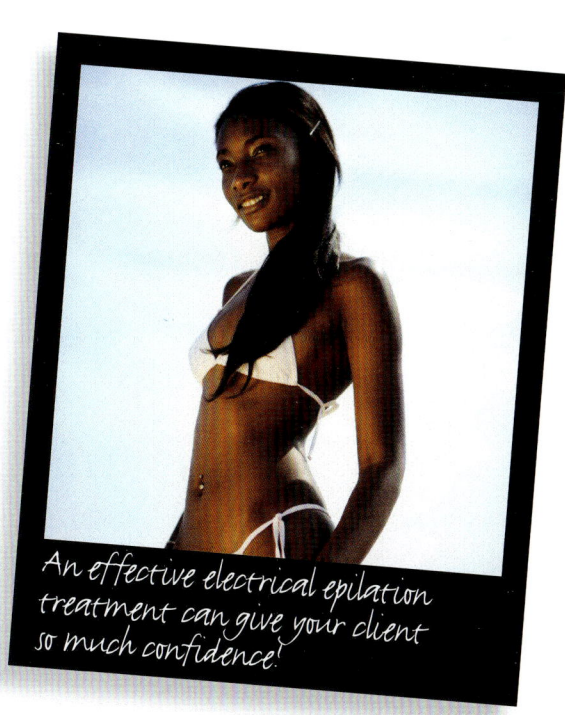

An effective electrical epilation treatment can give your client so much confidence!

What you must do
Practical observations descriptors table

This table shows what you need to do to achieve 1, 2 or 3 marks for the criteria indicated with * on pages 104 and 105.

	1 mark	2 marks	3 marks
2 Use suitable consultation techniques to identify treatment objectives	Basic consultation Examples: uses open and closed questions, checks for contra-indications and area to be treated.	Good consultation Examples: positive body language, uses open and closed questions to identify contra-indications and area to be treated, general health and expectations, identifies the treatment objectives and any factors that may limit or restrict the treatment.	Thorough consultation Examples: positive body language, uses open and closed questions to identify contra-indications and area to be treated, general health, age, cause of hair growth and expectations, explains the hair growth cycle, identifies any factors that may limit or restrict the treatment.
4 Provide clear recommendations to the client	A basic treatment plan is recommended Example: explains treatment procedure and area to be treated.	A good treatment plan is recommended Examples: explains treatment procedure and area to be treated and the method to be chosen including its advantages.	A thorough treatment plan is recommended Examples: explains treatment procedure and area to be treated and the method to be chosen including its advantages and the reason for the choice of needle, allows the client to ask questions about the treatment plan.

Continues on next page

"

Short wave diathermy takes 1–2 seconds, Blend a minimum of 5 seconds and Galvanic a maximum of 10 seconds per hair.

	1 mark	2 marks	3 marks
8 Select and use products, tools, equipment and techniques to suit the client treatment needs, skin type and conditions	Selects and uses correct products, tools, equipment, needle type and size, follows manufacturers' instructions regarding safe use of equipment, intensity is altered during treatment as necessary for different hair thicknesses.	Selects and uses correct products, tools, equipment, needle type and size, follows manufacturers' instructions regarding safe use of equipment, intensity is altered during treatment as necessary for different hair thickness, client is positioned correctly throughout the treatment, uses magnifying lamp, asks for and acts on relevant feedback from the client during treatment.	Selects and uses correct products, tools, equipment, needle type and size, follows manufacturers' instructions regarding safe use of equipment, intensity is altered during treatment as necessary for different hair thickness, client is positioned correctly throughout the treatment, uses magnifying lamp, varies techniques to minimise discomfort and maintain modesty, asks for and acts on relevant feedback from the client during treatment, needle and method are altered during the treatment as necessary.
10 Correctly insert the needle into the hair follicle with regard to depth and angle	The skin is stretched correctly and the needle is inserted into the follicle at the correct angle to a suitable depth.	The skin is stretched correctly and the needle is inserted into the follicle at the correct angle to a suitable depth. The working point is found within optimum time.	The skin is stretched correctly and the needle is inserted into the follicle at the correct angle to a suitable depth with confidence. The working point is found within optimum time.

Continues on next page

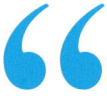

> *The treated hair should be gently released from the follicle with tweezers. If the hair has been properly treated, the hair should be lifted easily from the follicle.*

What you must do
Practical observations descriptors table (continued)

This table shows what you need to do to achieve 1, 2 or 3 marks for the criteria indicated with * on pages 104 and 105.

	1 mark	2 marks	3 marks
12 Complete the treatment to the satisfaction of the client	The treatment is completed within the agreed time and brought to a satisfactory close.	The treatment is completed within the agreed time, brought to a satisfactory close and positive feedback is gained from the client.	The treatment is completed within the agreed time, brought to a satisfactory close and positive feedback is gained from the client, shows the client the results of the treatment and encourages the client to ask questions.
14 Provide suitable aftercare advice	Basic aftercare advice Possible contra-actions, avoidance of touching the area and how to deal with re-growth.	Good level of aftercare advice Possible contra-actions, avoidance of touching the area, heat, make-up and perfumes and how to deal with re-growth, home care product.	Excellent aftercare advice Possible contra-actions, avoidance of touching the area, heat, make-up and perfumes, how to deal with re-growth, home care product and frequency of further treatments.

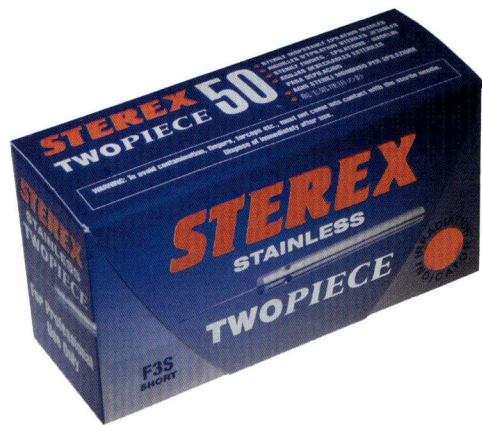

Image courtesy of Sterex

Comment form
Unit 308 Provide electrical epilation

This form can be used to record comments by you, your client, or your assessor.

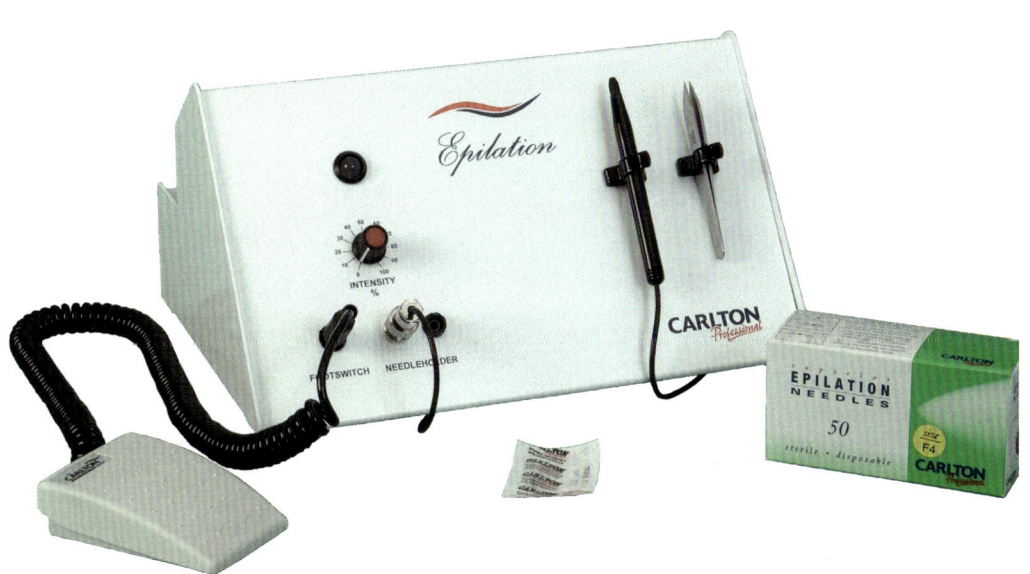

Image courtesy of Carlton Professional

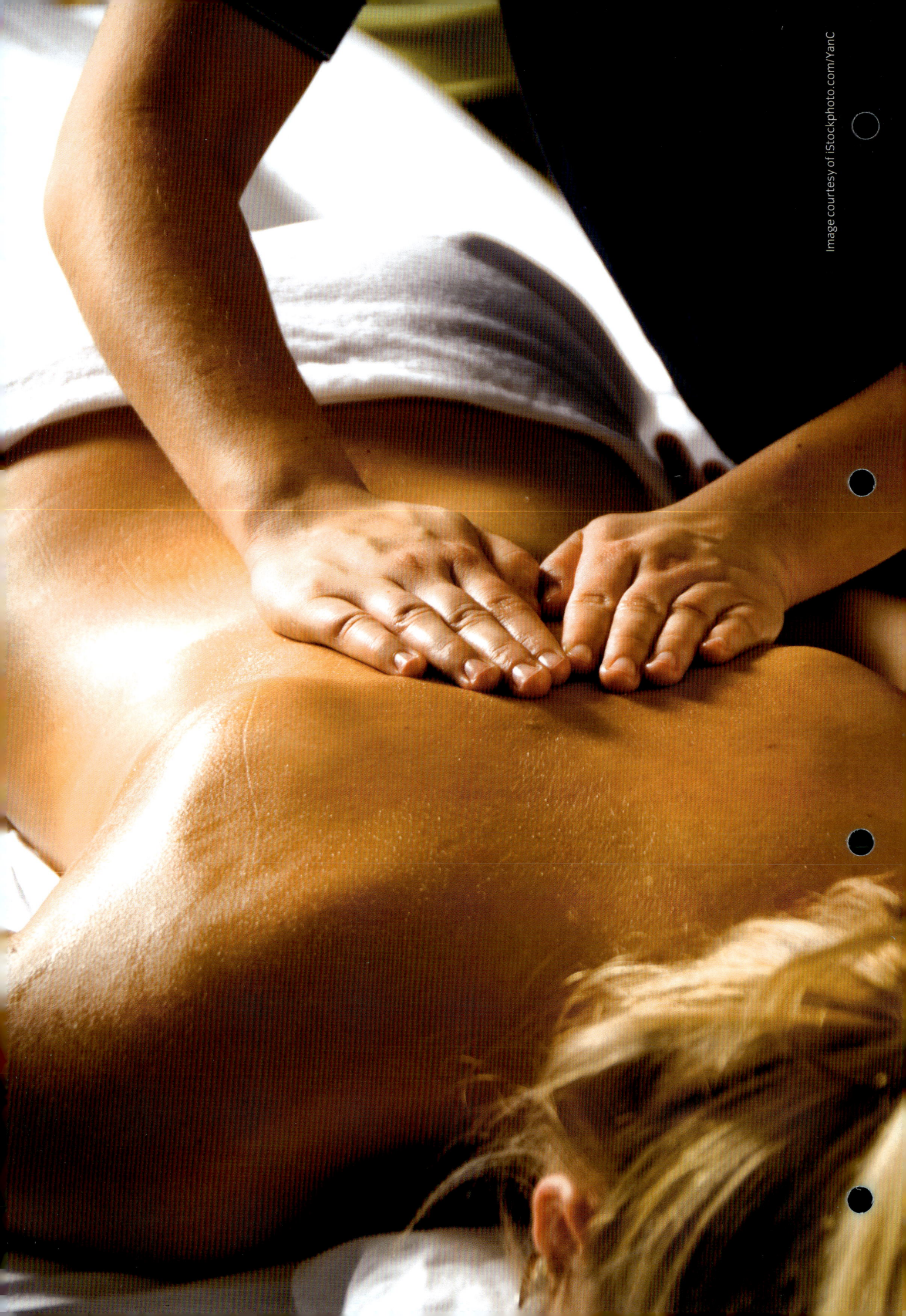

309

Provide massage using pre-blended aromatherapy oils

Massage using pre-blended aromatherapy oils uses a combination of specialised massage techniques and the fragrant, therapeutic oils extracted from plants. Depending on the blend you choose you can relax or uplift your client or stimulate their skin, body and senses. You will learn how to perform an aromatherapy routine for the body, face and scalp plus how to select the facial and body blends most suitable for your client's skin type and the treatment objective. You will also learn safety precautions that make this wonderful treatment not only enjoyable but also safe.

Assignment mark sheet
Unit 309 Provide massage using pre-blended aromatherapy oils

Your assessor will mark you on each of the practical tasks in this unit. This page is used to work out your overall grade for the unit. You must pass **all** parts of the tasks to be able to achieve a grade. For each completed practical task, a pass equals 1 point, a merit equals 2 points and a distinction equals 3 points.

What you must know	Tick when complete
Task 1a: produce an information sheet	
Task 1b: produce a fact sheet	
Task 1c: produce a fact sheet	
Task 1d: anatomy and physiology	
Or tick if covered by an online test	

What you must do	Grade	Points
Task 2: Provide massage using pre-blended aromatherapy oils		

Overall grade

Candidate name:

Candidate signature: Date:

Assessor signature: Date:

Quality assurance co-ordinator signature (where applicable): Date:

External Verifier signature (where applicable): Date:

What does it mean?
Some useful words are explained below

Acute toxicity
Essential oils being taken orally, or excessive use of essential oils on the skin, could lead to liver and kidney damage.

Carrier oils
Oily plant base used to dilute essential oils for use on the skin.

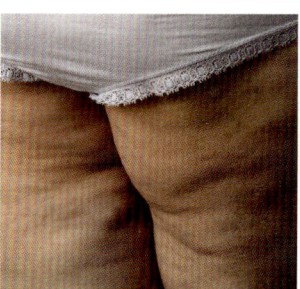

Cellulite
Congested tissue with a dimply 'orange peel' appearance. It is usually cold to the touch and found on the thighs and buttocks.

Chronic toxicity
This is when an essential oil has been overused repeatedly over a period of time.

Contra-indications
Conditions that prevent treatment from taking place, or make it necessary to modify the treatment.

Dehydrated skin
This is a lack of water or moisture within the skin as opposed to a lack of oil, and can occur on any skin type.

Effleurage
A stroking technique used to begin the massage and complete an area. It is also useful to link movements to provide flow and rhythm in the massage.

Limbic system
The area of the brain connected to instinct, memory and behaviour.

Mature skin
In beauty therapy terms, this is any skin over the age of 25. However, the skin is generally not classed as being mature until the signs of ageing are apparent.

Neuromuscular
A firm form of massage, used to stimulate nerves.

Olfactory system
The body system that provides us with the sense of smell.

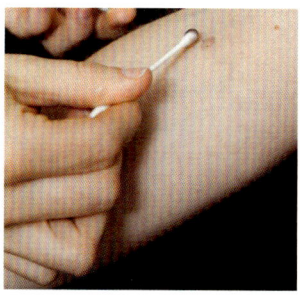

Patch testing
The application of the blend to be used either behind the ear, or in the crook of the elbow, 24 hours before treatment to check for skin reaction.

Petrissage
A technique that compresses the tissues of the body and lifts them away from the underlying structures.

Photo toxicity/sensitivity
The reaction of the skin when exposed to UV light in the presence of some essential oils, often resulting in pigmentation marks.

Physiological effects
The effect that massage has on the systems of the body.

Pre-blended essential oils
Essential oils, which have been pre-mixed in vegetable oil base by a professional experienced blender, in order to achieve specific effects.

Pressure points
Specific points on the body, which help to release blocked energy flow when stimulated.

Sensitive skin
Skin that reacts readily to products, heat or pressure. Whilst it can occur on any skin type, sensitive skin usually has a fine texture, thin epidermis, and blood vessels very close to the surface. This can result in blotchiness, redness, flushing, increased warmth and irritation if stimulated.

Treatment objectives
The desired outcome of the massage using pre-blended oils. These can be achieved through the blend selected and the massage movements carried out.

Vibrations
Fine trembling movements that can stimulate or relax nerves depending on how they are applied.

Volatility
The speed at which an essential oil evaporates.

> **Revision tip**
>
> Essential oils are absorbed through the skin during massage, and will also be inhaled, affecting both the respiratory system and the olfactory system.

What you must know
You must be able to:

1. Describe salon requirements for preparing themselves, the client and work area
2. Describe the environmental conditions suitable for body treatments using pre-blended aromatherapy oils
3. Describe the different consultation techniques used to identify treatment objectives
4. Describe how to select products and tools to suit client treatment needs, skin types and conditions
5. Outline the safety precautions associated with the range of pre-blended aromatherapy oils
6. Explain the contra-indications that prevent or restrict aromatherapy treatments
7. Explain how to communicate and behave in a professional manner
8. Describe health and safety working practices
9. Explain the importance of positioning themselves and the client correctly throughout the treatment
10. Explain the importance of using products, tools and techniques to suit client's treatment needs, skin types and conditions

Continues on next page

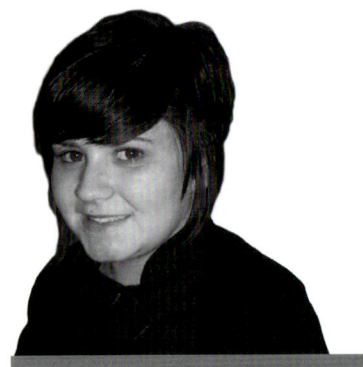

Follow in the footsteps of ... *Laura Stevens*

Laura is currently taking her Level 3 VRQ in Beauty Therapy at the Folkestone Academy. She loves giving massages with pre-blended oils because she enjoys adapting the treatment for her client's needs. When Laura finishes her qualification she would like to get a job in a Beauty salon, before progressing to a spa so she can gain as much experience of the industry as she can. Read on for Laura's massage tips!

11 Describe how treatments can be adapted to suit client treatment needs, skin types and conditions

12 State the contra-actions that may occur during and following treatments and how to respond

13 Explain the importance of completing the treatment to the satisfaction of the client

14 Explain the importance of completing treatment records

15 Describe the methods of evaluating the effectiveness of the treatment

16 Describe the aftercare advice that should be provided

17 Describe the structure and the main functions of the following body systems in relation to massage:
- skin
- skeletal
- muscular
- cardio-vascular
- lymphatic
- nervous
- digestive
- urinary
- endocrine

18 Describe the main diseases and disorders of body systems

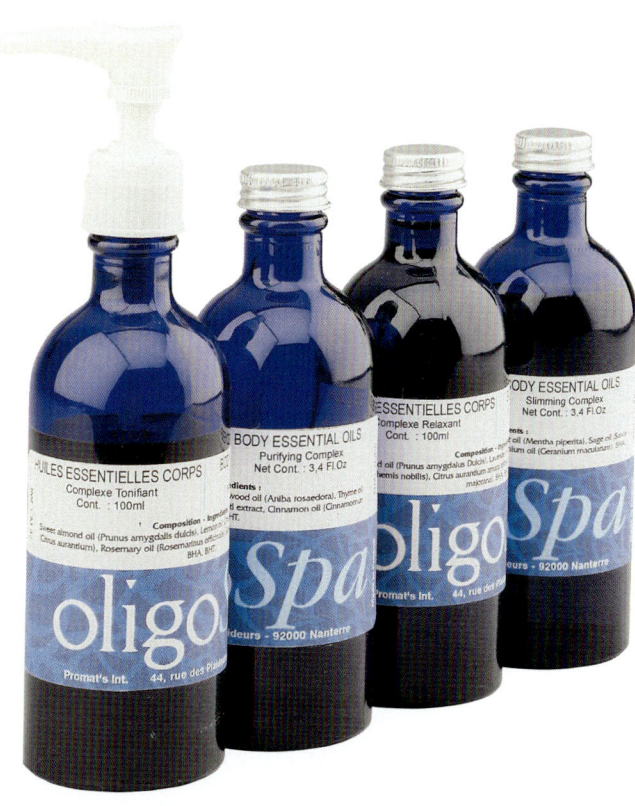

Image courtesy of House of Famuir

It's really important to check for allergies before deciding on the blend you intend to use. They may contain nuts or other ingredients that your client will react to.

Aroma

If your client has lower back pain when lying on the couch, place support under their knees to alleviate this.

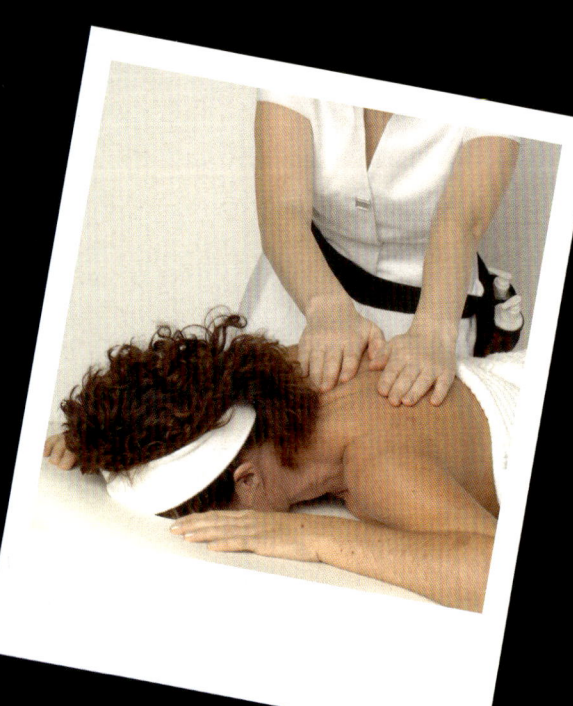

Image courtesy of www.therapyessentials.co.uk

> "Nearly anyone can have this treatment as it is so smooth and gentle.

Image courtesy of iStockphoto.com/nicolesy

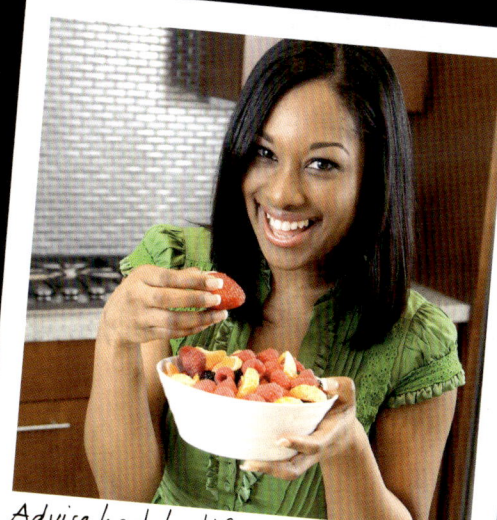

Advise healthy lifestyle changes to your client.

therapy

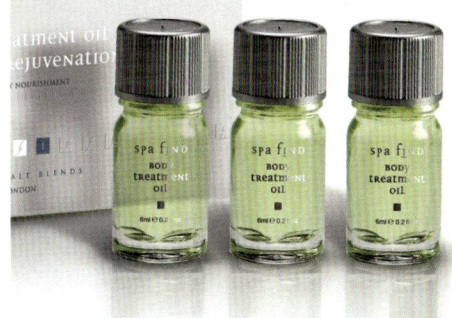

Pre-blended oils can treat a range of conditions.

Spa Find Skincare

What you must do
Practical observations

This page shows what you need to do during your practical task. You can look at it beforehand, but you're **not** allowed to have it with you while carrying out your practical task. You must achieve **all** the criteria; you can achieve 1 mark, 2 marks or 3 marks for the criteria indicated with *.

Conversion chart

Grade	Marks
Pass	12–14
Merit	15–20
Distinction	21–24

○ Please tick when all pre-observation requirements have been met

	Provide massage using pre-blended aromatherapy oils		
1 Prepare yourself, the client and the work area for massage treatment using pre-blended aromatherapy oils	1		
2 Use suitable consultation techniques to identify treatment objectives *	1	2	3
3 Advise the client how to prepare for the treatment	1		
4 Provide clear recommendations to the client *	1	2	3
5 Position yourself and the client correctly throughout the treatment	1		
6 Follow health and safety working practices	1		
7 Communicate and behave in a professional manner	1		
8 Select and use products to suit client's treatment needs, skin types and condition *	1	2	3
9 Use and adapt massage techniques to meet the needs of the client *	1	2	3
10 Complete the treatment to the satisfaction of the client *	1	2	3
11 Record and evaluate the results of the treatment	1		
12 Provide suitable aftercare advice *	1	2	3

Total

Grade

Candidate signature and date

Assessor signature and date

What you must do
Practical observations descriptors table

This table shows what you need to do to achieve 1, 2 or 3 marks for the criteria indicated with * on the previous page.

	1 mark	2 marks	3 marks
2 Use suitable consultation techniques to identify treatment objectives	Basic consultation Examples: uses open and closed questions, checks for contra-indications, identifies the treatment objectives correctly.	Good consultation Examples: positive body language, uses open and closed questions to identify contra-indications, general health, lifestyle and expectations; identifies the treatment objectives and any factors that may limit or restrict the treatment.	Thorough consultation Examples: positive body language, uses open and closed questions to identify contra-indications, general health, lifestyle and expectations, how client feels about their body and what improvement they would like to achieve; identifies the treatment objectives and any factors that may limit or restrict the treatment, allows the client to ask any questions to confirm understanding.
4 Provide clear recommendations to the client	A basic treatment plan is recommended Example: explains treatment procedure and any adaptations to meet client treatment needs.	A good treatment plan is recommended Examples: explains treatment procedure and any adaptations to meet client treatment needs based on factors identified during consultation (lifestyle, medication (if any), contra-indications, results of postural diagnosis), a choice of products to be used.	A thorough treatment plan is recommended Examples: explains treatment procedure and any adaptations to meet client treatment needs based on factors identified during consultation (lifestyle, medication (if any), contra-indications, results of postural diagnosis), a choice of products to be used, adaptation of massage movements to suit client treatment needs, allows the client to ask questions about the treatment plan.

Continues on next page

What you must do
Practical observations descriptors table (continued)

This table shows what you need to do to achieve 1, 2 or 3 marks for the criteria indicated with * on page 118.

	1 mark	**2 marks**	**3 marks**
8 **Select and use products to suit client's treatment needs, skin types and condition**	Selects appropriate pre-blended aromatherapy oils to suit client's skin type and conditions.	Selects appropriate pre-blended aromatherapy oils to suit client's skin type and conditions, taking into account client preference.	Selects appropriate pre-blended aromatherapy oils to suit client's skin type and conditions, taking into account client preference, lifestyle, general health and treatment objectives.
9 **Use and adapt massage techniques to meet the needs of the client**	Adapts the massage routine to suit client treatment objectives. Uses a variety of movements, movements are even and flowing, uses appropriate pressure for the client.	Adapts the massage routine to suit client treatment objectives, muscle and fat type. Carries out massage movements correctly and fully with even flow showing variations in rate and rhythm according to treatment objectives, uses appropriate pressure for the client.	Adapts the massage routine to suit client treatment objectives, muscle and fat type taking into account all factors. The whole routine flows throughout, uses appropriate pressure for the client, checks the client's comfort and wellbeing at appropriate times.
10 **Complete the treatment to the satisfaction of the client**	The treatment is completed within the agreed time and brought to a satisfactory close.	The treatment is completed within the agreed time, brought to a satisfactory close, excess massage medium is removed from the skin correctly.	The treatment is completed within the agreed time, brought to a satisfactory close, excess massage medium is removed from the skin correctly, the client is asked for feedback and is allowed sufficient time to get dressed.

Continues on next page

	1 mark	2 marks	3 marks
12 Provide suitable aftercare advice	Basic aftercare advice Examples: how to deal with possible contra-actions, product(s) to use, importance of rest and relaxation, future treatment needs.	Good level of aftercare advice Examples: how to deal with possible contra-actions, product(s) to use, importance of rest and relaxation, specific lifestyle advice (ie dealing with stress, fluid intake, healthy eating), future treatment needs.	Excellent aftercare advice Examples: how to deal with possible contra-actions, product(s) to use, importance of rest and relaxation, specific lifestyle advice (ie dealing with stress, fluid intake, healthy eating), advice to improve postural awareness, recommends future treatment programme (regular massage, introduction of new/alternative treatments).

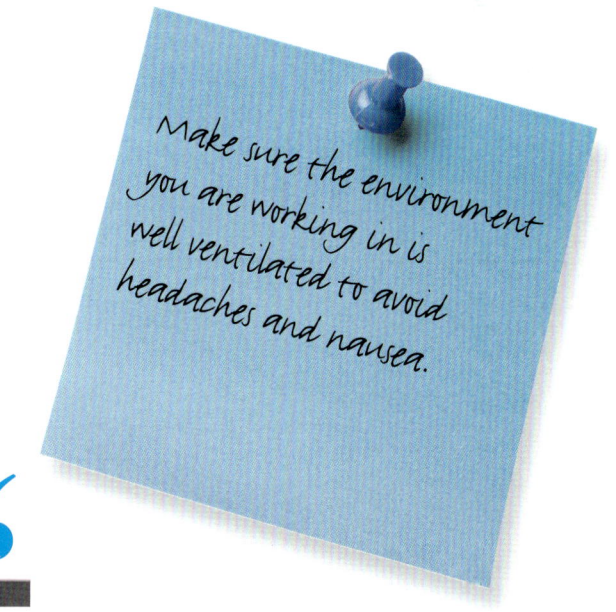

Make sure the environment you are working in is well ventilated to avoid headaches and nausea.

> *Study your anatomy and physiology books thoroughly as it helps to understand the effect massage has on the lymphatic system.*

Comment form
Unit 309 Provide massage using pre-blended aromatherapy oils

This form can be used to record comments by you, your client, or your assessor.

___

___

___

___

___

___

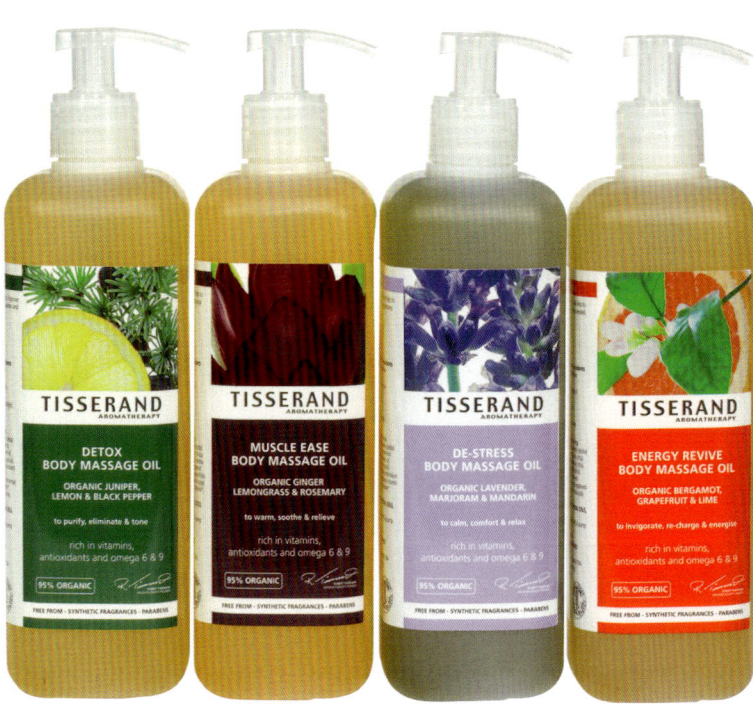

Image courtesy of Tisserand (www.tisserand.com)

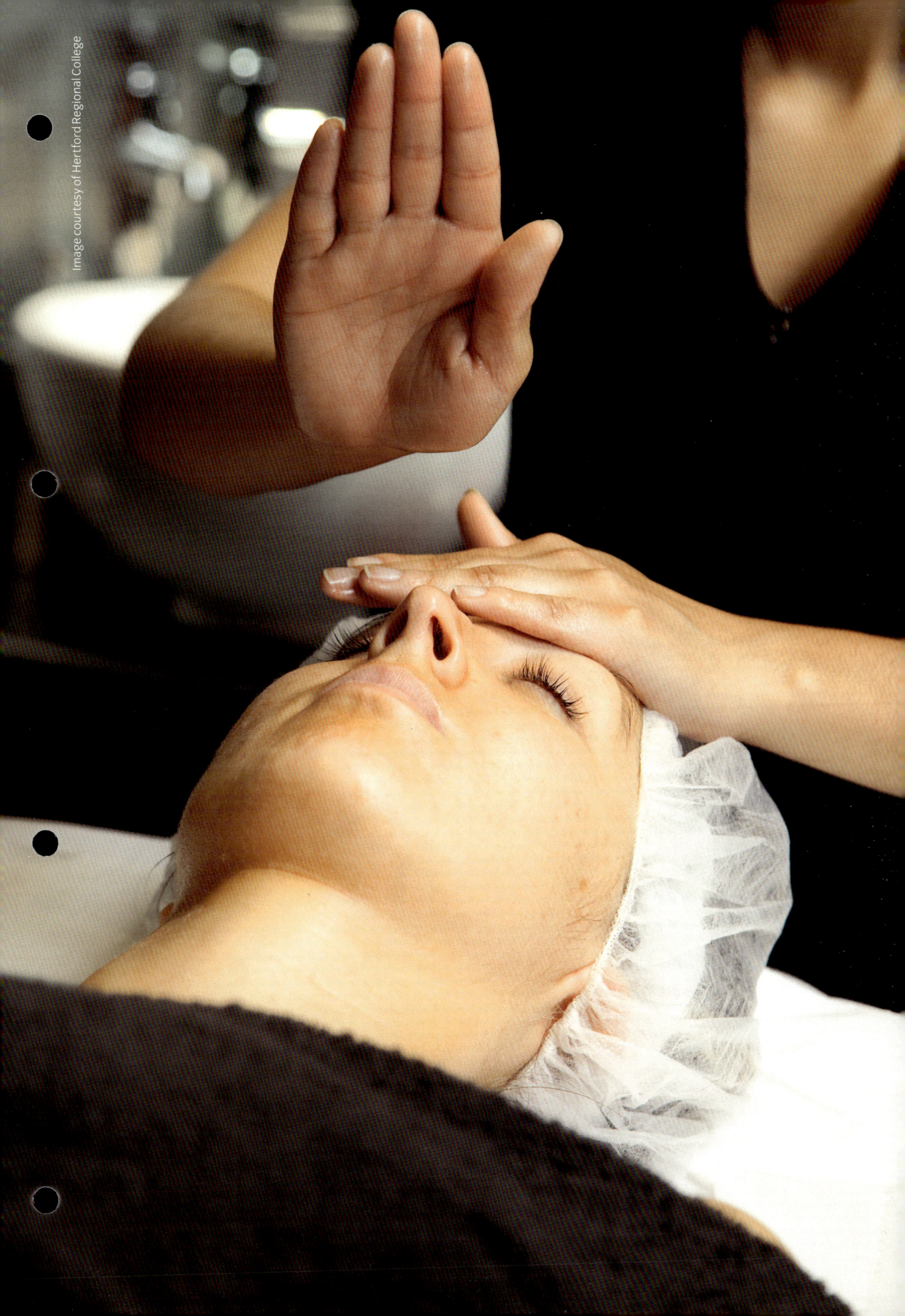

Image courtesy of Hertford Regional College

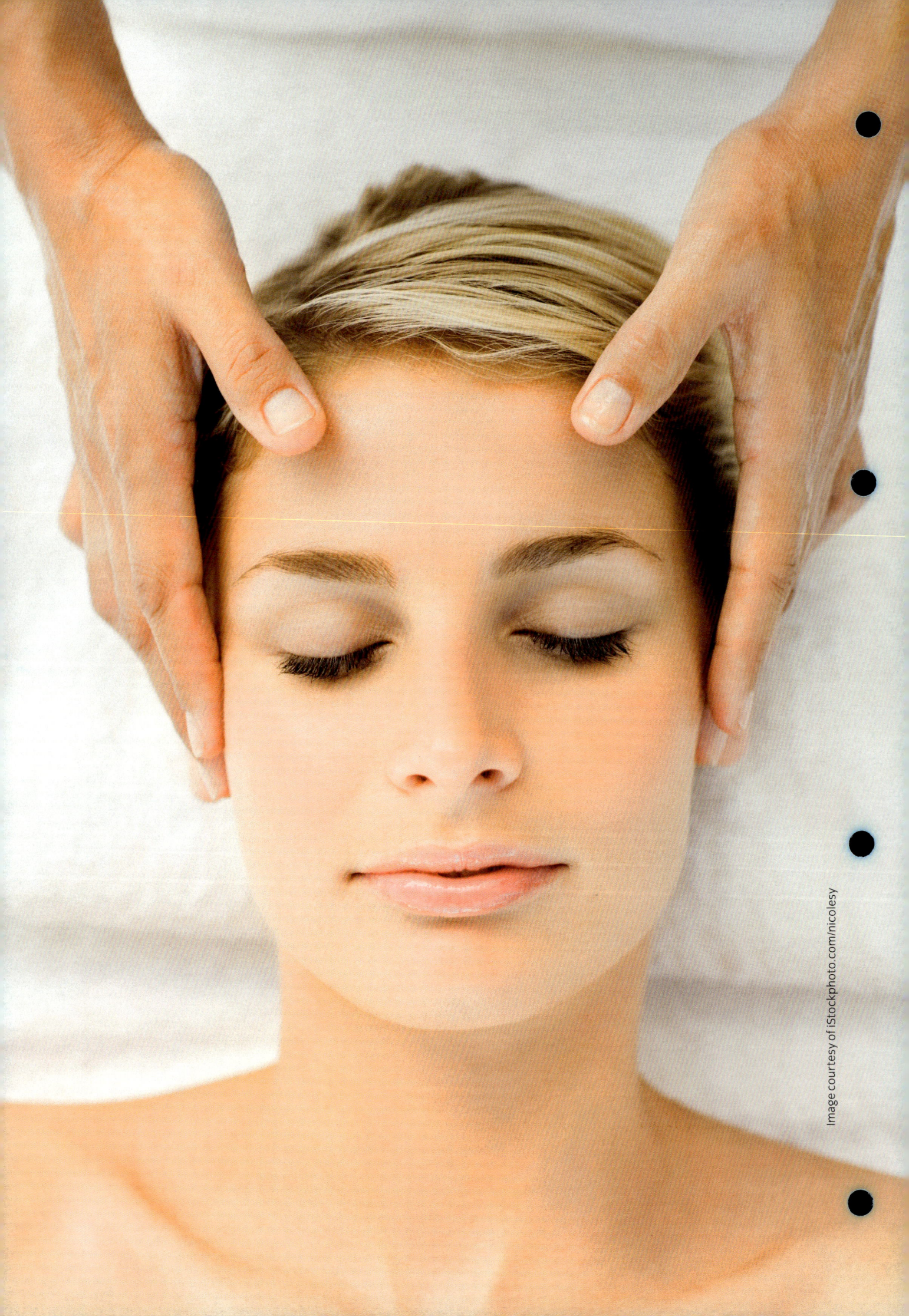

Image courtesy of iStockphoto.com/nicolesy

311

Provide Indian head massage

Indian head massage is an ancient art handed down through generations in India, as an integral part of family life. Its roots lie in the medicine system of Ayurveda, which aims to promote health, beauty and a long life. Depending on the techniques used, it can relax or invigorate. This unit will teach you how to select the most suitable medium for your client to improve scalp or hair condition, and how to adapt your treatment according to your client. You will learn what is meant by the chakras, as well as how the body systems work.

Assignment mark sheet
Unit 311 Provide Indian head massage

Your assessor will mark you on each of the practical tasks in this unit. This page is used to work out your overall grade for the unit. You must pass **all** parts of the tasks to be able to achieve a grade. For each completed practical task, a pass equals 1 point, a merit equals 2 points and a distinction equals 3 points.

What you must know	Tick when complete
Task 1a: produce an information sheet	
Task 1b: produce a report	
Task 1c: produce a fact sheet	
Task 1d: anatomy and physiology	
Or tick if covered by an online test	

What you must do	Grade	Points
Task 2: Provide Indian head massage		

Overall grade

Candidate name:

Candidate signature: Date:

Assessor signature: Date:

Quality assurance co-ordinator signature   Date:
(where applicable):

External Verifier signature   Date:
(where applicable):

The nourishing oils used, plus the massage, help to promote healthy hair growth.

Image courtesy of Paul Mitchell

What does it mean?
Some useful words are explained below

Alopecia
Partial or total hair loss. It can result from shock, trauma, illness, prolonged stress, or trichotillomania.

Ayurveda
A healing system describing how the mind, body and spirit must be in harmony to improve health and wellbeing.

Chakras
There are seven major chakras (energy centres without a physical form). They are a way of describing energies and energy flow and are the focal points for restoring balance to the body.

Dehydrated skin
A lack of water or moisture within the skin. It can occur on any skin type.

Effleurage
A stroking technique used to begin and end a massage. It is also useful to link movements to provide flow and rhythm in the massage.

Erythema
Redness of the skin, resulting from dilation of blood vessels, due to stimulation, irritation or allergy.

Mature skin
In beauty therapy terms, this is any skin over the age of 25. However, the skin is not usually described as mature until ageing is apparent.

Medium
The product used to give slip and glide during the massage, as well as to nourish the hair and scalp.

Mustard oil
A popular oil in India, which creates a warming sensation. It is good for tense, tight muscles and dryness of the scalp. Not for use on sensitive skins.

Osteoporosis
A disease in which the bones become extremely porous and are subject to fracture.

Petrissage
A technique that compresses the tissues of the body and lifts them away from the underlying structures.

Sesame oil
Used in Ayurveda, this has a high mineral content and is useful for nourishing the hair.

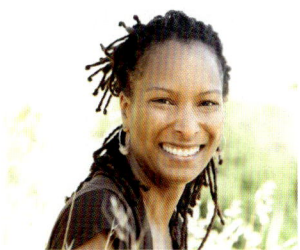

Skin type
A way of classifying the skin according to the amount of oil it produces. The skin types are normal, dry, oily and combination.

Tapotement
A rhythmic, stimulating movement performed to stimulate the skin and muscle tissues.

Tinea capitis
Ringworm of the scalp. A contagious fungal infection where there are circles of red itchy skin. On the scalp, it will result in hair breakage and loss.

Tinnitus
Sensation of a ringing, roaring, or buzzing sound in the ears or head, when no external sound is present.

Trichotillomania
A nervous habit where the sufferer has a compulsive urge to pull out hair from the scalp, brows or lashes.

Vibrations
Fine, trembling movements used by the therapist during massage that can stimulate or relax nerves.

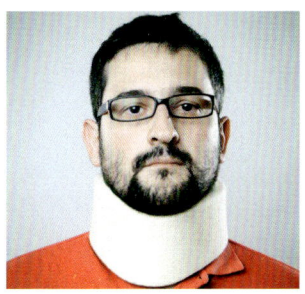

Whiplash
A condition produced when the muscles, ligaments, discs or nerves in the neck are damaged due to sudden trauma.

> **Revision tip**
>
> By relaxing the muscles of the head, neck and shoulders, Indian head massage can help with the relief of tension headaches.

What you must know
You must be able to:

1. Describe salon requirements for preparing yourself, the client and work area
2. Describe the environmental conditions suitable for Indian head massage
3. Describe the different consultation techniques used to identify treatment objectives
4. Explain the importance of carrying out relevant tests
5. Describe how to select products and equipment to suit client treatment needs
6. Explain the contra-indications that prevent or restrict Indian head massage
7. Explain how to communicate and behave in a professional manner
8. Explain health and safety working practices
9. Explain the importance of positioning yourself and the client correctly throughout the treatment
10. Explain the importance of using products, equipment and techniques to suit client's treatment need
11. Explain the effects and benefits of Indian head massage

Continues on next page

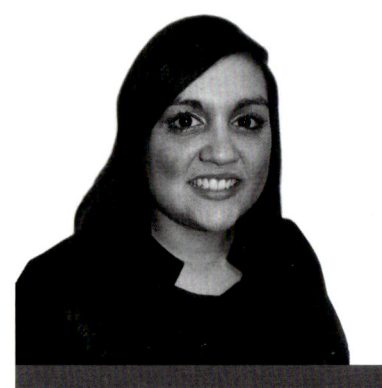

Follow in the footsteps of... *Jenny Smith*

"

Jenny has always known that she wanted to study Hair and Beauty. She completed her Level 2 and 3 in Hairdressing at Andover College, and during this course her secondary learning goal was Indian head massage. She soon realised her passion for Massage Therapy, and went on to do Level 2 Beauty Therapy, before progressing on to Level 3 Complementary Therapies. In the future she'd like to get a job in a salon where she can do both hair and beauty. **Read on for Jenny's top tips!**

12. Describe how treatments can be adapted to suit client treatment needs
13. State the contra-actions that may occur during and following treatments and how to respond
14. Explain the importance of completing the treatment to the satisfaction of the client
15. Explain the importance of completing treatment records
16. Describe the methods of evaluating the effectiveness of the treatment
17. Describe the aftercare advice that should be provided
18. Describe the structure and functions of the skin
19. Describe skin types, conditions, diseases and disorders
20. Describe the structure and function of the hair
21. Describe the structure of the head, neck, upper back and arms
22. Outline the position and actions of the muscles in the head, neck, upper back and arms
23. Describe the structure, function and supply of the blood and lymph to the head
24. Describe the location and function of chakras

To achieve a better massage use a lower backed chair, or even purchase a professional Indian head chair.

Revision tip

The hair shaft is made up of three main parts: the outer cuticle, the cortex and the medulla. The sebaceous gland is attached to the follicle, lubricating the hair.

> *Always remember to have a towel or a pillow to support the client's head and neck when working on the face.*

Indian hea

Poor posture can cause many conditions, including tension, poor circulation and headaches. Noting the client's posture, adapting the massage and then giving advice may provide relief.

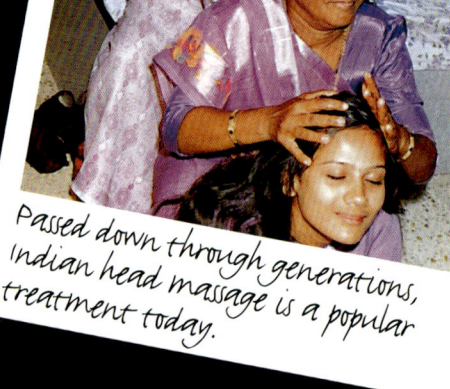

Passed down through generations, Indian head massage is a popular treatment today.

Image courtesy of London School of Indian Champissage

You need to check your pressure with the client during the massage. Start the massage by asking if the client prefers a light or deeper massage.

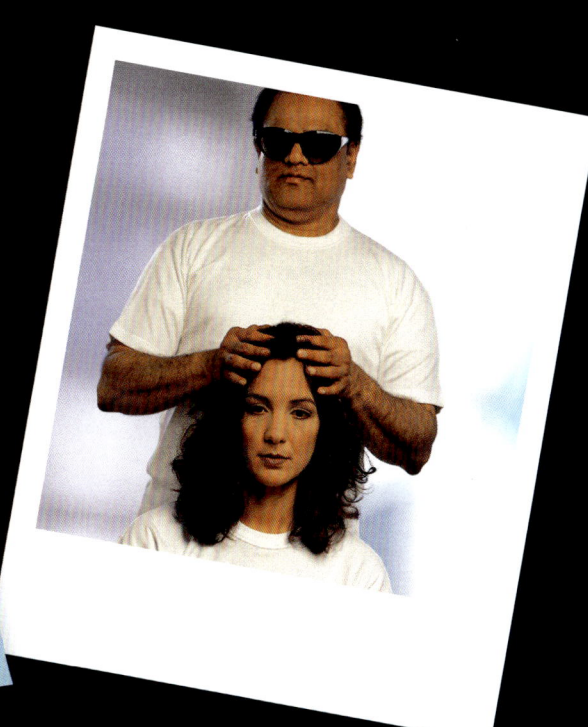

d massage

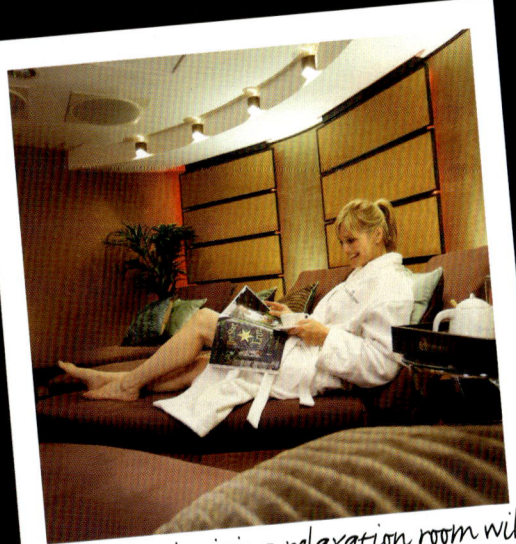

A warm, inviting relaxation room will help the client stay relaxed even after their treatment.

" *Pick the carrier oil to suit your client's needs, eg almond oil for dry skin.*

What you must do
Practical observations

This page shows what you need to do during your practical task. You can look at it beforehand, but you're **not** allowed to have it with you while carrying out your practical task. You must achieve **all** the criteria; you can achieve 1 mark, 2 marks or 3 marks for the criteria indicated with *.

Conversion chart

Grade	Marks
Pass	11–13
Merit	14–19
Distinction	20–23

○ Please tick when all pre-observation requirements have been met

	Provide Indian head massage		
1 Prepare yourself, the client and the work area for Indian head massage	1		
2 Use suitable consultation techniques to identify treatment objectives *	1	2	3
3 Provide clear recommendations to the client *	1	2	3
4 Position yourself and the client correctly throughout the treatment	1		
5 Follow health and safety working practices	1		
6 Communicate and behave in a professional manner	1		
7 Select and use products to suit client's treatment needs, skin and hair conditions *	1	2	3
8 Use and adapt massage techniques to meet the needs of the client *	1	2	3
9 Complete the treatment to the satisfaction of the client *	1	2	3
10 Record and evaluate the results of the treatment	1		
11 Provide suitable aftercare advice *	1	2	3
Total			
Grade			
Candidate signature and date			
Assessor signature and date			

What you must do
Practical observations descriptors table

This table shows what you need to do to achieve 1, 2 or 3 marks for the criteria indicated with * on the previous page.

	1 mark	2 marks	3 marks
2 Use suitable consultation techniques to identify treatment objectives	Basic consultation Examples: uses open and closed questions, checks for contra-indications, identifies the treatment objectives correctly.	Good consultation Examples: positive body language, uses open and closed questions to identify contra-indications, general health, lifestyle and expectations; identifies the treatment objectives and any factors that may limit or restrict the treatment.	Thorough consultation Examples: positive body language, uses open and closed questions to identify contra-indications, general health, lifestyle and expectations, how client feels about their body and what improvement they would like to achieve; identifies the treatment objectives and any factors that may limit or restrict the treatment, allows the client to ask any questions to confirm understanding.
3 Provide clear recommendations to the client	A basic treatment plan is recommended Example: explains treatment procedure and any adaptations to meet client treatment needs.	A good treatment plan is recommended Examples: explains treatment procedure and any adaptations to meet client treatment needs based on factors identified during consultation (lifestyle, medication (if any), contra-indications, hair and skin conditions), a choice of products to be used.	A thorough treatment plan is recommended Examples: explains treatment procedure and any adaptations to meet client treatment needs based on factors identified during consultation (lifestyle, medication (if any), contra-indications, hair and skin conditions), a choice of products to be used, adaptation of massage movements to suit client treatment needs, allows the client to ask questions about the treatment plan.

Continues on next page

What you must do
Practical observations descriptors table (continued)

This table shows what you need to do to achieve 1, 2 or 3 marks for the criteria indicated with * on page 132.

	1 mark	2 marks	3 marks
7 Select and use products to suit client's treatment needs, skin types and condition	Selects appropriate massage media to suit client's skin and hair conditions.	Selects appropriate massage media to suit client's skin and hair conditions, taking into account client preference.	Selects appropriate massage media to suit client's skin and hair conditions, taking into account client preference, lifestyle, general health and treatment objectives.
8 Use and adapt massage techniques to meet the needs of the client	Adapts the massage routine to suit client treatment objectives. Uses a variety of movements, movements are even and flowing, uses appropriate pressure for the client.	Adapts the massage routine to suit client treatment objectives, skin and hair conditions. Carries out massage movements correctly and fully with even flow, showing variations in rate and rhythm according to treatment objectives, uses appropriate pressure for the client.	Adapts the massage routine to suit client treatment objectives, hair and skin conditions, taking into account all factors. The whole routine flows throughout, uses appropriate pressure for the client, checks the client's comfort and wellbeing at appropriate times.
9 Complete the treatment to the satisfaction of the client	The treatment is completed within the agreed time and brought to a satisfactory close.	The treatment is completed within the agreed time, brought to a satisfactory close, and feedback is gained from the client.	The treatment is completed within the agreed time, brought to a satisfactory close, feedback is gained from the client, and client is allowed sufficient time to get dressed and is provided with tools (eg comb and mirror) to neaten the hair.

Continues on next page

	1 mark	2 marks	3 marks
11 Provide suitable aftercare advice	Basic aftercare advice Examples: how to deal with possible contra-actions, product(s) to use, importance of rest and relaxation, future treatment needs.	Good level of aftercare advice Examples: how to deal with possible contra-actions, product(s) to use, importance of rest and relaxation, specific lifestyle advice (ie dealing with stress, fluid intake, healthy eating), future treatment needs.	Excellent aftercare advice Examples: how to deal with possible contra-actions, product(s) to use, importance of rest and relaxation, specific lifestyle advice (ie dealing with stress, fluid intake, healthy eating), advice to improve postural awareness, recommends future treatment programme (regular Indian head massage, introduction of new/alternative treatments).

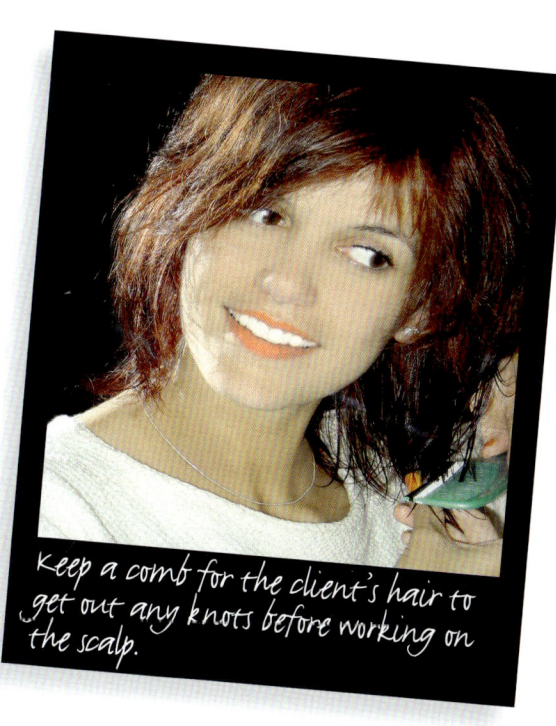

Keep a comb for the client's hair to get out any knots before working on the scalp.

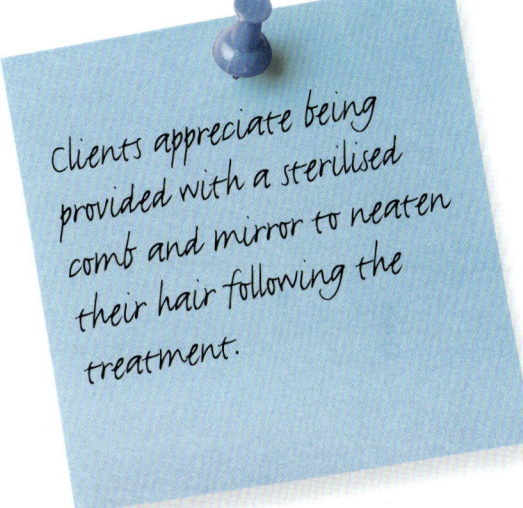

Clients appreciate being provided with a sterilised comb and mirror to neaten their hair following the treatment.

Provide Indian head massage **Unit 311**

Comment form
Unit 311 Provide Indian head massage

This form can be used to record comments by you, your client, or your assessor.

_____

_____

_____

_____

_____

_____

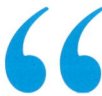

Keep nails short and tidy for when working with the pressure points – you don't want to hurt your client.

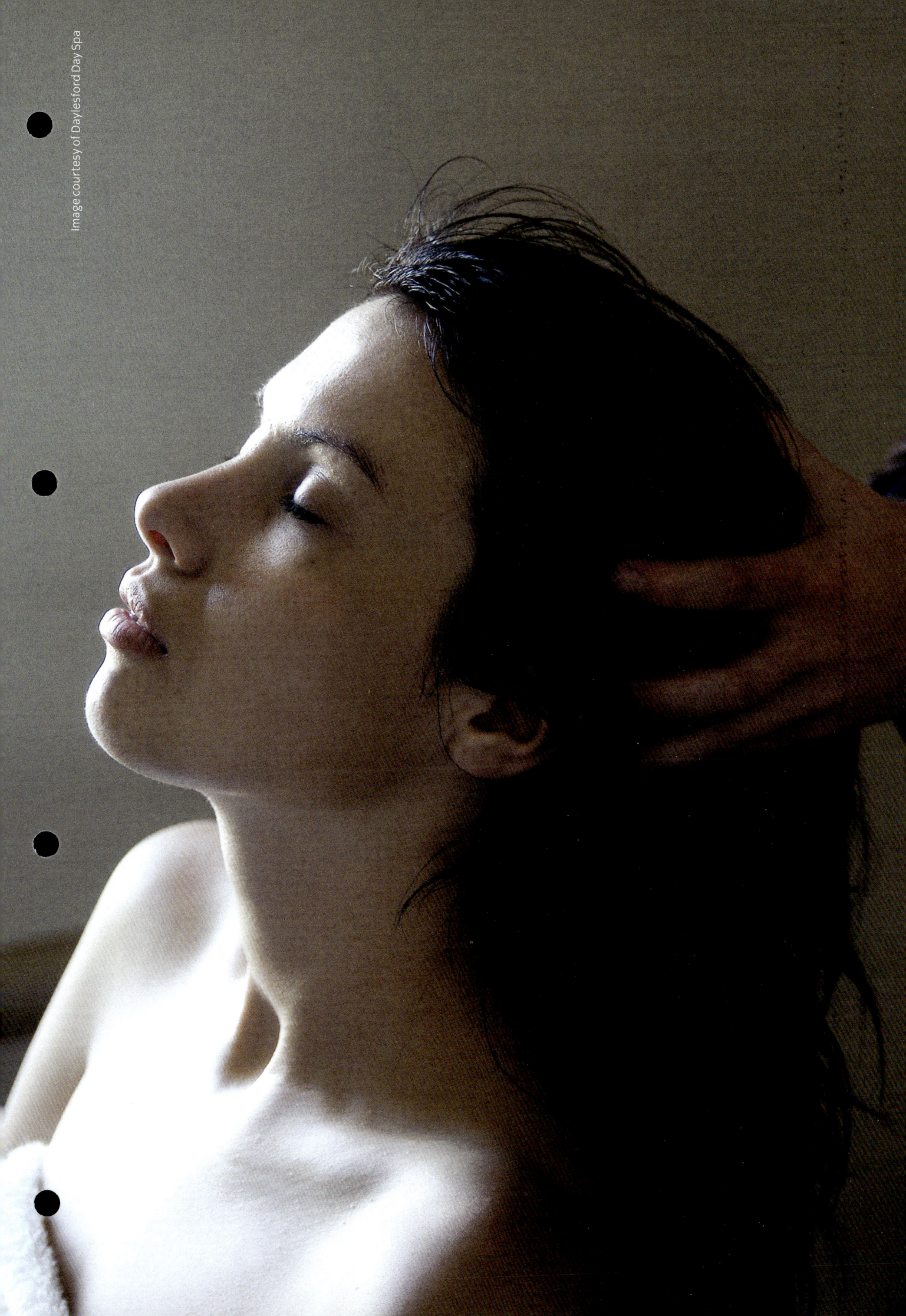

Image courtesy of Daylesford Day Spa

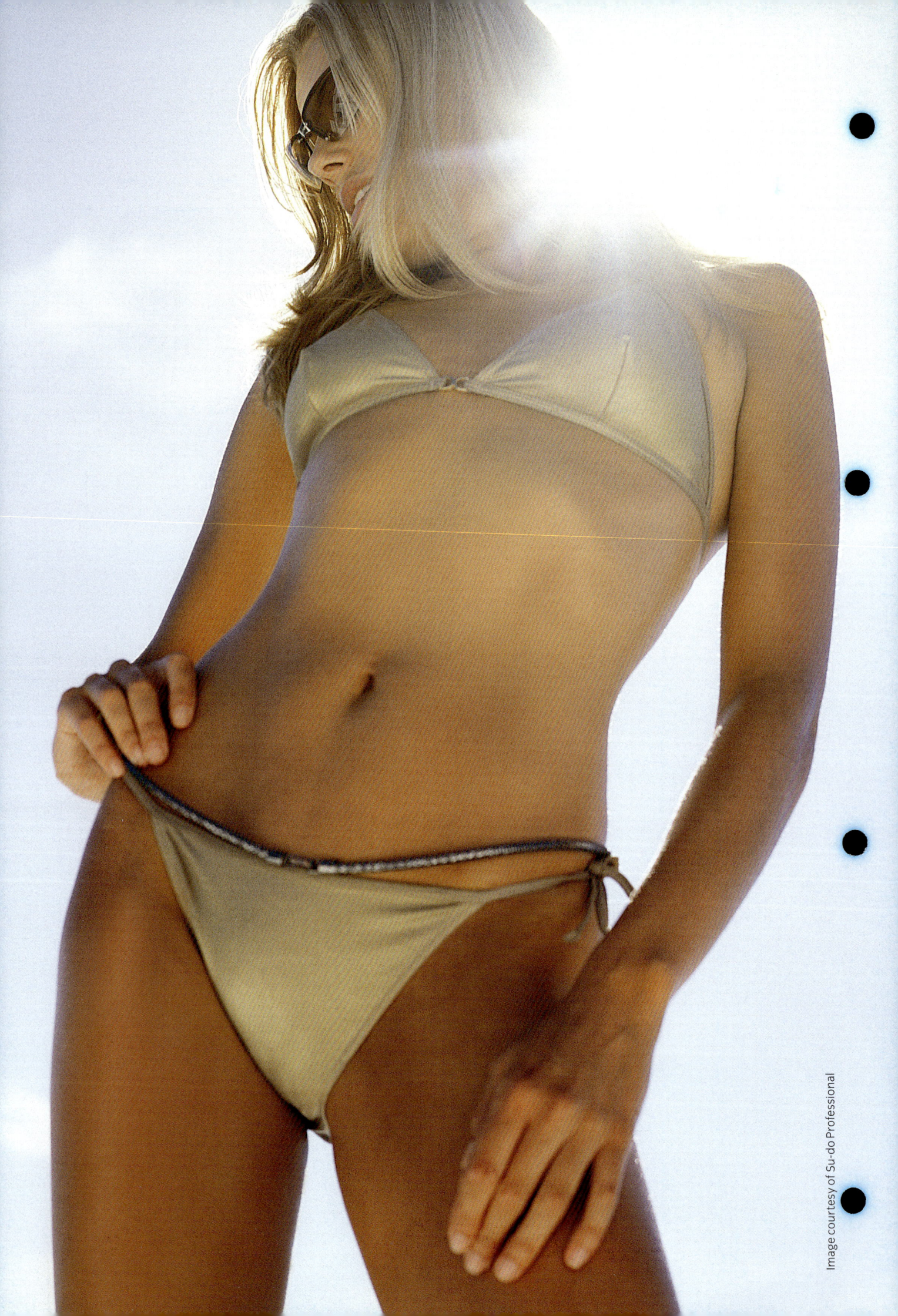

Image courtesy of Su-do Professional

313

Provide self tanning

Bronzed skin makes many people feel healthier and more attractive. However, these days getting a natural or sun bed tan is becoming unpopular as awareness grows that UV rays age the skin and can result in skin cancer. An even, all-over sun-kissed look can be difficult to achieve at home, meaning more and more people look for the results only a professional can achieve. In this unit you will learn how to apply the perfect tan to the body and face. You will also learn how to advise clients about preparing for the treatment, as well as the home care they can follow to preserve the colour and care for their skin.

Assignment mark sheet
Unit 313 Provide self tanning

Your assessor will mark you on each of the practical tasks in this unit. This page is used to work out your overall grade for the unit. You must pass **all** parts of the tasks to be able to achieve a grade. For each completed practical task, a pass equals 1 point, a merit equals 2 points and a distinction equals 3 points.

What you must know	Tick when complete
Task 1a: produce an information sheet	
Task 1b: produce an information sheet	
Task 1c: produce a fact sheet	
Task 1d: anatomy and physiology	
Or tick if covered by an online test	

What you must do	Grade	Points
Task 2: Provide self tanning		
Overall grade		

Candidate name:

Candidate signature: Date:

Assessor signature: Date:

Quality assurance co-ordinator signature (where applicable): Date:

External Verifier signature (where applicable): Date:

What does it mean?
Some useful words are explained below

Chloasma
A hyper-pigmentation disorder resulting in darker patches of skin.

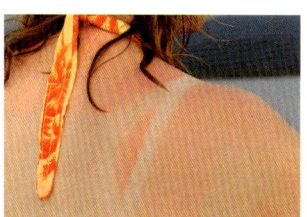

Contra-indications
Conditions that prevent a treatment from taking place or may require the therapist to modify the treatment.

Dehydrated skin
This is a lack of water or moisture within the skin as opposed to a lack of oil, and can occur on any skin type.

Development time
The length of time a product should be left on before the self tan produces the desired effect.

Dihydroxyacetone (DHA)
A sugar found in self tanning products, which reacts with the amino acids in the skin to produce a tanned effect.

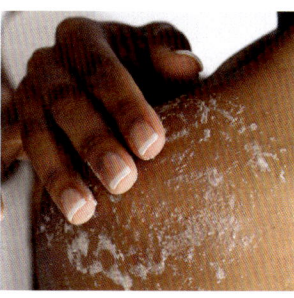

Exfoliation
The removal of dead skin cells from the surface of the skin to leave it smooth and even, prior to the application of the self tan.

Guide colour
The colour of the product when it is first applied to the skin. When washed off following the development time, the true colour will be visible. This will be unique to each client.

Hyper-pigmentation
Increased melanin production, causing darker areas of skin.

Hypo-pigmentation
Decreased melanin production on areas of the skin, resulting in paler patches.

Longevity of tan
The length of time that the tan lasts before fading.

Mature skin
In beauty therapy terms this is any skin over the age of 25. However, the skin is generally not classed as being mature until the signs of ageing are apparent.

Melanin
The pigment formed in skin by melanocytes. It gives the skin colour and provides natural protection against UV rays. It also has the function of absorbing heat from the sun.

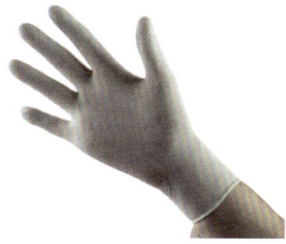

PPE
Equipment, such as gloves, aprons and respiratory equipment, that is intended to be worn or held by a person at work to protect them against one or more risks to their health and safety.

Skin analysis
A careful assessment of the skin to determine its type, condition and colour.

Skin patch test
A test where a small amount of product is applied to the skin and left on for 24 hours to check whether the client will react to the product.

SPF
Stands for sun protection factor. It is present in sunscreen products applied to protect the skin from the effects of the sun's rays. Professionals recommend wearing a minimum of SPF 15 regularly.

Ventilation
A ventilation system circulates air within a building to remove stale air and fumes, and replaces it with fresh air.

Vitiligo
A hypo-pigmentation disorder resulting in areas of very pale skin.

Revision tip

Wearing gloves during the application of a self tan not only prevents your hands from becoming stained, but also reduces the risk of contact dermatitis, irritation or allergy.

What you must know
You must be able to:

1 Describe salon requirements for preparing yourself, the client and work area

2 Describe the environmental conditions suitable for self tanning treatments

3 Describe the different consultation techniques used to identify treatment objectives

4 Explain the importance of carrying out a skin analysis

5 Describe how to select products and equipment to suit client treatment needs and skin conditions

6 Explain the contra-indications that prevent or restrict self tanning treatments

7 Compare the benefits of self tanning treatments with UV tanning treatments

8 Explain how to communicate and behave in a professional manner

9 Describe health and safety practices

Continues on next page

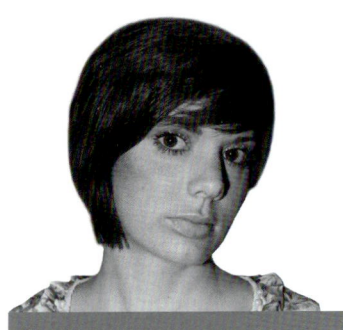

Follow in the footsteps of... *Lauren Key*

After achieving her Level 3 Diploma in Beauty Therapy at the Bournemouth and Poole College, Lauren went on to work at the UK's most prestigious spa hotel, The Chewton Glen. After four years at Chewton Glen she opened her own salon, LaSpa Health and Beauty. LaSpa has been established for three years, providing professional treatments to a strong and regular client base. Whilst running her salon Lauren completed her teacher training in Beauty Therapy. In the future her goal is to combine the two professions. **Read on for Lauren's self tanning tips!**

10 Explain the importance of positioning yourself and client correctly throughout the treatment

11 Explain the importance of using products, equipment and techniques to suit client's treatment needs and skin condition

12 Describe the effects and benefits of self tanning treatments and products on the skin

13 Describe the structure and function of the skin

14 Describe the contra-actions that might occur during or following treatments and how to respond

15 Explain the importance of completing the treatment to the satisfaction of the client

16 Explain the importance of completing treatment records

17 Describe the methods of evaluating the effectiveness of the treatment

18 Describe the aftercare advice that should be provided

Tell your clients to exfoliate and moisturise their skin every morning a few days before they apply self tan.

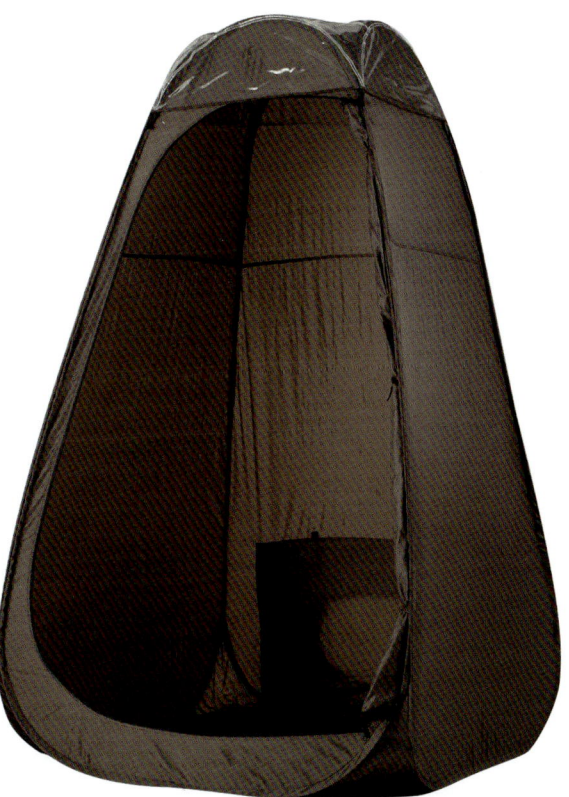

> "Dilute the self tanner with an equal amount of moisturiser for feet, ankles, elbows and knees.

Self ta

The client's privacy and modesty is very important during self tanning. Build a rapport with your client during the consultation so that they don't feel too self-conscious.

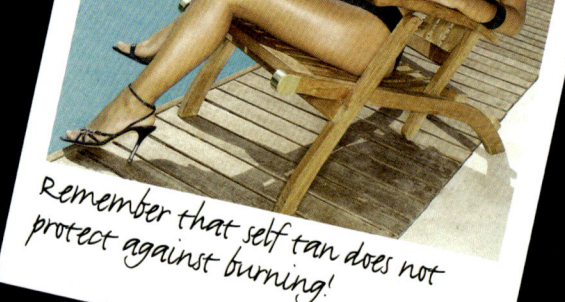

Remember that self tan does not protect against burning!

Image courtesy of Germaine de Capuccini

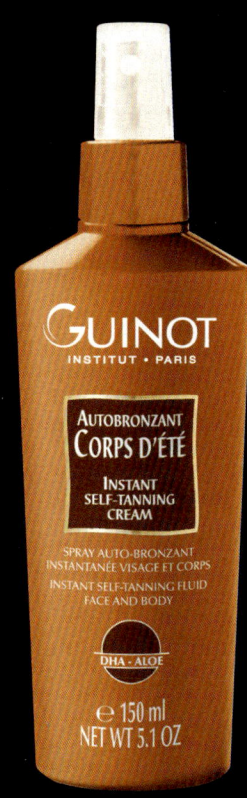
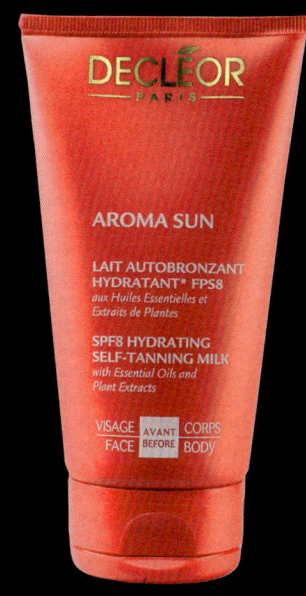

nning

"*Experiment with a variety of product ranges to find your client's perfect shade. Unless their natural skin tone is very dark, start off with a product that has a lower concentration of DHA, and give them two or three applications, spread out over a few days.*

A thorough exfoliation prior to the application of self tan will result in a more even and longer-lasting end result.

What you must do
Practical observations

This page shows what you need to do during your practical task. You can look at it beforehand, but you're **not** allowed to have it with you while carrying out your practical task. You must achieve **all** the criteria; you can achieve 1 mark, 2 marks or 3 marks for the criteria indicated with *.

Conversion chart

Grade	Marks
Pass	12–14
Merit	15–20
Distinction	21–24

○ Please tick when all pre-observation requirements have been met

	Provide self tanning treatment		
1 Prepare yourself, the client and the work area for self tanning treatment	1		
2 Use suitable consultation techniques to identify treatment objectives *	1	2	3
3 Carry out a skin analysis	1		
4 Advise the client on how to prepare for the treatment *	1	2	3
5 Provide clear recommendations to the client *	1	2	3
6 Position yourself and the client correctly throughout the treatment	1		
7 Follow health and safety working practices	1		
8 Communicate and behave in a professional manner	1		
9 Select and use products, equipment and techniques to suit client's treatment needs and skin conditions *	1	2	3
10 Complete the treatment to the satisfaction of the client *	1	2	3
11 Record and evaluate the results of the treatment	1		
12 Provide suitable aftercare advice *	1	2	3
Total			
Grade			
Candidate signature and date			
Assessor signature and date			

What you must do
Practical observations descriptors table

This table shows what you need to do to achieve 1, 2 or 3 marks for the criteria indicated with * on the previous page.

	1 mark	2 marks	3 marks
2 Use suitable consultation techniques to identify treatment objectives	Basic consultation Examples: uses open and closed questions, checks for contra-indications, identifies the treatment objectives correctly.	Good consultation Examples: positive body language, uses open and closed questions to identify contra-indications, general health, lifestyle and expectations with regard to depth of colour and longevity of tan and reasons/occasion for having tan; identifies the treatment objectives and any factors that may limit or restrict the treatment.	Thorough consultation Examples: positive body language, uses open and closed questions to identify contra-indications, general health, lifestyle and expectations with regard to depth of colour and longevity of tan and reasons/occasion for having tan, identifies the treatment objectives and any factors that may limit or restrict the treatment, allows the client to ask any questions to confirm understanding.
4 Advise the client on how to prepare for the treatment	Advises the client on the items of clothing and jewellery that need to be removed, gives basic information on how the equipment and products are used.	Advises the client on the items of clothing and jewellery that need to be removed, gives detailed information on how the equipment and products are used and how the client should be positioned during the treatment, explains the treatment procedure.	Advises the client on the items of clothing and jewellery that need to be removed, gives detailed information on how the equipment and products are used and how the client should be positioned during the treatment, explains the treatment procedure, makes the client feel at ease by explaining how their privacy will be ensured during the treatment, allows the client to ask questions.

Continues on next page

What you must do
Practical observations descriptors table (continued)

This table shows what you need to do to achieve 1, 2 or 3 marks for the criteria indicated with * on page 146.

	1 mark	2 marks	3 marks
5 Provide clear recommendations to the client	A basic treatment plan is recommended. Example: explains treatment procedure and any adaptations to meet client treatment needs.	A good treatment plan is recommended. Examples: explains treatment procedure and any adaptations to meet client treatment needs, takes into account client lifestyle and expectations.	A thorough treatment plan is recommended. Examples: explains treatment procedure and any adaptations to meet client treatment needs, takes into account client lifestyle and expectations and skin colouring characteristics, identifies any necessary modifications.
9 Select and use products, equipment and techniques to suit client's treatment needs and skin conditions	Correctly selects equipment and applies the tanning products according to treatment objective.	Correctly selects equipment and applies the tanning products according to treatment objective. Takes into account the client's natural skin tone and colouring characteristics, and considers the depth of colour, longevity of tan required and occasion for application.	Correctly selects equipment and applies the tanning products according to treatment objective. Takes into account the client's natural skin tone and colouring characteristics, and considers the depth of colour, longevity of tan required and occasion for application, adapts and modifies the techniques used as necessary, correctly explains the treatment throughout.
10 Complete the treatment to the satisfaction of the client	The treatment is completed within the agreed time and brought to a satisfactory close.	The treatment is completed within the agreed time, brought to a satisfactory close, the product is allowed to dry and client is given sufficient time to get dressed.	The treatment is completed within the agreed time and brought to a satisfactory close, the product is allowed to dry and client is given sufficient time to get dressed, the client is asked for feedback.

Continues on next page

	1 mark	2 marks	3 marks
12 Provide suitable aftercare advice	Basic aftercare advice Examples: how to deal with possible contra-actions, product(s) to use, future treatment needs.	Good level of aftercare advice Examples: how to deal with possible contra-actions, product(s) to use, specific lifestyle advice (ie SPF information), future treatment needs.	Excellent aftercare advice Examples: how to deal with possible contra-actions, product(s) to use/avoid, specific lifestyle advice (ie SPF information), provides information on how to prolong/maintain tan, recommends future treatment programme (a course of tanning treatments, introduction of new/alternative treatments).

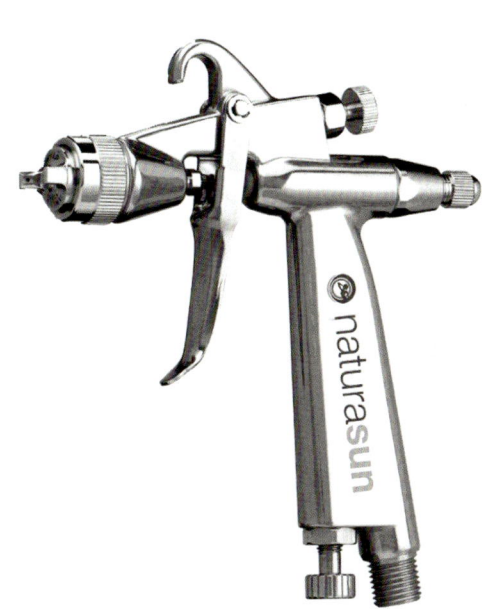

Image courtesy of naturasun

> *Advise your clients to prolong their tan by moisturising the skin daily.*

Provide self tanning **Unit 313**

Comment form
Unit 313 Provide self tanning

This form can be used to record comments by you, your client, or your assessor.

_____

_____

_____

_____

_____

_____

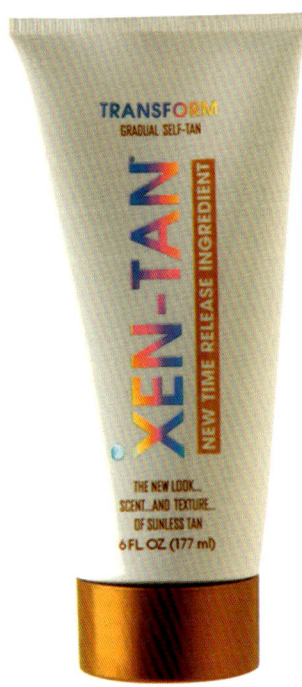

Image courtesy of Xen-Tan

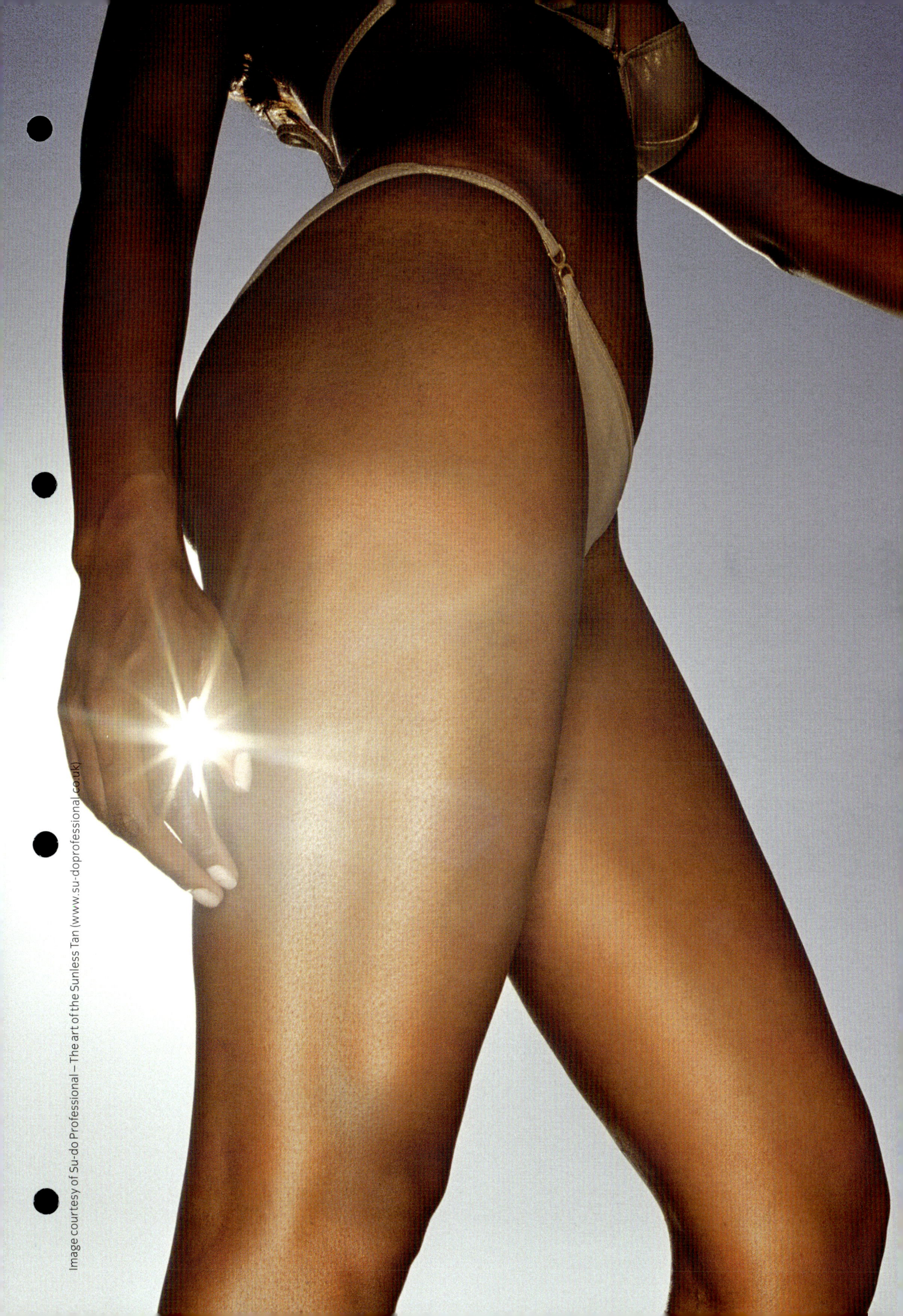

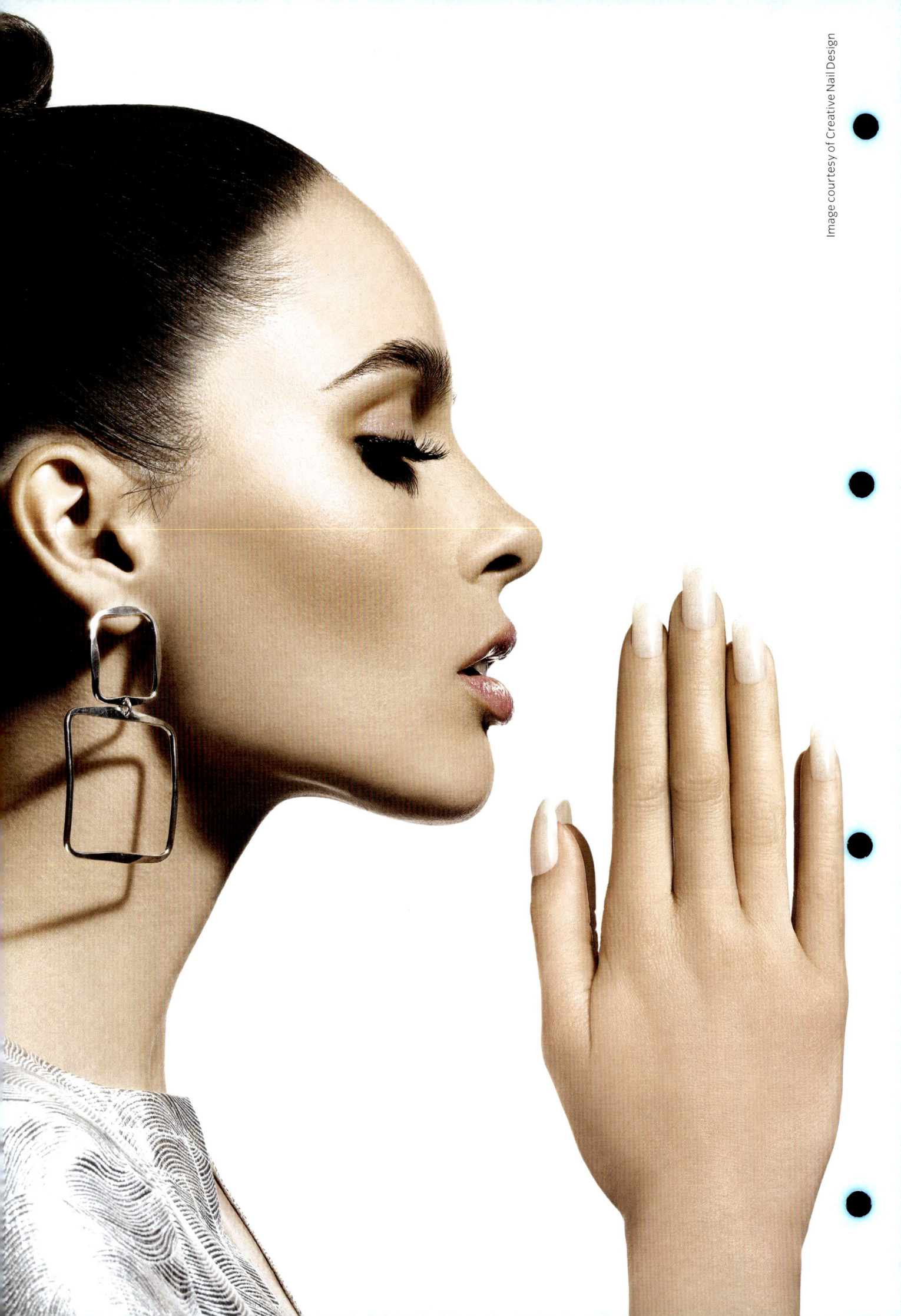

Image courtesy of Creative Nail Design

314

Apply and maintain nail enhancements

The application of nail enhancements requires high levels of skill, dexterity and care; it's an art form in itself. Techniques and products have advanced greatly in recent years and there are many different techniques that can be used to apply a beautiful set of balanced nail enhancements. They can be used to help mask imperfections, help to create a perfect finish and even elongate the nail bed. This unit covers the techniques you will learn, practise and perfect in order to achieve a high professional standard. Whichever system, product or manufacturer you choose you should always work in line with the Habia code of practice for nail services, follow manufacturer's instructions and observe hygiene, health and safety at all times.

Assignment mark sheet
Unit 314 Apply and maintain nail enhancements

Your assessor will mark you on each of the practical tasks in this unit. This page is used to work out your overall grade for the unit. You must pass **all** parts of the tasks to be able to achieve a grade. For each completed practical task, a pass equals 1 point, a merit equals 2 points and a distinction equals 3 points.

Conversion chart

Grade	Points
Pass	1–1.5
Merit	1.6–2.5
Distinction	2.6–3

What you must know	Tick when complete
Task 1a: produce an information sheet	
Task 1b: produce a fact sheet	
Task 1c: produce a fact sheet	
Task 1d: anatomy and physiology	
Or tick if covered by an online test	

What you must do	Grade	Points
Task 2a: Apply nail enhancements using liquid and powder		
Task 2b: Apply nail enhancements using UV gel		
Task 2c: Apply nail enhancements using wraps		
Task 2d: Maintenance service on one system		

Total points for graded tasks	
Divided by	÷ 4
= Average grade for tasks	
Overall grade (see conversion chart)	

Candidate name:

Candidate signature: Date:

Assessor signature: Date:

Quality assurance co-ordinator signature (where applicable):   Date:

External Verifier signature (where applicable):   Date:

> **Revision tip**
>
> Never overload your brush when applying gel so that it does not run onto the cuticle and surrounding skin. This could cause overexposure, which could lead to an allergic reaction or lifting of the overlay.

What does it mean?
Some useful words are explained below

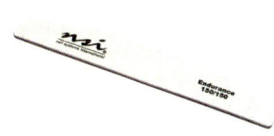

Abrasives
The term used to describe nail files and buffers.

Acrylates
The family of chemicals that nail enhancements are created from.

Activator
This liquid speeds up the polymerisation process for a cyanacrylate resin and is used within the wrap system.

Adhesive
Chemicals that cause two surfaces to bond together.

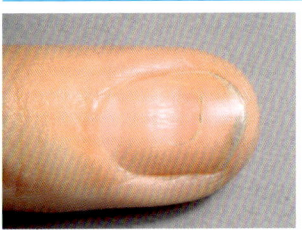

Beau's lines
Horizontal lines on the nail plate.

Breathing zone
The area surrounding the nail technician's air supply.

Catalyst
Chemical within a substance that controls the speed of the chemical reaction.

C-curve
The curvature of the nail plate from sidewall to sidewall.

Copolymer
A polymer made by a reaction of two or more different monomers.

Cross links
Chemical bonds between the polymer chains.

Curing
The process of polymerisation, ie turning a liquid or semi-liquid into a solid.

Cyanacrylate
A family of chemicals known as 'acrylates' that are used in adhesives and resins.

Dehydrator
This product is used at the beginning of a nail enhancements service to dehydrate excess oil and moisture from the nail plate.

Ethyl methacrylate (EMA)
This monomer is used in nail systems.

Exothermic reaction
A heat reaction that can occur during polymerisation.

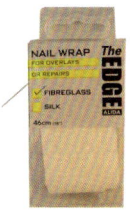

Fibreglass
A fine mesh fabric that has a glass content, used to create strength within the wrap system.

Forms
These are applied under the free edge while the nail enhancement is built onto it.

Initiator
The chemical that starts the process of polymerisation.

Lifting
The separation of the overlay from the natural nail plate.

Liquid and powder
Often referred to as acrylic but its correct term is liquid and powder. This system is a two component system that uses monomer (liquid) and a polymer (powder) mixed together to create a chemical reaction (polymersation) that produces a solid structure.

Lower arch
The curve of the lower underside of the free edge when checking the nail from the side profile.

Maintenance
The term used when the client returns to the salon every 2 to 3 weeks and has the nails reshaped, rebalanced, infilled, possibly repaired and the tip is repositioned, if appropriate.

Continues on next page

What does it mean?
Some useful words are explained below (continued)

Monomer
A molecule or one individual chemical unit that can react to form a polymer.

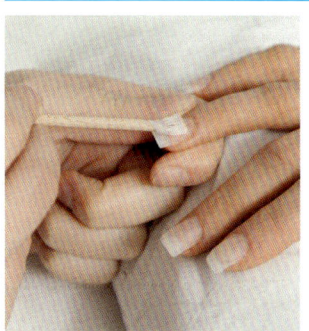

Nail wraps
Fabrics such as fibreglass and silk with an application resin are used to overlay the natural nail. This is often referred to as the three or several component system.

Oligomer
Monomer chains that are considerably shorter than a polymer.

Optical brightener
This is added to nail products to make colours look brighter and to enhance the white products to make them look crisp, clean and bright.

Overlay
An artificial coating applied to the natural nail that can also be used to extend it.

Photo initiator
This comes in the form of a UV light that acts as a catalyst to 'kickstart' the polymerisation process. This is commonly used with the gel system and also with certain brands of liquid and powder.

Polymer
Many units of chemically bonded monomers that form very long chains.

Polymerisation
A chemical reaction that turns the liquid or semi-liquid into a solid by creating polymer chains from monomers or oligomers.

Primer
This substance is used to improve adhesion between the nail plate and the nail enhancement.

Sculptured nail
This nail enhancement technique extends the nail plate by building it onto a nail form.

Smile line
The curve that is naturally created by the hyponychium. This can be simulated by the use of a natural coloured tip, a nail varnish or a coloured gel or liquid powder.

Solvent
A substance capable of dissolving other substances. Acetone is commonly used for this purpose.

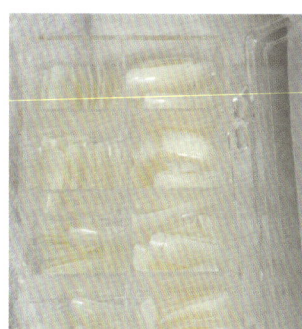

Stop point
This is the part where the tip fits around the free edge of the natural nail plate.

Upper arch
This refers to the curve of the nail from the cuticle area to the free edge.

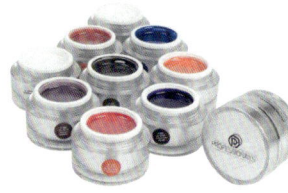

UV gel
A pre-mixed, semi-liquid that uses UV light to cure it. It requires no other product to activate it and has different viscosities, depending on type. It can also be used over the top of other systems to add shine.

Vapours
Chemical molecules in the air created by evaporation of a substance.

Continues on next page

What does it mean?
Some useful words are explained below (continued)

Ventilation
The interchanging of fresh air to remove odours and vapours from the air.

Viscosity
The density of a liquid.

Zones
Areas of the nail plate that are split into three sections:
Zone one – the free edge
Zone two – the apex area
Zone three – the cuticle area.

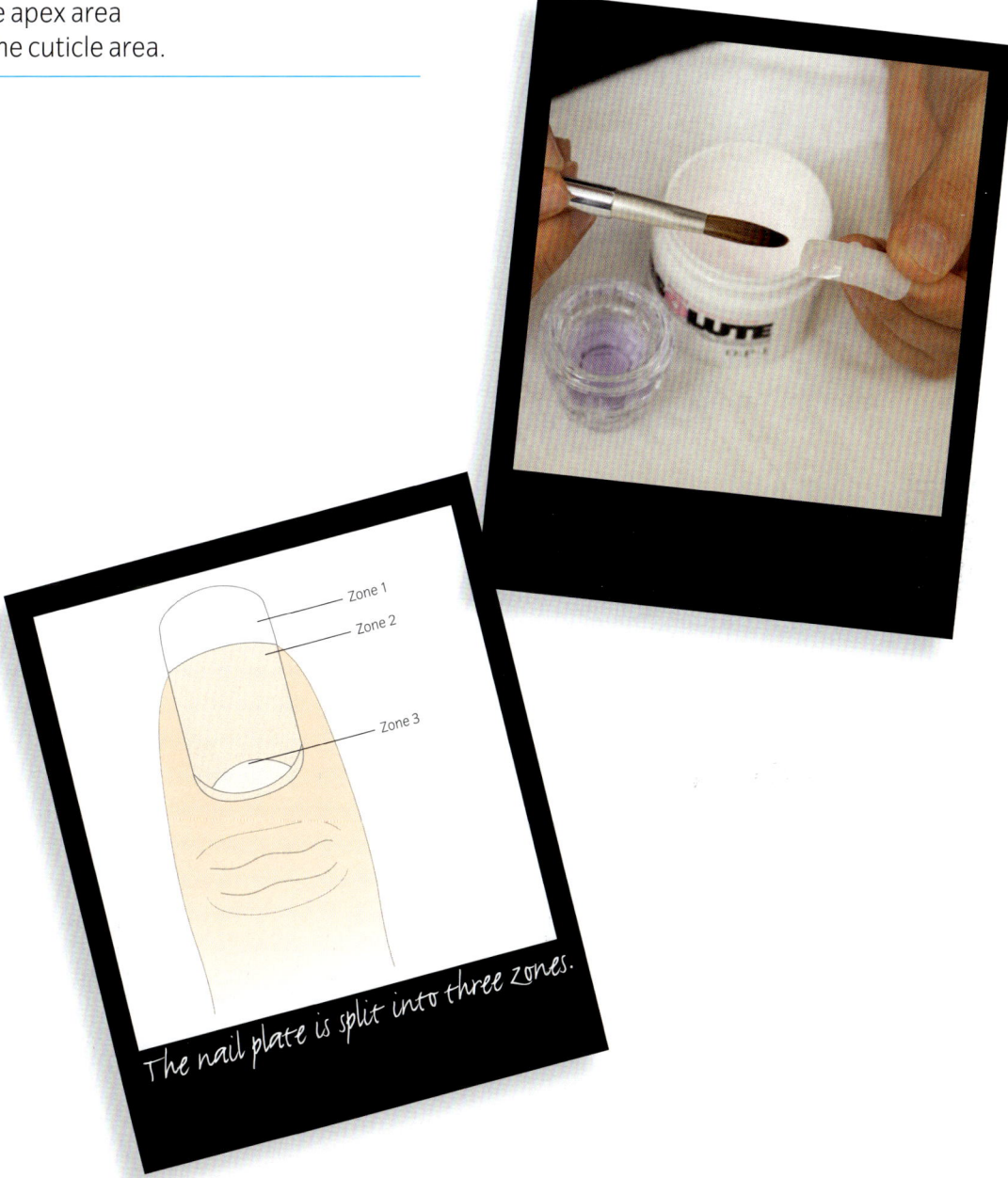

Image courtesy of Central Sussex College

The nail plate is split into three zones.

Apply and maintain nail enhancements Unit 314

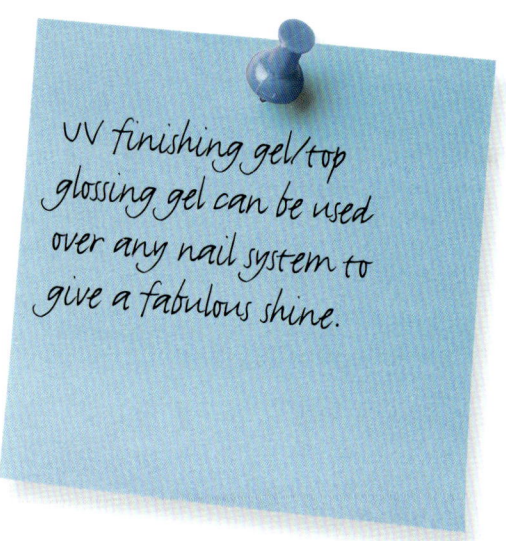

UV finishing gel/top glossing gel can be used over any nail system to give a fabulous shine.

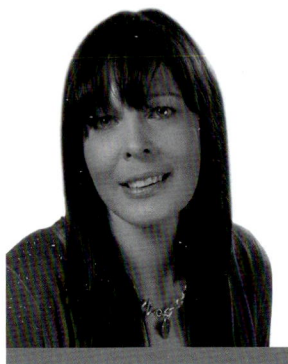

Follow in the footsteps of...
Samantha Watkinson

After studying Beauty Therapy it became clear that Samantha had a talent for creative work on the hands and feet and that nails was the industry for her. She attended a number of nail courses and over the years her career has taken her all over the world, working in education management, competing nationally and internationally gaining industry awards, competition judging, working on photo shoots, at various high profile events and with celebrities. She is now back in the classroom as a tutor at Derby College, and enjoys sharing her passion and knowledge with others. **Look for the blue quote marks to see what she has to say to you!**

What you must know
You must be able to:

1. Describe salon requirements for preparing themselves, the client and the work area
2. Describe the environmental conditions suitable for nail enhancement services
3. Describe the different consultation techniques used to identify treatment objectives
4. Explain the importance of carrying out a detailed nail and skin analysis
5. Describe how to select products, tools and equipment to suit client treatment needs, skin types and nail conditions
6. Describe the different skin and nail conditions
7. Explain the contra-indications that prevent or restrict manicure treatments
8. Explain how to communicate and behave in a professional manner
9. Describe health and safety working practices and industry Code of Practice for nail services
10. Explain the importance of positioning themselves and the client correctly throughout the service

Continues on next page

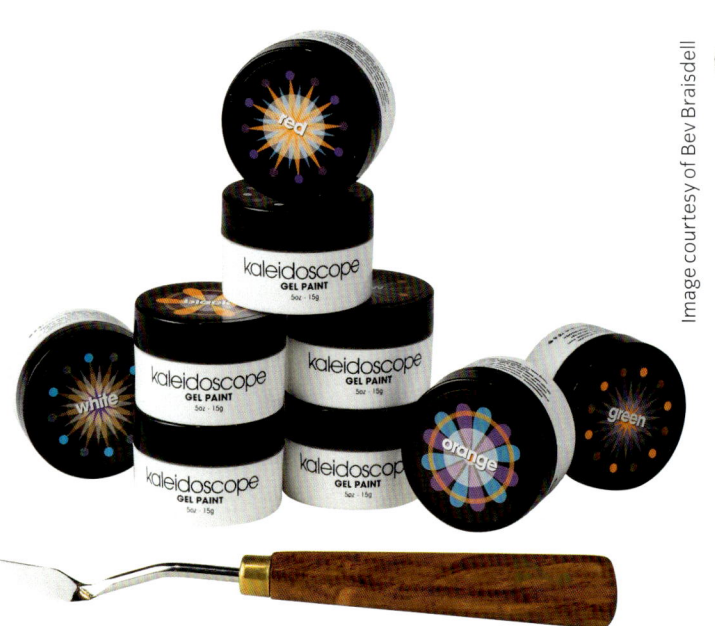

Image courtesy of Bev Braisdell

11 Explain the importance of using products, tools, equipment and techniques to suit client's service needs, nail and skin conditions

12 Describe how services can be adapted to suit client service needs, nail and skin conditions

13 Describe how to maintain and remove nail enhancements

14 State the contra-actions that may occur during and following the service and how to respond

15 Explain the importance of completing the service to the satisfaction of the client

16 Explain the importance of completing the treatment records

17 Describe the methods of evaluating the effectiveness of the treatment

18 Describe the chemical process involved in the nail enhancement systems

19 Describe the structure and functions of the nail and skin

20 Describe the different natural nail shapes

> *Keep up to date with new technology and continually practise all your skills to provide your clients with the best service possible.*

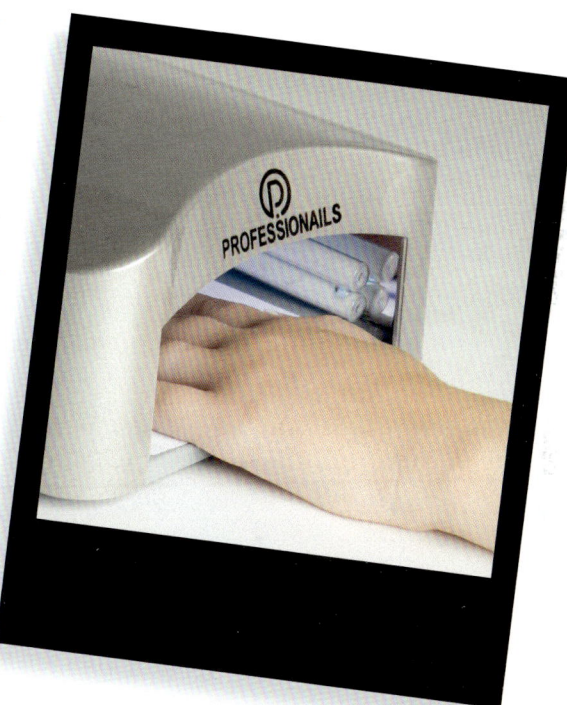

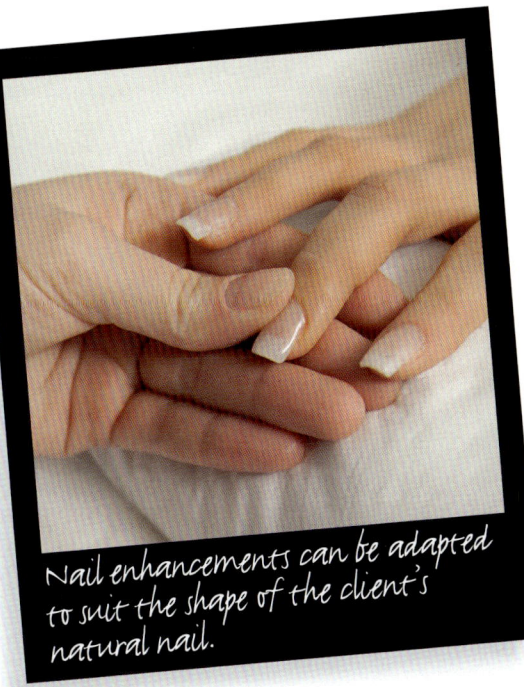

Nail enhancements can be adapted to suit the shape of the client's natural nail.

Revision tip

Take your time when learning the mix ratio of liquid to powder, product pick-up and placement. Once these aspects have been mastered it will be easier to apply the enhancements.

Use your time effectively during the service – educate your clients about their enhancements and how they should look after them.

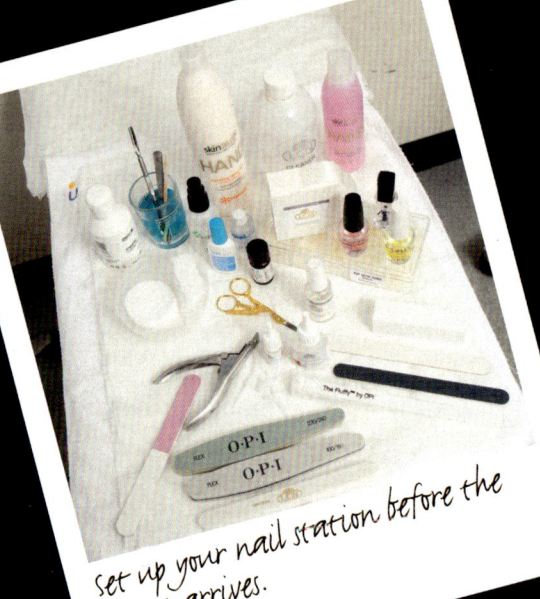

Set up your nail station before the client arrives.

Nail enha

The wrap system is excellent for repairs to natural nails. A stress strip may be used to reinforce the vulnerable area where the nail is broken.

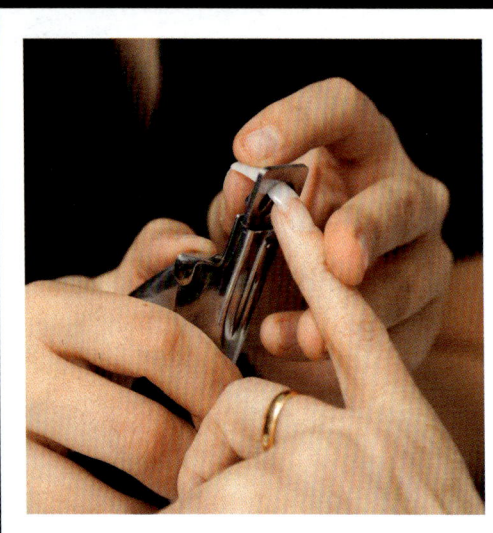

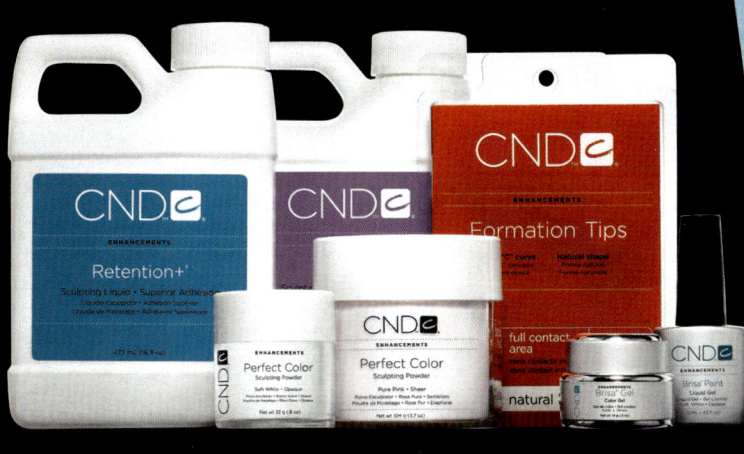

Specific products within the gel and liquid powder system are available to mask imperfections within the natural nail plate.

ncements

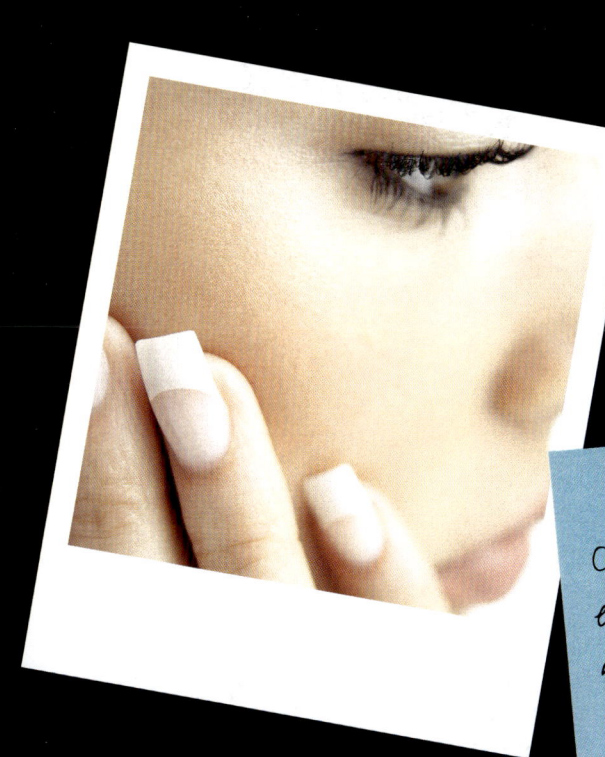

Coloured powders can be easily blended to create a customised colour that would mask imperfections and be matched perfectly to a client's skin tone to individualise the treatment.

What you must do
Practical observations

This page shows what you need to do during your practical task. You can look at it beforehand, but you're **not** allowed to have it with you while carrying out your practical task. You must achieve **all** the criteria; you can achieve 1 mark, 2 marks or 3 marks for the criteria indicated with *.

Conversion chart

Grade	Marks
Pass	11–13
Merit	14–18
Distinction	19–21

○ Please tick when all pre-observation requirements have been met.

	Nail enhancement service			
	a Liquid and powder	b UV gel	c Wrap	d Maintenance service on one system
1 Prepare yourself, client and work area for nail enhancement service	1	1	1	1
2 Use suitable consultation techniques to identify treatment objectives *	1 2 3	1 2 3	1 2 3	1 2 3
3 Carry out nail and skin analysis	1	1	1	1
4 Provide clear recommendations to the client *	1 2 3	1 2 3	1 2 3	1 2 3
5 Position yourself and the client correctly throughout the service	1	1	1	1
6 Follow health and safety working practices	1	1	1	1
7 Communicate and behave in a professional manner	1	1	1	1
8 Select and use correct products, tools, equipment and techniques to suit client service needs, nail and skin conditions *	1 2 3	1 2 3	1 2 3	1 2 3
9 Complete the treatment to the satisfaction of the client *	1 2 3	1 2 3	1 2 3	1 2 3
10 Record and evaluate the results of the treatment	1	1	1	1
11 Provide suitable aftercare advice *	1 2 3	1 2 3	1 2 3	1 2 3
Total				
Grade				
Candidate signature and date				
Assessor signature and date				

What you must do
Practical observations descriptors table

This table shows what you need to do to achieve 1, 2 or 3 marks for the criteria indicated with * on the previous page.

	1 mark	2 marks	3 marks
2 Use suitable consultation techniques to identify treatment objectives	Basic consultation Examples: uses open and closed questions, checks for contra-indications, identifies the treatment objectives correctly.	Good consultation Examples: positive body language, uses open and closed questions to identify contra-indications, lifestyle and expectations; identifies the treatment objectives and any factors that may limit or restrict the treatment.	Thorough consultation Examples: positive body language, uses open and closed questions to identify contra-indications, lifestyle and expectations, identifies the treatment objectives and any factors that may limit or restrict the treatment, allows the client to ask any questions to confirm understanding.
4 Provide clear recommendations to the client	A basic treatment plan is recommended Examples: explains service procedure and any adaptations to meet client service needs, equipment to be used.	A good treatment plan is recommended Examples: explains service procedure and any adaptations to meet client service needs, equipment to be used based on factors identified during consultation (lifestyle, natural nail shape, client wishes, results of skin and nail analysis, contra-indications), a choice of products to be used.	A thorough treatment plan is recommended Examples: explains service procedure and any adaptations to meet client service needs, equipment to be used based on factors identified during consultation (lifestyle, natural nail shape, client wishes, results of skin and nail analysis, contra-indications), a choice of products to be used, explains effects and benefits of the type of products/techniques used and the adaptation/modification to suit client service needs, allows the client to ask questions about the treatment plan.

Continues on next page

What you must do
Practical observations descriptors table (continued)

This table shows what you need to do to achieve 1, 2 or 3 marks for the criteria indicated with * on page 162.

	1 mark	2 marks	3 marks
8 Select and use correct products, tools, equipment and techniques to suit client service needs, nail and skin conditions	Selects and uses correct products, tools, equipment and techniques, nails have a uniform length.	Selects and uses correct products, tools, equipment and techniques, nails have a uniform length, no over-exposure to products, all nails are evenly balanced.	Selects and uses correct products, tools, equipment and techniques, nails have a uniform length, no over-exposure to products, all nails are evenly balanced, curvature of each nail has a uniform thickness.
9 Complete the treatment to the satisfaction of the client	The treatment is completed within the agreed time and brought to a satisfactory close.	The treatment is completed within the agreed time, brought to a satisfactory close and positive feedback is gained from the client.	The treatment is completed within the agreed time, brought to a satisfactory close and positive feedback is gained from the client, shows the client the results of the treatment and allows the client to ask questions.
11 Provide suitable aftercare advice	Basic aftercare advice Examples: how to deal with possible contra-actions, product(s) to use, future treatment needs.	Good level of aftercare advice Examples: how to deal with possible contra-actions, product(s) to use, specific advice (ie what to avoid immediately after the service, lifestyle), future service needs.	Excellent aftercare advice Examples: how to deal with possible contra-actions, product(s) to use, specific advice (ie what to avoid immediately after the service, lifestyle), recommends future service programme (maintenance and regular service, introduction of new/alternative services/treatments).

Comment form
Unit 314 Apply and maintain nail enhancements

This form can be used to record comments by you, your client, or your assessor.

Revision tip

Some clients and nail technicians may be sensitive to the resin activator in the spray format, which will touch the skin. To help prevent this, a brush-on version is available.

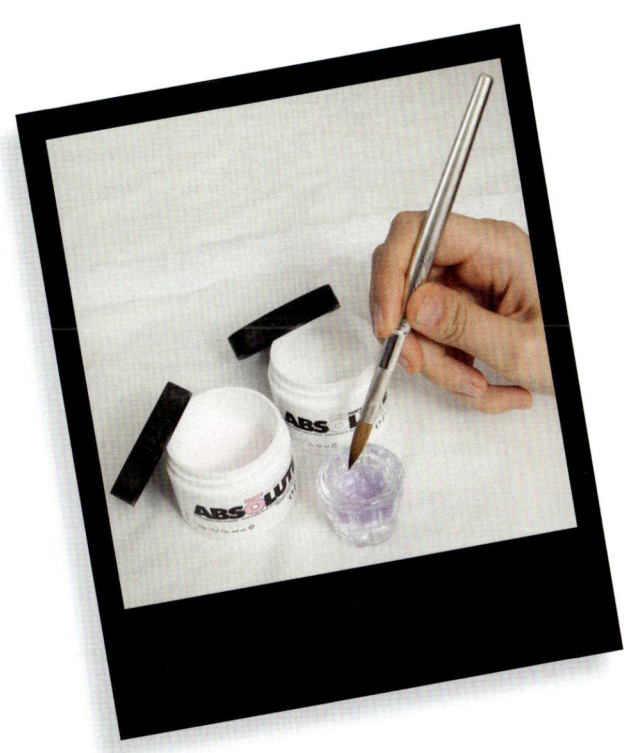

Image courtesy of Central Sussex College

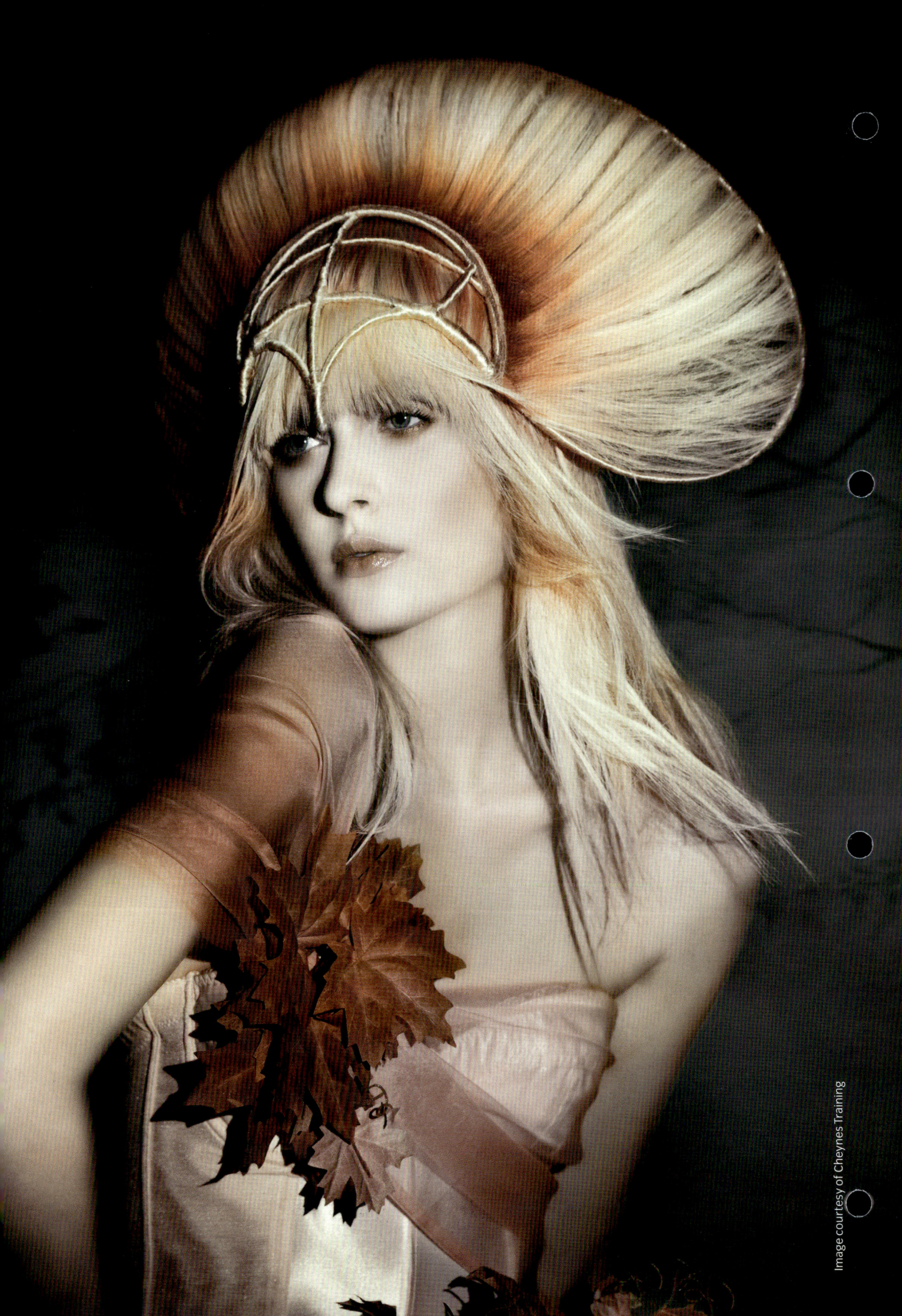

Image courtesy of Cheynes Training

316

Creative hairdressing design skills

Hairdressing is about imagination, vision and creativity. In this unit, you will produce images of your work for hair shows, photographic sessions or competition work. You will need to carry out research and planning in order to create an image that demonstrates the range of your skills. You will need to have the belief and confidence to explore new complex creative dressing techniques. This unit is about developing your creative hairdressing design skills in a way that enhances your own personal profile. Let's see how far your imagination can go, and it could be your pictures that are in this logbook next!

Assignment mark sheet
Unit 316 Creative hairdressing design skills

Your assessor will mark you on each of the practical tasks in this unit. This page is used to work out your overall grade for the unit. You must pass **all** parts of the tasks to be able to achieve a grade. For the practical task, a pass equals 1 point, a merit equals 2 points and a distinction equals 3 points.

What you must know	Tick when complete
Task 1a: produce a report	
Task 1b: produce a design plan	
Or tick if covered by an online test	

What you must do	Grade	Points
Task 2: Creative hair design		

Overall grade

Candidate name:

Candidate signature: Date:

Assessor signature: Date:

Quality assurance co-ordinator signature   Date:
(where applicable):

External Verifier signature   Date:
(where applicable):

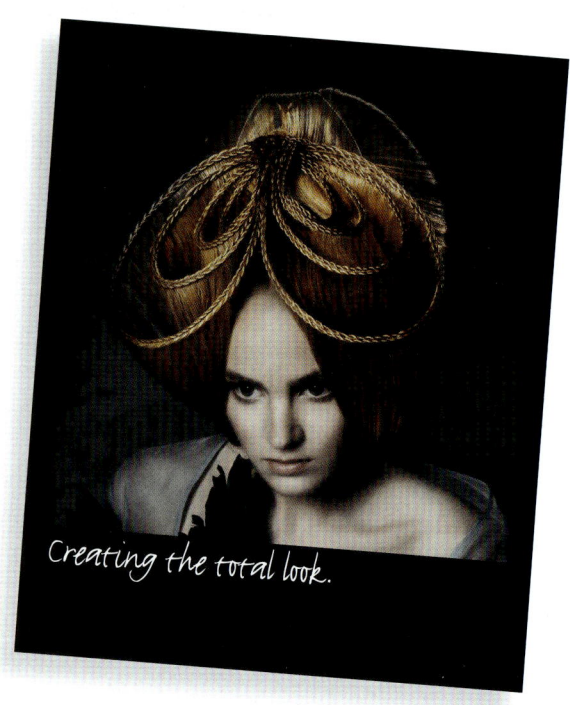

Creating the total look.

Image courtesy of Cheynes Training

What does it mean?
Some useful words are explained below

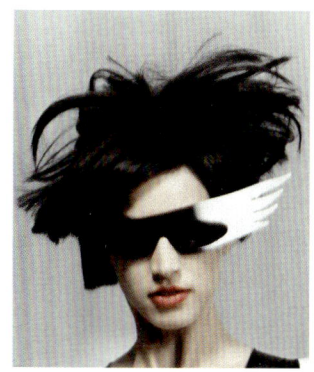

Avant-garde
A style, look or image that is ahead of the times, usually worn or produced by the leaders of fashion, before it becomes fashionable.

Evaluation
Actively seek feedback from a number of people (line manager, colleagues, audience, judges, models, photographer) on the impact of your image.

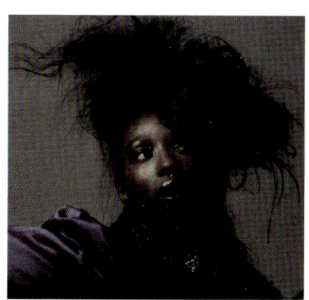

The image
The image is the total look. This includes hair, make-up, clothes, and jewellery. This can be avant-garde, based on a theme, or a commercial look.

Media
This is the make-up, ornamentations, accessories, video, photographs, and clothes that you use.

Mood board
A type of poster that consists of colours, images, text, and samples of materials, etc. You will produce a mood board to help develop your image concept, and to communicate the concept to others.

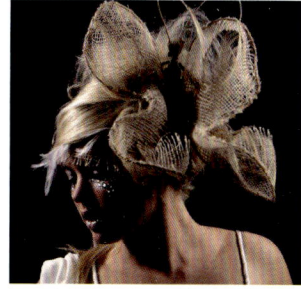

Ornamentation
An object used to complement a style, which adds interest and detail to the finished look.

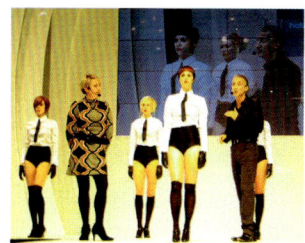

Planning
It is crucial that you carry out good planning before a photo shoot, hair show, or other event. Poor planning results in poor performance.

Risk assessment
This is a careful examination of what could cause harm to people in a particular location, such as a photo shoot set. You should do this so you can weigh up whether you have taken enough precautions or should do more to prevent harm.

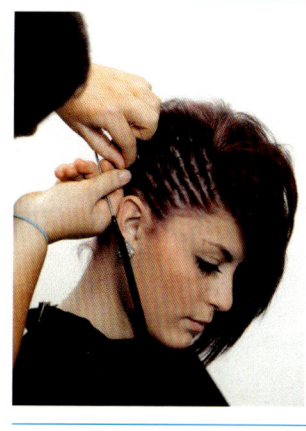

Techniques
These are the different methods used to create the finished image, for example, pin curling, finger waving, twisting, knotting, plaiting, weaving, and added hair.

Traction alopecia
Hair thinning or loss due to excessive tension on the hair follicle.

Creative hairdressing design skills Unit 316 169

Revision tip

Excessive pulling/tension of the hair at the root could result in traction alopecia.

What you must know
You must be able to:

1. Explain how to research and develop ideas for creating an image for a total look
2. Describe ways of combining styling, dressing and finishing techniques to create the completed total look
3. Explain ways of presenting a created image and look effectively
4. Describe methods of evaluating the design plan
5. Describe the potential commercial benefits of developing and creating design work
6. State the importance of accurate planning, attention to detail and working to timescales
7. Explain how the venue could affect design plans
8. Describe how to remedy problems that may occur with the different opportunities for creating an image
9. Explain the safety considerations that must be taken into account
10. Outline the skills required for presenting the image
11. Explain how other services can develop and complement the image and look
12. Outline safe and hygienic working practices
13. State how to communicate and behave within a salon environment

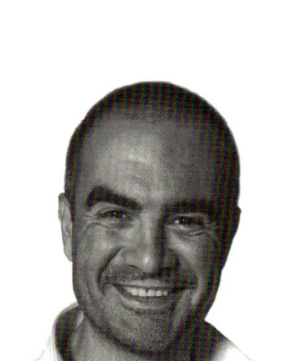

Be the next ...
Andrew Barton

Andrew Barton is known as hairdressing royalty, with his own flagship London salon, product range, electrical tools and a reputation as a TV makeover guru. **Follow the blue quotes for his creative design tips!**

Learn from the best and ask questions: never accept OK as a standard and you'll never be known for OK standards!

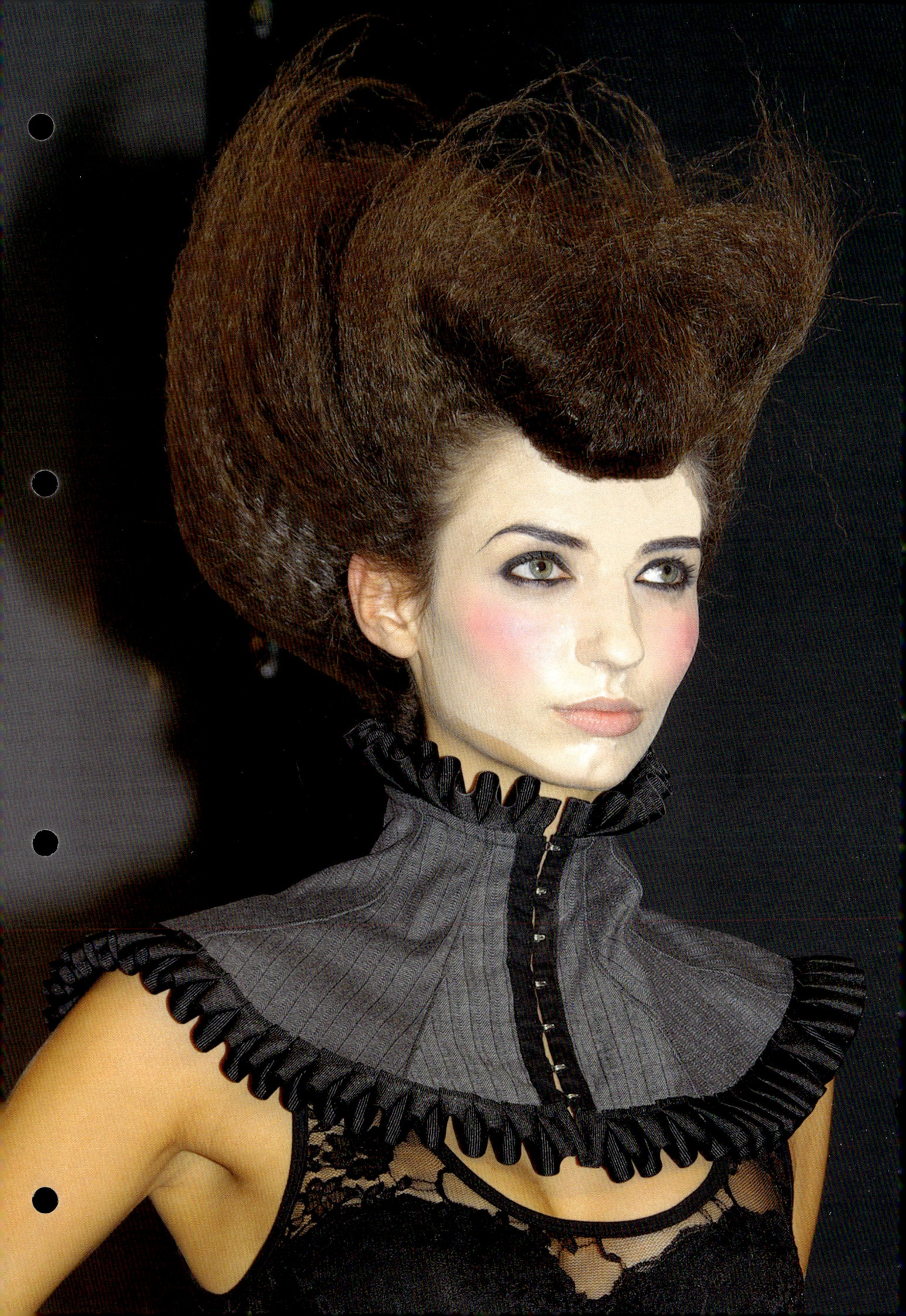

Hairpieces, accessories and ornamentation can enhance the overall appearance of the style.

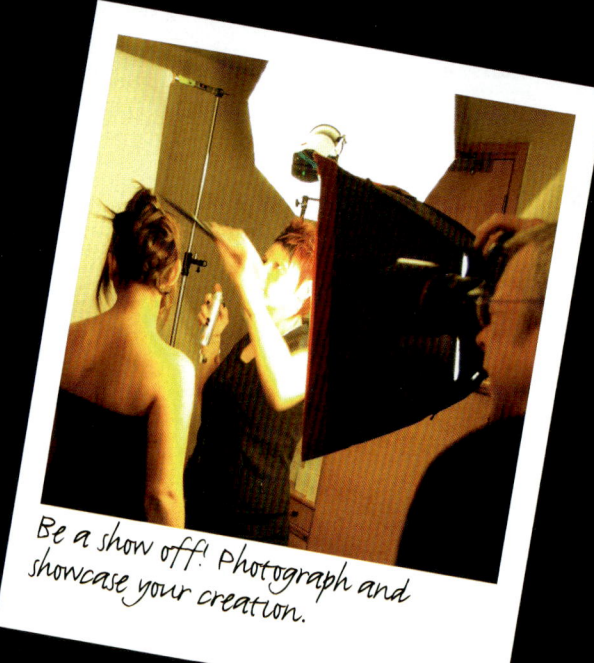

Be a show off! Photograph and showcase your creation.

Creative h

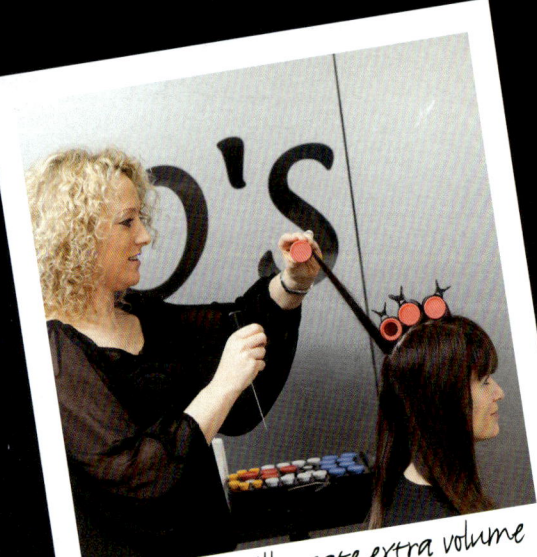

Dry setting will create extra volume for the finished look.

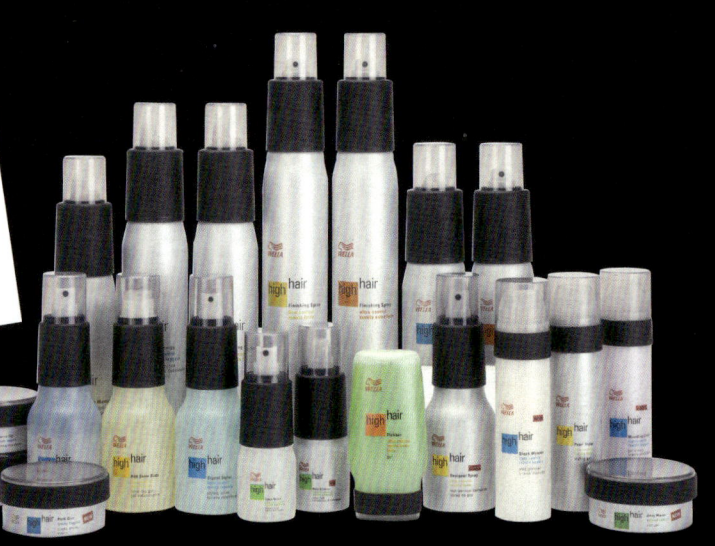

Image courtesy of Balmain

Image courtesy of Cheynes Training

Image courtesy of Wella

airdressing

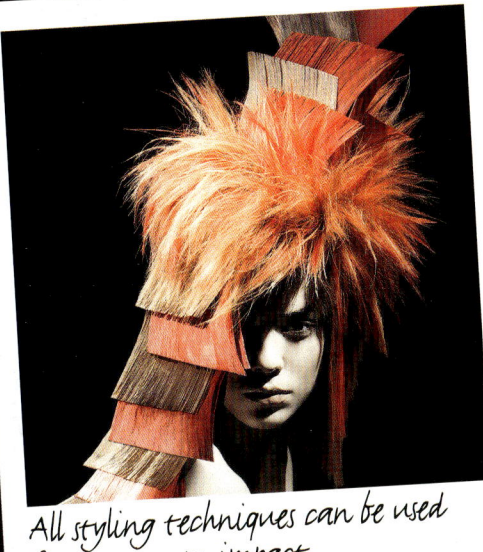

All styling techniques can be used for maximum impact.

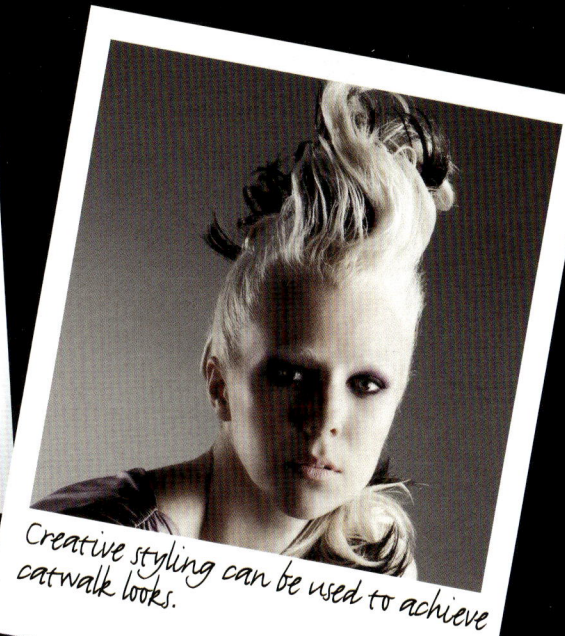

Creative styling can be used to achieve catwalk looks.

> Creative hairdressing is an artistic form of expression, personal to each creator. Ideas come from many sources, but primarily start with a strong understanding of classic hairdressing. We call them the rules, but creative hairdressing is often about breaking the rules and expressing your creativity.

After the event it is important to gain as much feedback as possible to evaluate the image.

What you must do
Practical observations

This page shows what you need to do during your practical task. You can look at it beforehand, but you're **not** allowed to have it with you while carrying out your practical task. You must achieve **all** the criteria; you can achieve 1 mark, 2 marks or 3 marks for the criteria indicated with *.

Conversion chart

Grade	Marks
Pass	8
Merit	9–10
Distinction	11–12

	Creative hair design		
1 Prepare self, the model and work area for hair design	1		
2 Select and use products, tools and equipment required to achieve and present the image	1		
3 Use and combine techniques and skills to present the image *	1	2	3
4 Create the finished image to the satisfaction of the client	1		
5 Record the creative hair design using media	1		
6 Evaluate the results of the finished look	1		
7 Follow safe and hygienic working practices	1		
8 Communicate and behave in a professional manner *	1	2	3
Totals			
Grade			
Candidate signature and date			
Assessor signature and date			

Revision tip

Accurate planning is important when creating an image to make sure you have all the necessary resources and you don't go over budget.

Inspiration is all around us, in fashion, art, multimedia or nature. It's vital that you are open to these stimuli and record them in photographs, sketch books or mood boards. Use your camera to record what you see and then think how it can inspire you as a creative hairdresser.

What you must do
Practical observations descriptors table

This table shows what you need to do to achieve 1, 2 or 3 marks for the criteria indicated with * on the previous page.

	1 mark	2 marks	3 marks
3 Style hair creatively incorporating a range of styling techniques	Uses a limited range of styling techniques. Example: two styling techniques without ornamentation	Uses a good range of styling techniques. Example: three styling techniques, and ornamentation	Uses an excellent variety of styling techniques. Example: five styling techniques, ornamentation and accessories
8 Communicate and behave in a professional manner	Satisfactory communication and behaviour. Examples: polite, friendly, positive body language, speaks clearly	Good communication and behaviour. Examples: polite, friendly, positive body language, speaks clearly, respectful to colleagues and clients, listens and responds to client needs	Excellent communication and behaviour. Examples: polite, friendly, positive body language, speaks clearly, respectful to colleagues and clients, listens and responds to client's needs, shows a reassuring and confident manner

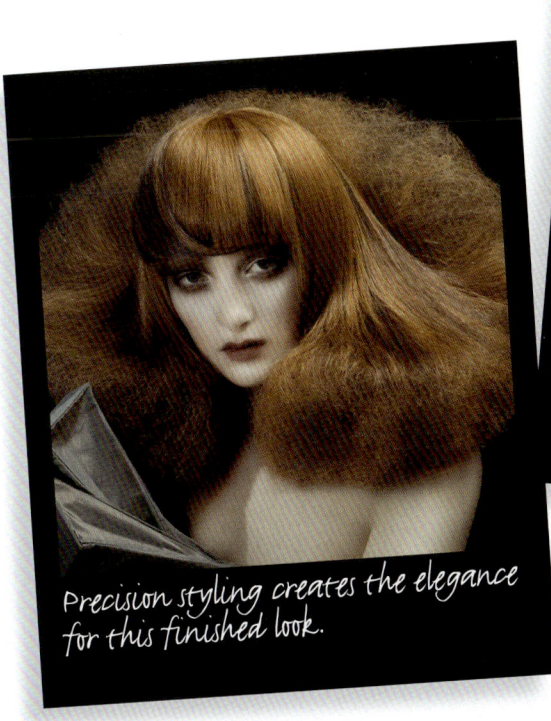

Precision styling creates the elegance for this finished look.

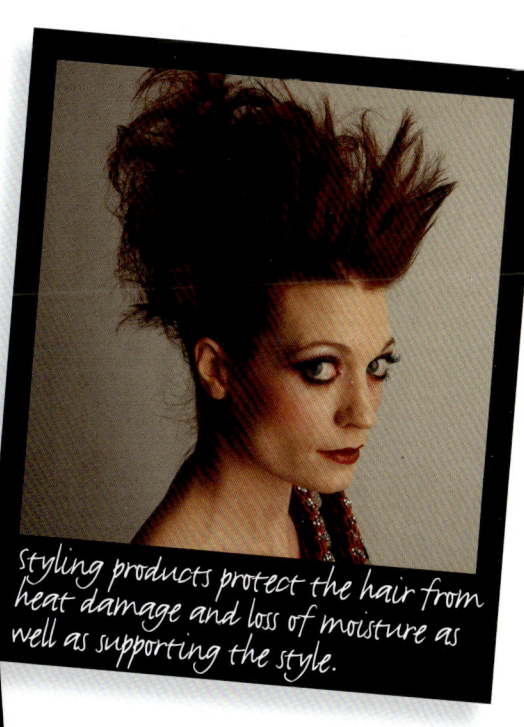

Styling products protect the hair from heat damage and loss of moisture as well as supporting the style.

Image courtesy of Desmond Murray

Comment form
Unit 316 Creative hairdressing design skills

This form can be used to record comments by you, your client, or your assessor.

___

___

___

___

___

___

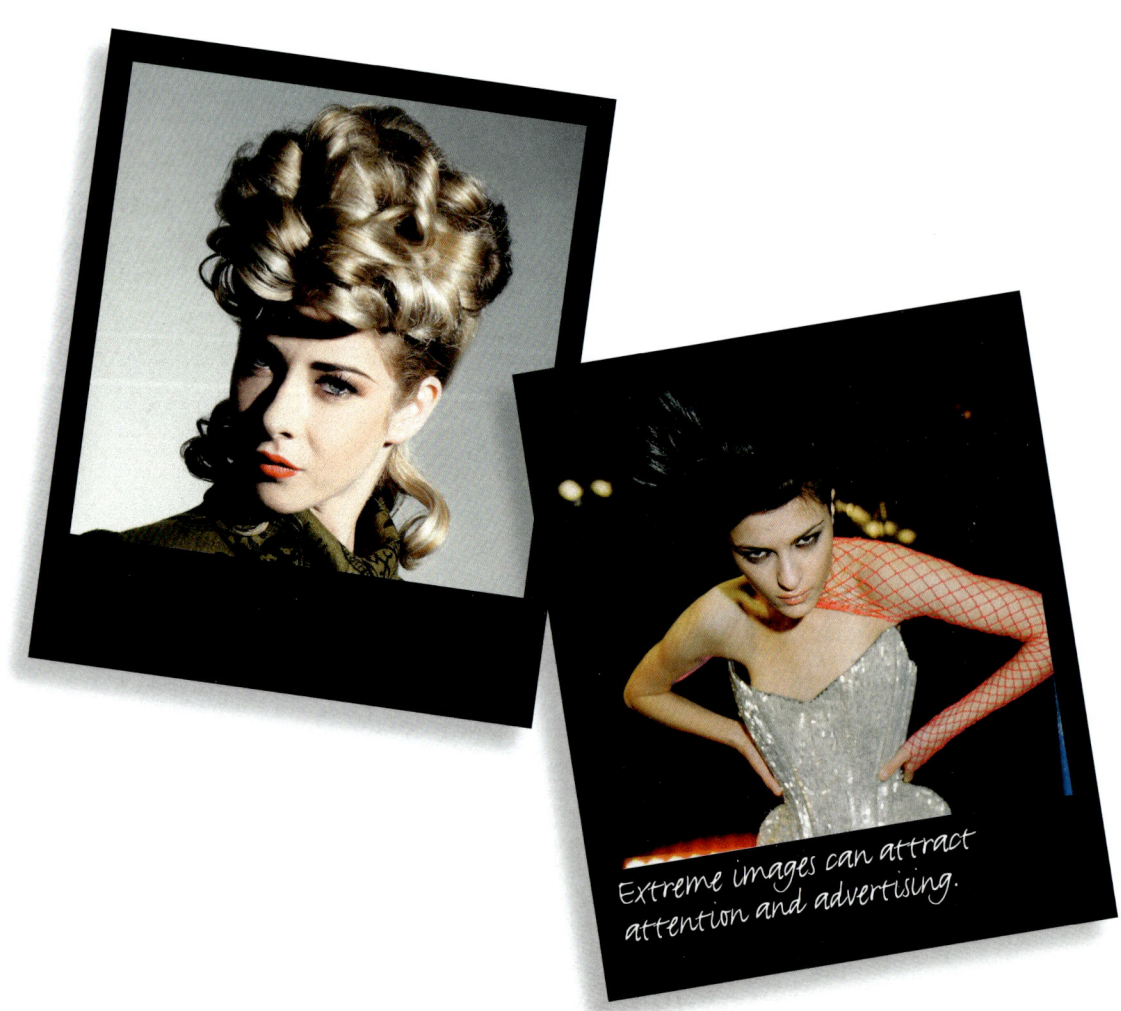

Extreme images can attract attention and advertising.

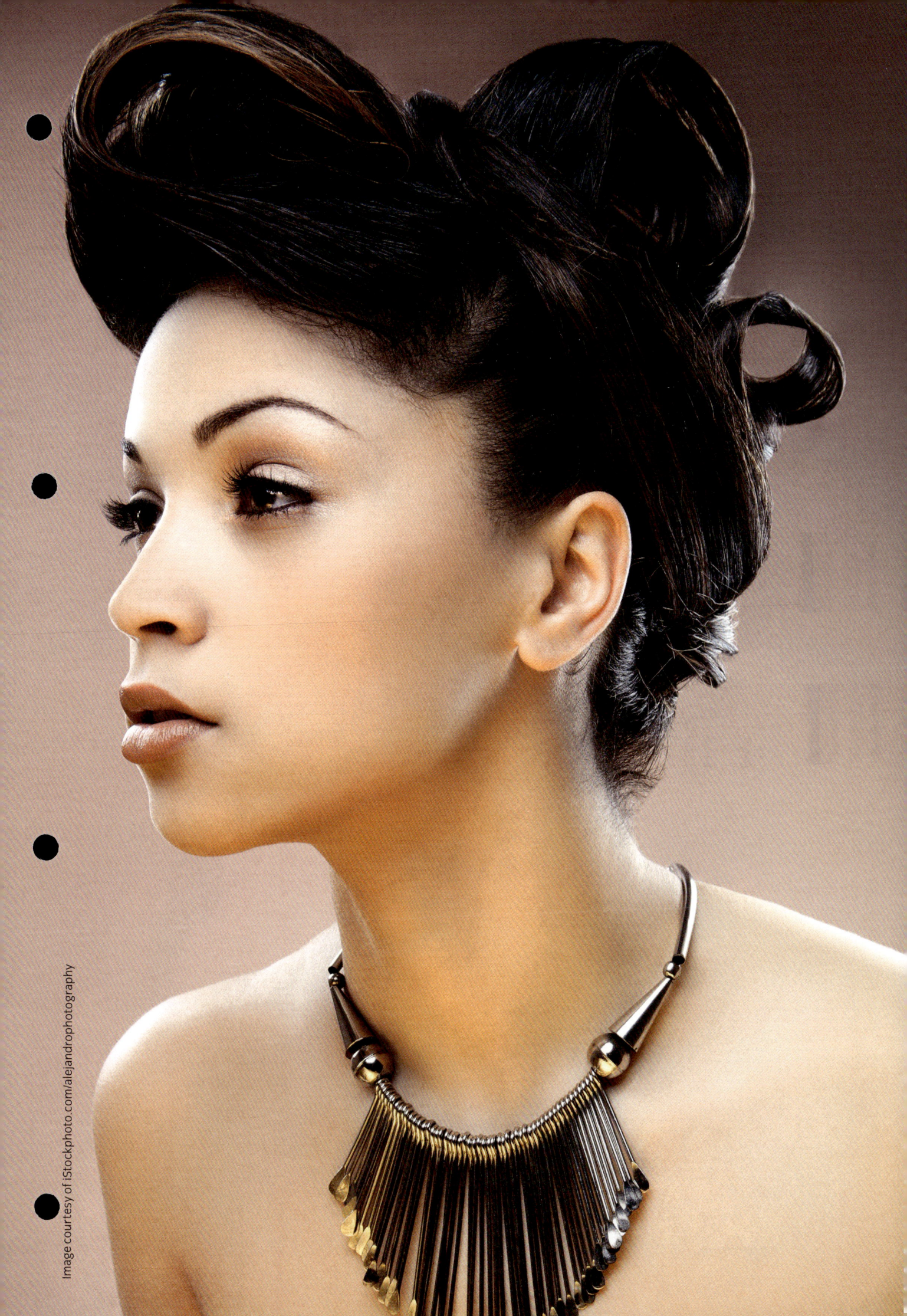

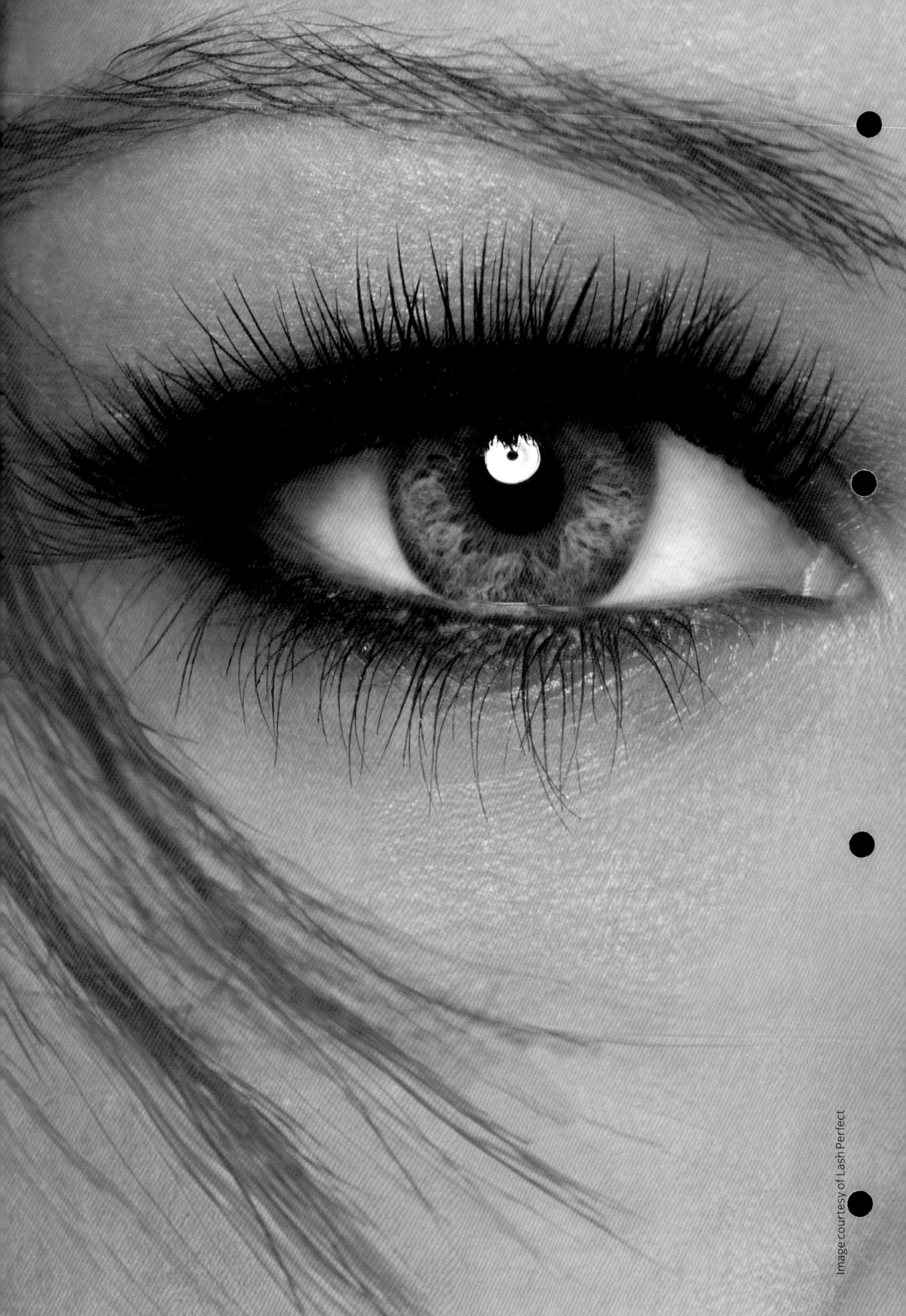

Image courtesy of Lash Perfect

317

Apply individual permanent lashes

Lashes have come a long way! For centuries, women have tried to enhance and beautify their lashes. The Egyptians blended kohl with crocodile dung, water and honey to create the first mascara, and around 400 BC Ancient Greek women rubbed powdery black incense into their eyelashes. These days a trip to the salon is an easier and longer-lasting solution. In this unit you will learn how to select the correct lashes for your client, and will master the techniques of applying and layering long, thick, luxurious lashes for a show-stopping look!

Assignment mark sheet
Unit 317 Apply individual permanent lashes

Your assessor will mark you on each of the practical tasks in this unit. This page is used to work out your overall grade for the unit. You must pass **all** parts of the tasks to be able to achieve a grade. For each completed practical task, a pass equals 1 point, a merit equals 2 points and a distinction equals 3 points.

What you must know	Tick when complete
Task 1a: produce an information sheet	
Task 1b: produce an information sheet	
Task 1c: produce a fact sheet	
Task 1d: anatomy and physiology	
Or tick if covered by an online test	

What you must do	Grade	Points
Task 2: Apply individual permanent lashes		

Overall grade

Candidate name:

Candidate signature: Date:

Assessor signature: Date:

Quality assurance co-ordinator signature (where applicable):   Date:

External Verifier signature (where applicable):   Date:

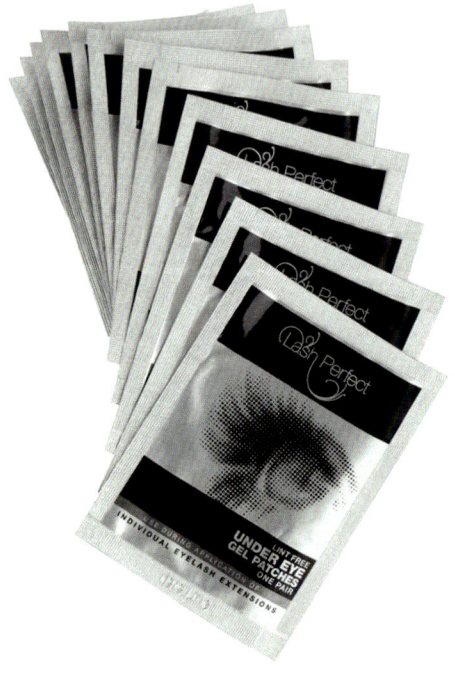

Image courtesy of Lash Perfect

180 Unit 317 Level 3 VRQ Beauty Therapy

What does it mean?
Some useful words are explained below

Alopecia
Hair loss that can affect people of any age, resulting in full or partial loss of hair anywhere on the face or body.

Anagen hair
The active stage of hair growth where the hair is still attached to its blood supply. As the hair grows out, so will the extension.

Blepharitis
Inflammation of the eyelid or eyelid rim. The eyes look red and feel irritated and itchy. Dandruff-like crusts can appear on the eyelashes.

Conjunctiva
The outermost layer of the eye and the inner surface of the eyelids.

Conjunctivitis
An inflammation of the conjunctiva, resulting in redness, discharge, itching and in some cases light sensitivity. It can occur in one eye or both. The cause of conjunctivitis can be viral or bacterial infection, or may be down to an irritant or allergy.

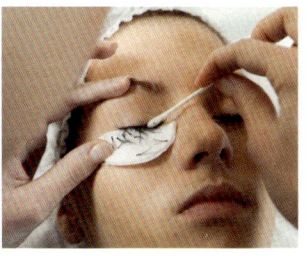

Flare lashes
A cluster of synthetic lashes applied to the natural lashes. They use a different adhesive from permanent lashes and do not last as long.

Hair growth cycle
The stages of growth, transition and inactivity in the hair follicle.

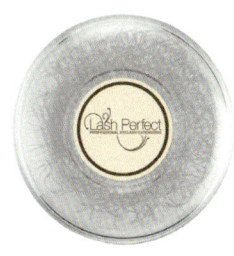

Individual permanent lashes
A process where a single synthetic lash is applied on to a single natural lash using a medical grade long-lasting adhesive.

Lash perming
Only available professionally, this treatment adds curl and uplift to the lashes.

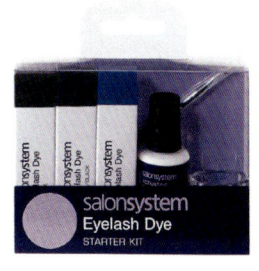

Lash tinting
A treatment where the eyelashes are coloured to give them emphasis.

Patch/sensitivity test
A test where a small amount of product is applied to the skin and left on for 24 hours to check whether the client reacts to the product.

Repetitive strain injury
Soft tissue injury, usually in the wrists as a result of overuse.

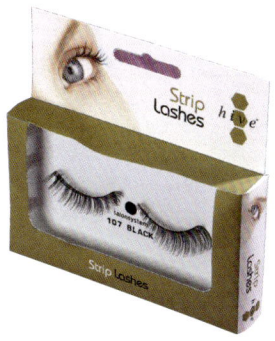

Strip lashes
Available in pairs, these run the entire length of the eyelid, and are applied to the skin just above the lash line. They are available in a variety of lengths, styles, and thicknesses, and are designed to be removed nightly.

Stye
An infection of the eyelash follicle.

Terminal hair
Thick, coarse hair with a deep root and rich blood supply.

Trichotillomania
A disorder or habit where the sufferer has repeated urges to pull out scalp, lash, facial or brow hair, which can result in bald patches.

Y-type lashes
Lashes that split in two at the tapered end, giving the effect of double the number of lashes.

What you must know
You must be able to:

1. Describe salon requirements for preparing themselves, the client and work area
2. Describe the environmental conditions suitable for individual permanent lash extension treatments
3. Describe the different consultation techniques used to identify treatment objectives
4. Describe the types of tests that are carried out before providing lash extension treatments
5. Explain the importance of carrying out tests prior to the treatment and accurately recording the results
6. Explain the contra-indications that prevent or restrict individual permanent lash extension treatments
7. Describe how to select products, tools and equipment to suit client treatment needs
8. Describe the types of eyelash treatments available and their benefits
9. Explain the importance of assessing facial characteristics prior to carrying out eyelash treatments
10. Explain how to communicate and behave in a professional manner

Continues on next page

> **Revision tip**
> Remember to check if your client has had the recommended patch test to comply with manufacturers' instructions and insurance guidelines.

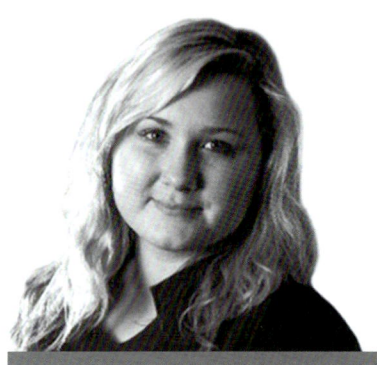

Follow in the footsteps of… *Leanne Darbinson*

From a young age Leanne realised that working in the Make-Up industry was what she wanted to do. After doing a Level 1 course in Personal Therapies and a Level 2 course in Beauty Therapy, she is now doing a Level 3 in Media Make-Up. She loved doing lash extensions because they can enhance the natural eye shape and can also be used to perfect many other looks, such as a make-up treatment. Leanne hopes to go to university to get a degree in Make-Up for the lens based industries. Follow the blue quote marks to find out what Leanne has to say!

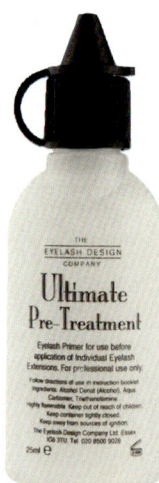

Image courtesy of Lash Perfect

11 Describe health and safety working practices

12 Explain the importance of positioning themselves and the client correctly throughout the treatment

13 Explain the importance of using products, tools, equipment and techniques to suit client's treatment needs and facial characteristics

14 Describe how treatments can be adapted to suit client treatment needs and facial characteristics

15 State the contra-actions that may occur during and following treatments and how to respond

16 Explain the importance of completing the treatment to the satisfaction of the client

17 Explain the importance of completing treatment records

18 Describe the methods of evaluating the effectiveness of the treatment

19 Describe the aftercare advice that should be provided

20 Describe the structure of the hair and hair growth cycle

21 Describe the main diseases and disorders of the hair

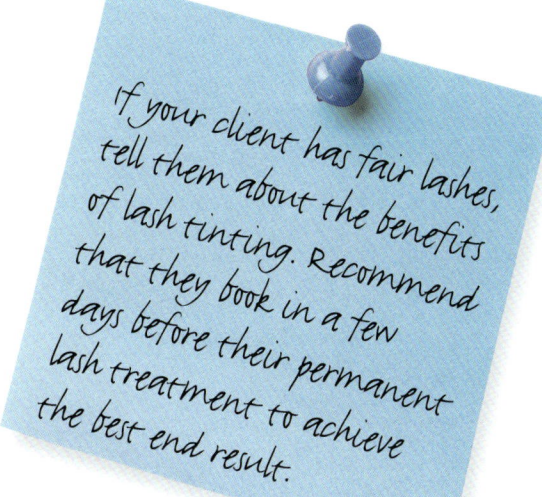

If your client has fair lashes, tell them about the benefits of lash tinting. Recommend that they book in a few days before their permanent lash treatment to achieve the best end result.

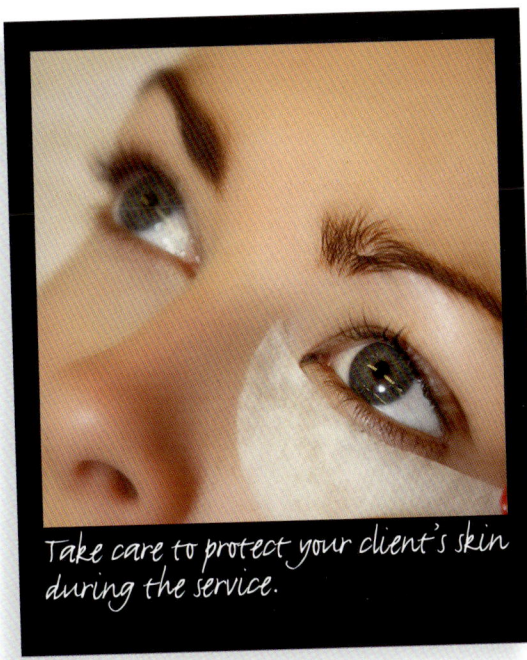

Take care to protect your client's skin during the service.

Image courtesy of Maria Retter

❝

Always make sure that you have clean, glue-free tweezers.

> *Always have a tidy and organised station. This will help you to remember the order of the treatment.*

Las

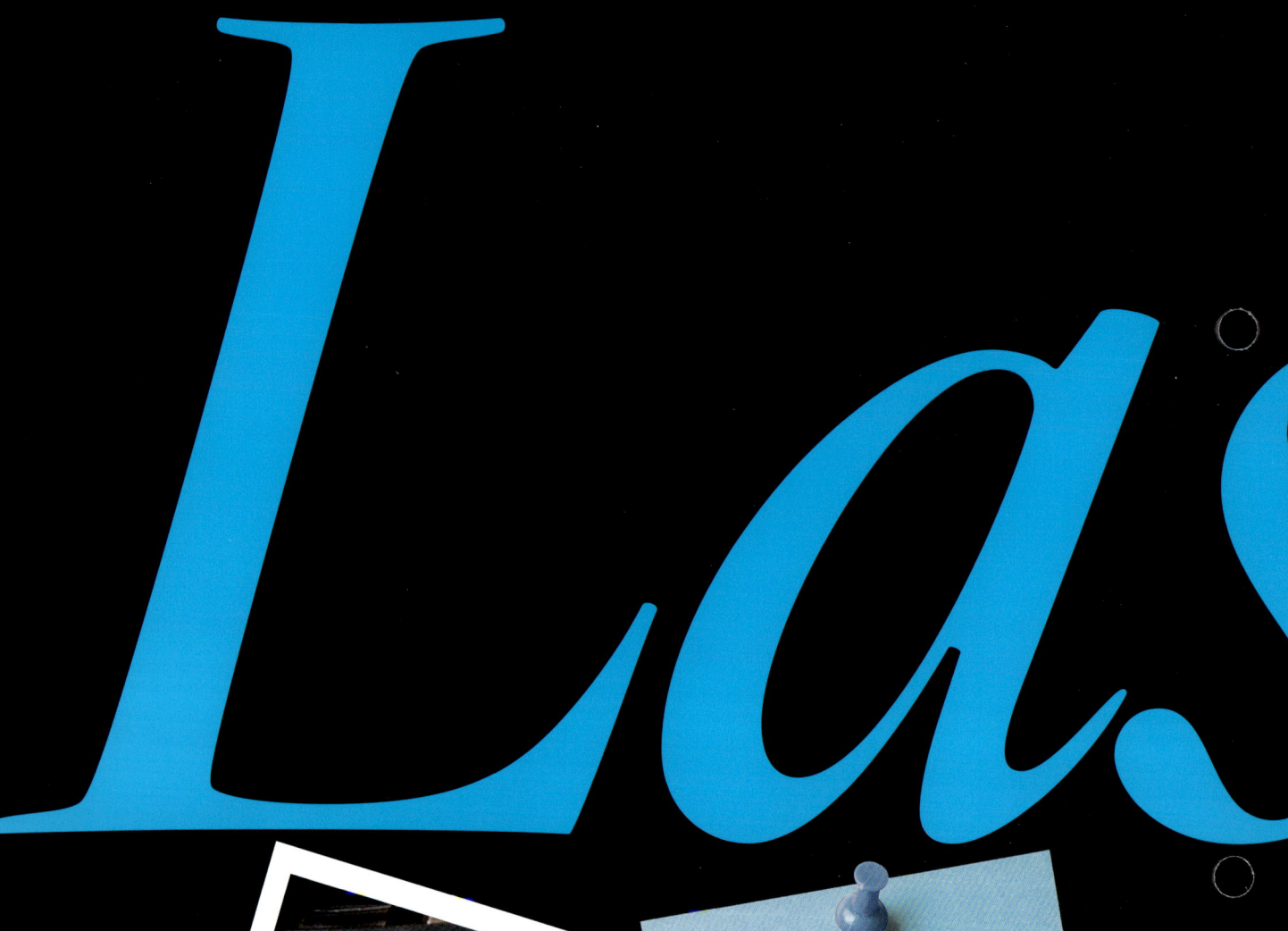

Applying individual lashes takes time to master.

To ensure that the lashes stick properly, make sure you stroke the adhesive down the length of the natural lash before placement.

...shes

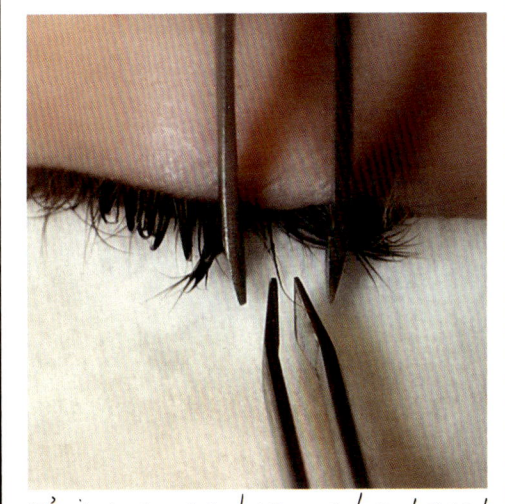

It's important to keep your hand steady when inserting individual lashes.

Before applying individual permanent lashes, consider the thickness of the client's own lashes. Very thick lashes look stunning but they won't last long if the client's own lashes can't support them!

> " Start at the outer corners on the eye, applying one lash on each eye at a time. This will help to prevent the eyelashes from sticking together.

What you must do
Practical observations

This page shows what you need to do during your practical task. You can look at it beforehand, but you're **not** allowed to have it with you while carrying out your practical task. You must achieve **all** the criteria; you can achieve 1 mark, 2 marks or 3 marks for the criteria indicated with *.

Conversion chart

Grade	Marks
Pass	11–13
Merit	14–18
Distinction	19–21

○ Please tick when all pre-observation requirements have been met

	Apply individual permanent lashes		
1 Prepare yourself, the client and the work area for individual permanent lash extension treatment	1		
2 Use suitable consultation techniques to identify treatment objectives *	1	2	3
3 Interpret and accurately record the result of the test carried out prior to the treatment	1		
4 Provide clear recommendations to the client *	1	2	3
5 Position yourself and the client correctly throughout the treatment	1		
6 Select and use products, tools, equipment and techniques to suit client's treatment needs *	1	2	3
7 Communicate and behave in a professional manner	1		
8 Follow health and safety working practices	1		
9 Complete the treatment to the satisfaction of the client *	1	2	3
10 Record and evaluate the results of the treatment	1		
11 Provide suitable aftercare advice *	1	2	3

Total

Grade

Candidate signature and date

Assessor signature and date

What you must do
Practical observations descriptors table

This table shows what you need to do to achieve 1, 2 or 3 marks for the criteria indicated with * on the previous page.

	1 mark	2 marks	3 marks
2 Use suitable consultation techniques to identify treatment objectives	Basic consultation carried out. Example: uses open and closed questions throughout, questioning covers contra-indications.	Good consultation carried out. Examples: uses open and closed questions, positive body language, questioning covers contra-indications, general health, lifestyle and expectations of end result.	Thorough consultation carried out. Examples: open and closed questions, effective use of body language, questioning covers contra-indications, expectations of end result. Candidate is able to accurately identify adaptations to suit client lifestyle and expectations.
4 Provide clear recommendations to the client	A basic treatment plan is recommended. Examples: contra-indications and objectives of the treatment identified.	A good treatment plan is recommended. Examples: contra-indications and objectives of the treatment, taking into account client lifestyle and expectations of end result.	A thorough treatment plan is recommended. Examples: contra-indications and objectives of the treatment, taking into account client lifestyle and expectations of end result, lashes of a suitable length and thickness are recommended.
6 Select and use products, tools, equipment and techniques to suit client's treatment needs	A basic application of un-layered lashes is applied.	An application of layered lashes is applied. Lash thickness is chosen according to client's own lash characteristics and treatment objectives.	An application of layered lashes is applied of the correct thickness and differing lengths according to client's own lash characteristics, facial characteristics and treatment objectives.

Continues on next page

Apply individual permanent lashes **Unit 317**

What you must do
Practical observations descriptors table (continued)

This table shows what you need to do to achieve 1, 2 or 3 marks for the criteria indicated with * on page 186.

	1 mark	2 marks	3 marks
9 Complete the treatment to the satisfaction of the client	The treatment is completed within the agreed time and brought to a satisfactory close.	The treatment is completed within the agreed time, brought to a satisfactory close, the product is allowed to dry and client is shown the end result in the mirror.	The treatment is completed within the agreed time, brought to a satisfactory close, result is adapted if necessary, the client is shown the end result in the mirror, and positive client feedback is gained.
11 Provide suitable aftercare advice	Basic aftercare advice is provided including possible contra-actions.	Good level of aftercare advice is provided including possible contra-actions, maintenance requirements and frequency of further treatments.	A good level of aftercare advice is provided including possible contra-actions, maintenance requirements and frequency of further treatments, the importance of professional removal and beneficial home care products.

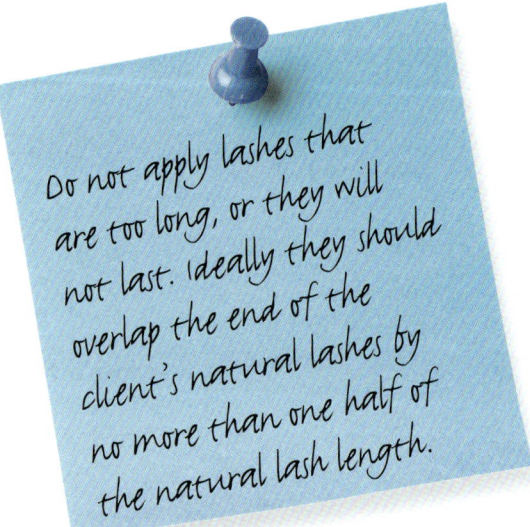

Do not apply lashes that are too long, or they will not last. Ideally they should overlap the end of the client's natural lashes by no more than one half of the natural lash length.

Comment form
Unit 317 Apply individual permanent lashes

This form can be used to record comments by you, your client, or your assessor.

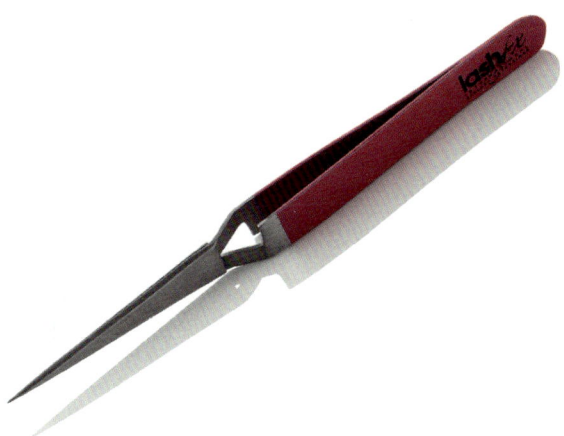

Image courtesy of Lash Perfect

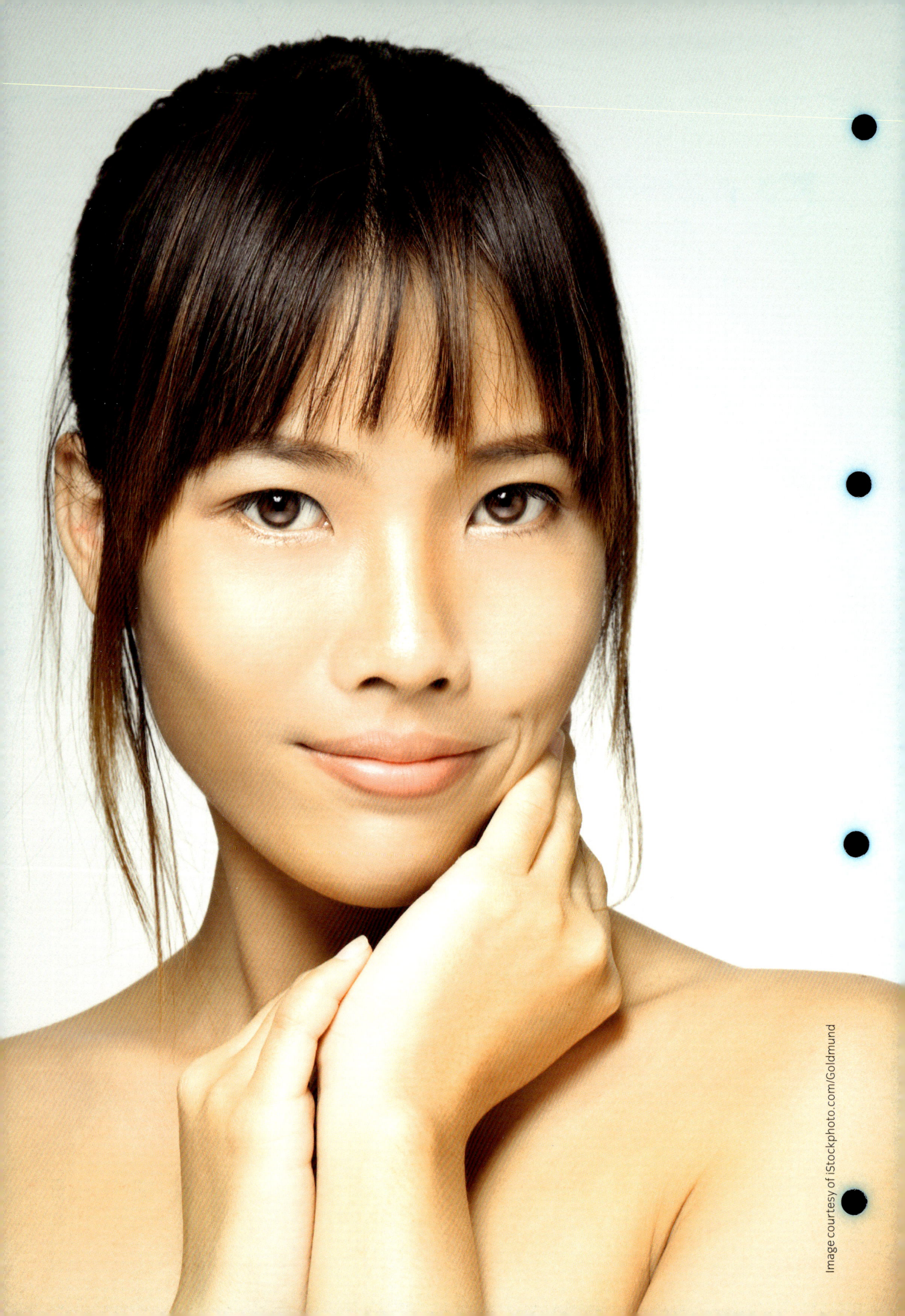

Image courtesy of iStockphoto.com/Goldmund

321

Apply micro-dermabrasion techniques

Micro-dermabrasion uses a controlled flow of crystals to mechanically exfoliate the surface of the skin. It gently removes surface layers to uncover a brighter, smoother skin. Whilst it is quite an easy treatment to carry out, it is important to have proper training, as it can cause damage if done incorrectly. Clients love having it because it leaves the skin feeling soft and smooth. The unit covers the skin types and conditions you are likely to come across in facial work, plus how to advise clients on product usage and lifestyle changes in order to make the most of their complexion.

Assignment mark sheet
Unit 321 Apply micro-dermabrasion techniques

Your assessor will mark you on each of the practical tasks in this unit. This page is used to work out your overall grade for the unit. You must pass **all** parts of the tasks to be able to achieve a grade. For each completed practical task, a pass equals 1 point, a merit equals 2 points and a distinction equals 3 points.

What you must know	Tick when complete
Task 1a: produce an information sheet	
Task 1b: produce a fact sheet	
Task 1c: produce a fact sheet	
Task 1d: anatomy and physiology	
Or tick if covered by an online test	

What you must do	Grade	Points
Task 2: Provide skin treatment using micro-dermabrasion		

Overall grade _____

Candidate name:

Candidate signature: Date:

Assessor signature: Date:

Quality assurance co-ordinator signature (where applicable):   Date:

External Verifier signature (where applicable):   Date:

What does it mean?
Some useful words are explained below

Accutane
An oral medication used for the treatment of severe acne. A side effect is thinned and sensitised skin, so is a contra-indication to micro-dermabrasion.

Acid mantle
The layer of sebum and sweat on the skin's surface that provides lubrication and protects against bacteria.

Chloasma
A hyper-pigmentation disorder resulting in darker patches of skin.

Contra-indications
Condition that prevent treatment from taking place or make it necessary to modify the treatment.

Dehydrated skin
This is a lack of water or moisture within the skin as opposed to a lack of oil, and can occur on any skin type.

Disposal of contaminated waste
It will be necessary to check the correct disposal of the crystals with your local council, as occasional 'pin prick' bleeding may occur.

Erythema
Redness of the skin resulting from dilation of blood vessels, due to stimulation, irritation or allergy.

Flow
The rate at which the crystals flow through the applicator on to the skin.

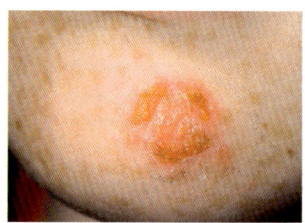

Impetigo
A bacterial skin infection where small blisters break open and then crust over to form honey coloured scabs.

Keloid scar
A raised scar that grows above skin level due to overproduction of collagen.

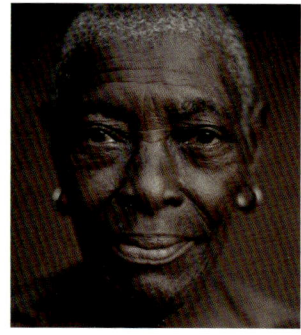

Mature skin
In beauty therapy terms this is any skin over the age of 25. However, the skin is generally not classed as being mature until the signs of ageing are apparent.

Normal skin
An uncommon skin type with small pores and a smooth texture, an even colouring, and no blemishes, flaky or oily patches present.

Retin A
A topical cream derived from vitamin A, prescribed for its anti-ageing effects or the treatment of moderate acne. As it thins the skin, it is a contra-indication to micro-dermabrasion.

Ringworm
A contagious fungal infection where there are circles of red, itchy skin, which heal from the centre.

Skin analysis
A careful assessment of the skin to determine its type and condition, taking into account contributory factors.

Skin type
A way of classifying the skin according to the amount of oil it produces. The skin types are normal, dry, oily and combination.

Sterilisation
The complete destruction of micro-organisms and their spores.

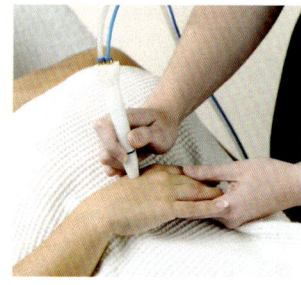

Vacuum flow
The pressure of the vacuum at the applicator head. The higher the pressure of vacuum, the more aggressive the treatment.

What you must know
You must be able to:

1. Describe salon requirements for preparing themselves, the client and work area
2. Describe the environmental conditions suitable for micro-dermabrasion skin treatment
3. Describe the different consultation techniques used to identify treatment objectives
4. Describe how to select products and tools to suit client treatment needs, skin types and conditions
5. Describe known contra-indications that may restrict or prevent micro-dermabrasion treatment
6. Describe the importance of carrying out a skin analysis
7. Describe the effects and benefits of a micro-dermabrasion treatment
8. Explain how to communicate and behave in a professional manner
9. Describe health and safety working practices
10. Explain the importance of positioning themselves and the client correctly throughout the treatment

Continues on next page

Revision tip

It is really important to carry out a thorough consultation and skin analysis before carrying out micro-dermabrasion as existing medical conditions, medications and sensitivity may contra-indicate the treatment.

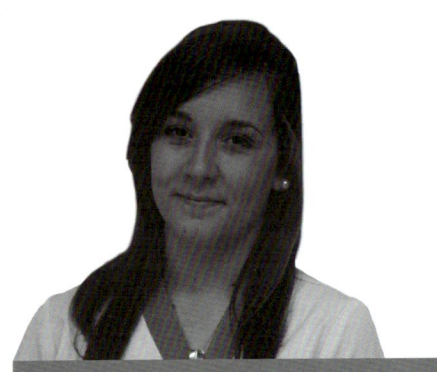

Follow in the footsteps of...
Rebecca Sommerfeld

Rebecca is currently taking her Level 3 VRQ in Beauty Therapy at Bexley College. She loves all areas of Beauty Therapy because she enjoys carrying out treatments to her clients' satisfaction, although micro-dermabrasion is her favourite. Rebecca's plans for the future are always changing, but she is considering a career in physiotherapy. Read on for Rebecca's micro-dermabrasion tips!

11 Explain the importance of using products, tools and techniques to suit client's treatment needs, skin types and conditions

12 Describe how treatment can be adapted to suit client treatment needs

13 State the contra-actions that may occur during and following treatments and how to respond

14 Explain the importance of completing the treatment to the satisfaction of the client

15 Explain the importance of completing treatment records

16 Describe the methods of evaluating the effectiveness of the treatment

17 Describe the aftercare advice that should be provided

18 Describe the structure and function of the skin

19 Describe the main diseases and disorders of the skin

20 Describe skin types, conditions and characteristics

21 Describe the growth cycle and repair of the skin

22 Explain how natural ageing, lifestyle and environmental factors affect the condition of the skin

Store crystals in an airtight container in dry conditions, or they will absorb moisture and be unfit for use.

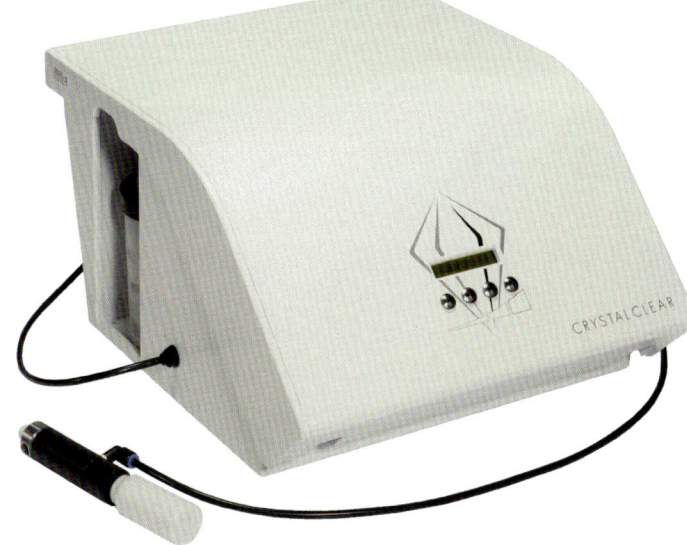

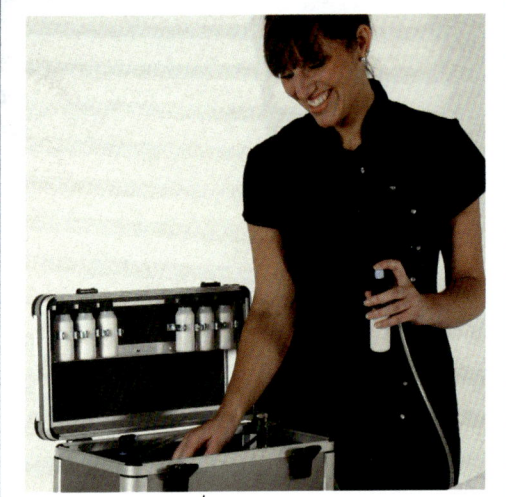

Micro-dermabrasion is an easy treatment to perform but you must know your equipment.

Micro-der

> "Remind clients not to exfoliate for a week after the micro-dermabrasion treatment.

Always use a fresh disposable applicator head for each client for hygiene reasons.

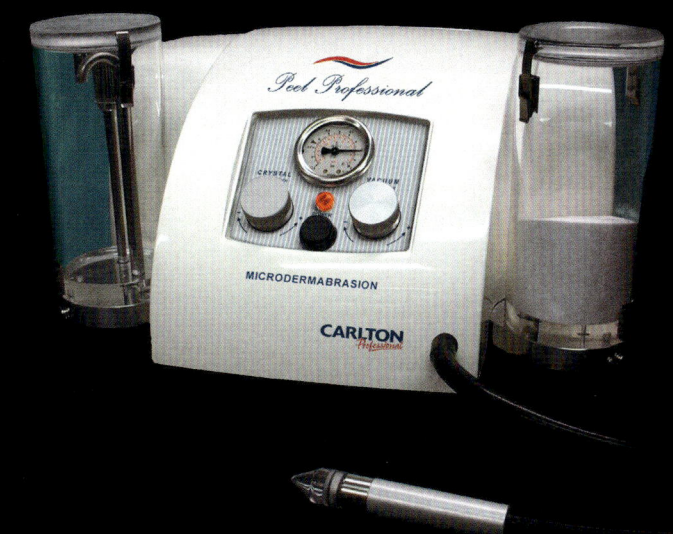

Image courtesy of Carlton Professional

mabrasion

> " Try using a cooling masque on your client after the treatment.

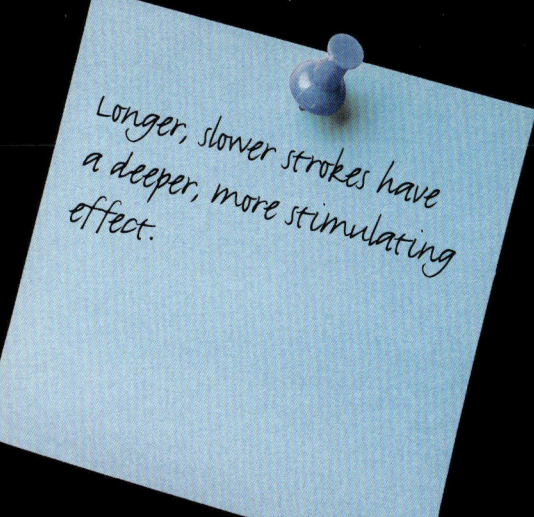

Longer, slower strokes have a deeper, more stimulating effect.

What you must do
Practical observations

This page shows what you need to do during your practical task. You can look at it beforehand, but you're **not** allowed to have it with you while carrying out your practical task. You must achieve **all** the criteria; you can achieve 1 mark, 2 marks or 3 marks for the criteria indicated with *.

Conversion chart

Grade	Marks
Pass	12–14
Merit	15–20
Distinction	21–24

○ Please tick when all pre-observation requirements have been met

	Apply micro-dermabrasion techniques		
1 Prepare yourself, the client and the work area for skin treatment using micro-dermabrasion	1		
2 Use suitable consultation techniques to identify treatment objectives *	1	2	3
3 Advise the client on how to prepare for the treatment	1		
4 Carry out a skin analysis *	1	2	3
5 Provide clear recommendations to the client *	1	2	3
6 Position yourself and the client correctly throughout the treatment	1		
7 Select and use products, tools, equipment and techniques to suit client's treatment needs, skin type and conditions *	1	2	3
8 Communicate and behave in a professional manner	1		
9 Follow health and safety working practices	1		
10 Complete the treatment to the satisfaction of the client *	1	2	3
11 Record and evaluate the results of the treatment	1		
12 Provide suitable aftercare advice *	1	2	3

Total

Grade

Candidate signature and date

Assessor signature and date

What you must do
Practical observations descriptors table

This table shows what you need to do to achieve 1, 2 or 3 marks for the criteria indicated with * on the previous page.

	1 mark	2 marks	3 marks
2 Use suitable consultation techniques to identify treatment objectives	Basic consultation Examples: uses open and closed questions, checks for contra-indications, identifies the treatment objectives correctly.	Good consultation Examples: positive body language, uses open and closed questions to identify contra-indications, general health, lifestyle and expectations, identifies the treatment objectives and any factors that may limit or restrict the treatment.	Thorough consultation Examples: positive body language, uses open and closed questions to identify contra-indications, general health, lifestyle and expectations, how client feels about their skin and what improvement they would like to achieve, identifies the treatment objectives and any factors that may limit or restrict the treatment, allows the client to ask any questions to confirm understanding.
4 Carry out a skin analysis	Skin cleansed, magnifier and light used. Some recording of skin characteristics.	Skin cleansed, magnifier and light used, good observations of skin characteristics recorded.	Skin is cleansed thoroughly, magnifier and light used, detailed observations of skin characteristics recorded.

Continues on next page

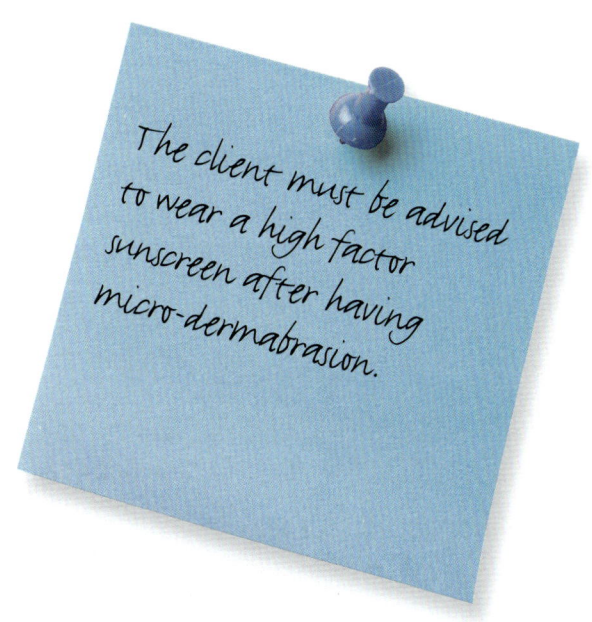

The client must be advised to wear a high factor sunscreen after having micro-dermabrasion.

What you must do
Practical observations descriptors table (continued)

This table shows what you need to do to achieve 1, 2 or 3 marks for the criteria indicated with * on page 198.

	1 mark	2 marks	3 marks
5 Provide clear recommendations to the client	A basic treatment plan is recommended. Examples: explains treatment procedure and any adaptations to meet client treatment needs, equipment to be used.	A good treatment plan is recommended. Examples: explains treatment procedure and any adaptations to meet client treatment needs, equipment to be used based on factors identified during consultation (lifestyle, medication (if any), contra-indications, results of skin analysis), a choice of products to be used.	A thorough treatment plan is recommended. Examples: explains treatment procedure and any adaptations to meet client treatment needs, equipment to be used based on factors identified during consultation (lifestyle, medication (if any), contra-indications, results of skin analysis), a choice of products to be used, explains effects and benefits of the type of equipment used and the adaptation/modification to suit client treatment needs, allows the client to ask questions about the treatment plan.
7 Select and use products, tools, equipment and techniques to suit client's treatment needs, skin type and conditions	Selects and uses the correct equipment, tools, techniques and basic products based on factors identified in skin analysis.	Selects and uses the correct equipment, tools, techniques and a variety of products based on factors identified in skin analysis, explains effects and benefits of the products and equipment to the client as appropriate throughout.	Selects and uses the correct equipment, tools, techniques and a variety of products based on factors identified in skin analysis, explains effects and benefits of the products and equipment to the client as appropriate throughout, adapts and modifies the techniques used, explains the treatment to the client as appropriate throughout.

Continues on next page

	1 mark	2 marks	3 marks
10 Complete the treatment to the satisfaction of the client	The treatment is completed within the agreed time and brought to a satisfactory close.	The treatment is completed within the agreed time, brought to a satisfactory close and positive feedback is gained from the client.	The treatment is completed within the agreed time, brought to a satisfactory close and positive feedback is gained from the client, shows the client the results of the treatment and allows the client to ask questions.
12 Provide suitable aftercare advice	Basic aftercare advice Examples: how to deal with possible contra-actions, product(s) to use, future treatment needs.	Good level of aftercare advice Examples: how to deal with possible contra-actions, product(s) to use, specific advice (ie what to avoid immediately after the treatment, fluid intake, healthy eating), future treatment needs.	Excellent aftercare advice Examples: how to deal with possible contra-actions, product(s) to use, specific advice (ie what to avoid immediately after the treatment, fluid intake, healthy eating), recommends future treatment programme (regular treatments, introduction of new/alternative treatments).

Advise your client to purchase an SPF 30 moisturiser to protect the skin after micro-dermabrasion.

Comment form
Unit 321 Apply micro-dermabrasion techniques

This form can be used to record comments by you, your client, or your assessor.

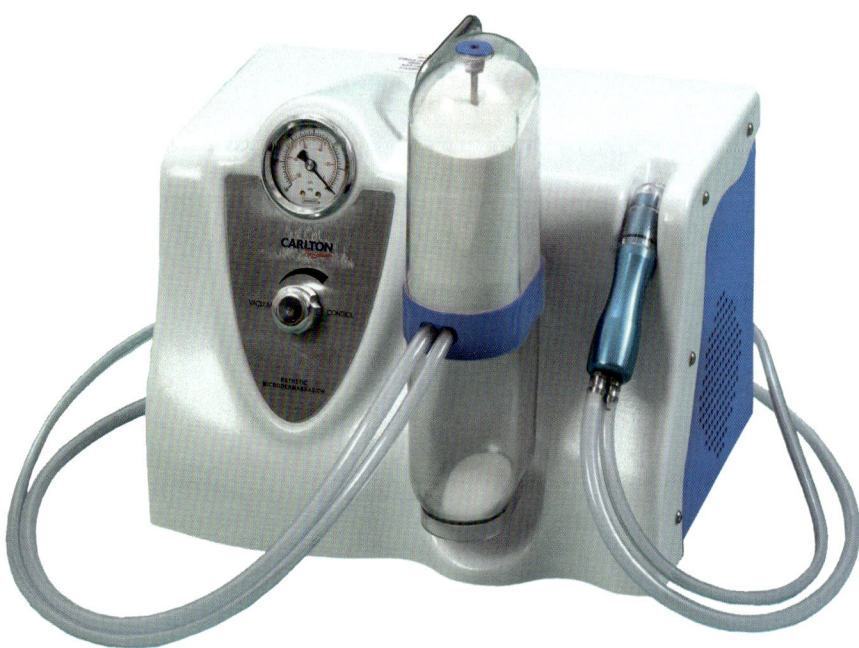

Image courtesy of Carlton Professional

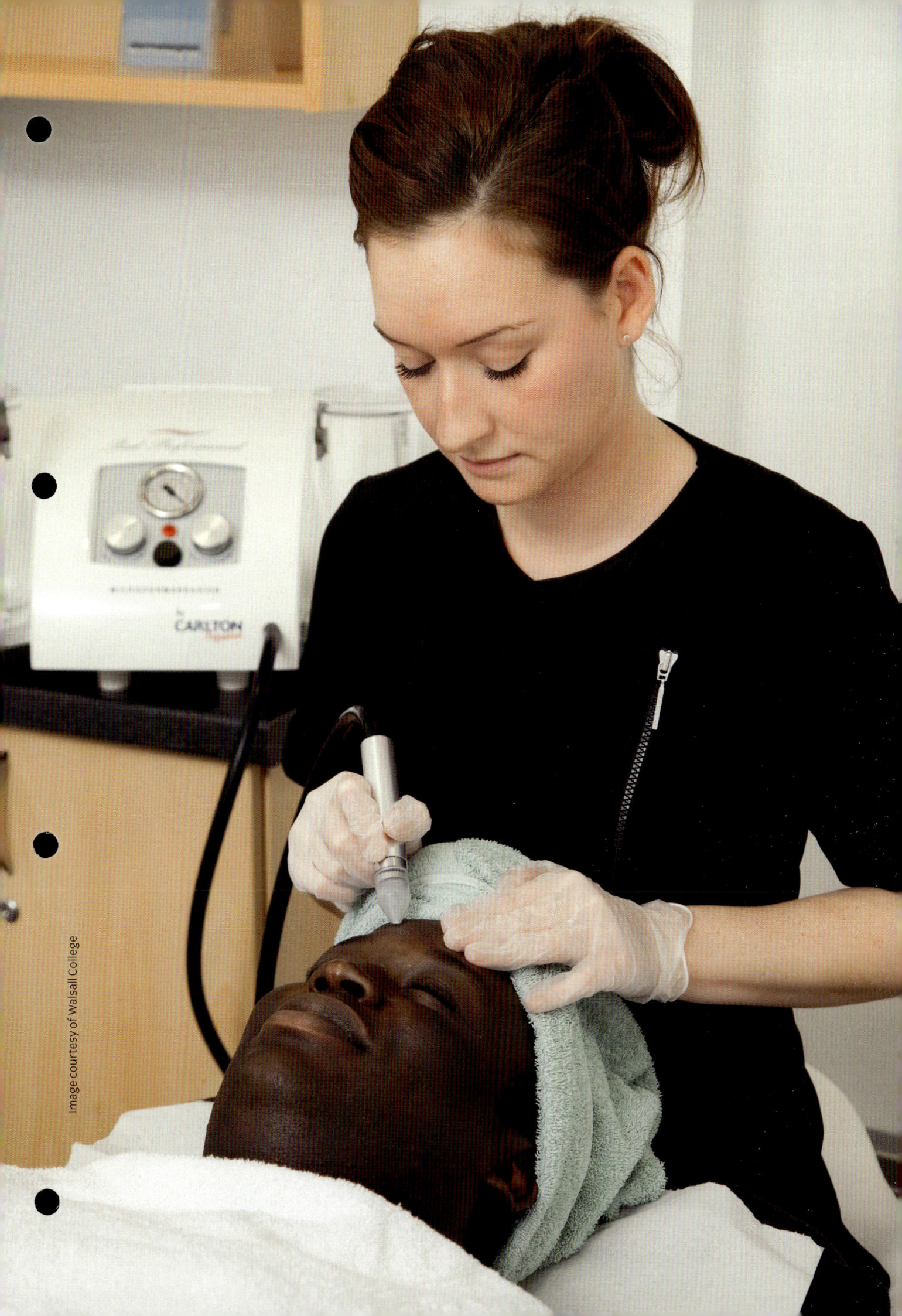

Image courtesy of Walsall College

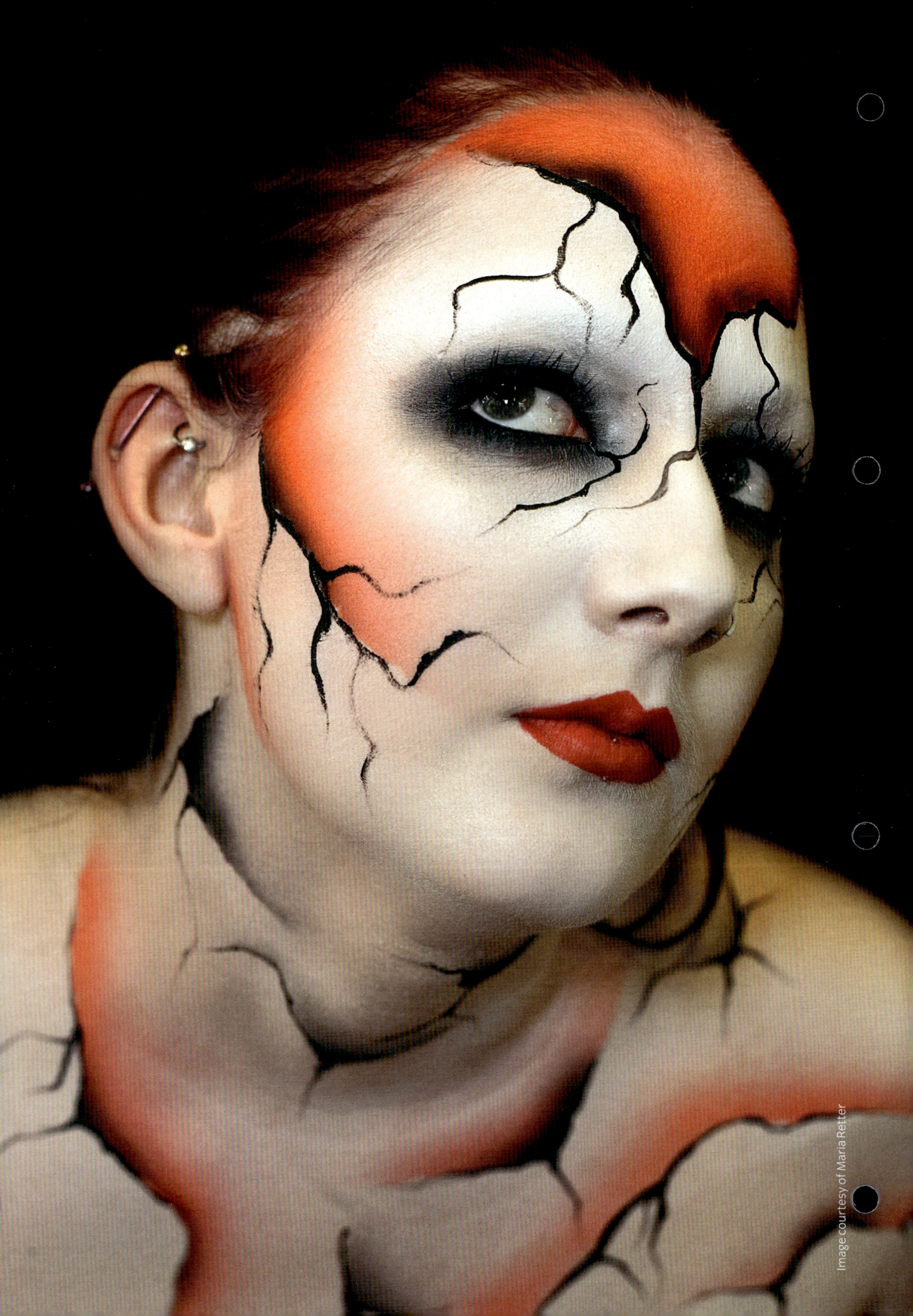
Image courtesy of Maria Retter

323

Design and apply face and body art

Face and body art is the creation of temporary designs applied to the skin, and has existed in many cultures, from the blue dyes used by the Picts of ancient Northern Britain, to the clays and pigments used by the Native Americans. In this unit, you will learn the artistic skills and techniques used to create different effects. You will need to research ideas in order to create the design plans and then apply them using a range of media, such as oil and water based paints and additional adornments such as body gems, sequins and glitter. Finally you will need to record and evaluate your finished design.

Assignment mark sheet
Unit 323 Design and apply face and body art

Your assessor will mark you on each of the practical tasks in this unit. This page is used to work out your overall grade for the unit. You must pass **all** parts of the tasks to be able to achieve a grade. For the practical task a pass equals 1 point, a merit equals 2 points and a distinction equals 3 points.

What you must know	Tick when complete
Task 1a: produce an information sheet	
Task 1b: produce a fact sheet	
Task 1c: anatomy and physiology	
Or tick if covered by an online test	

What you must do	Grade	Points
Task 2: Apply face and body art design		

Overall grade

Candidate name:

Candidate signature: Date:

Assessor signature: Date:

Quality assurance co-ordinator signature (where applicable): Date:

External Verifier signature (where applicable): Date:

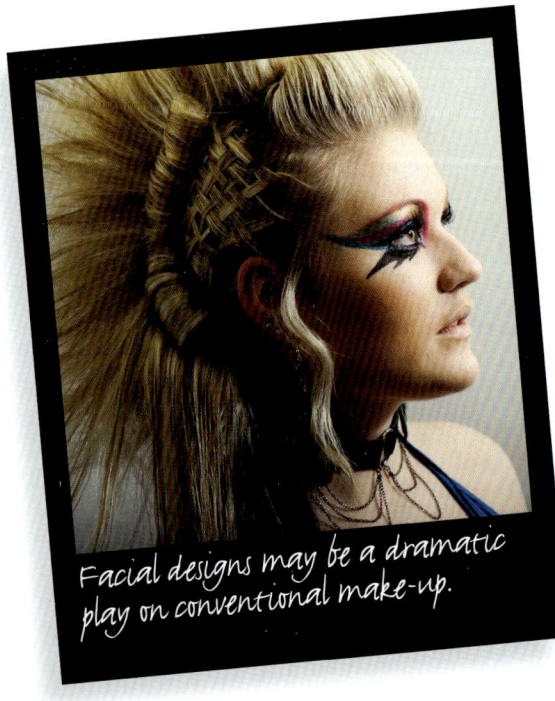

Facial designs may be a dramatic play on conventional make-up.

Image courtesy of www.peteralvey.co.uk

What does it mean?
Some useful words are explained below

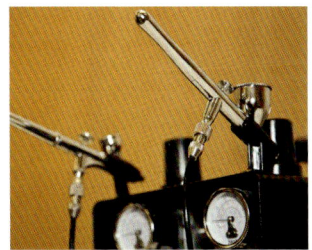

Airbrushing
Using a compressor to spray a fine mist of product onto a surface. Air brush tools consist of a trigger, compressor and reservoir.

Body language
Gestures, facial expressions, eye contact and postures which are often used unconsciously.

Communication
The giving and receiving of, and responding to, information. This may include thoughts and feelings.

Conjunctivitis
An inflammation of the conjunctiva, resulting in redness, discharge, itching and in some cases light sensitivity. It can occur in one eye or both. The cause of conjunctivitis can be a viral or bacterial infection, or may be down to an irritant or an allergy.

Contra-actions
A reaction caused by the service. Some of these are a natural reaction, but others are down to poor practice.

Contra-indications
A condition that prevents treatment from taking place or makes it necessary to modify the treatment.

Dehydrated skin
A lack of water or moisture within the skin as opposed to a lack of oil. This can occur on any skin type.

Design objective
The aim or desired end result of the make-up.

Erythema
Redness of the skin resulting from dilation of blood vessels, due to stimulation, irritation or allergy.

Freehand
Manipulation of the airbrush medium, air pressure being sprayed without shields or stencils.

Hyperkeratosis
Thickening of the skin, common on elbows and knees.

Impetigo
A bacterial skin infection where small blisters break open and then crust over to form scabs.

Make-up artist
An individual who uses make-up and specialised techniques to alter or enhance the appearance.

Manual body art techniques
Methods of applying the media by hand using sponges and brushes.

Media
The make-up products used to create the effect.

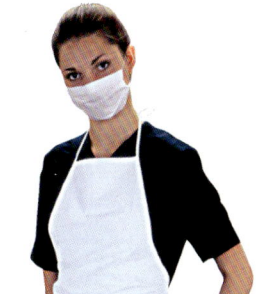

Personal Protective Equipment (PPE)
Clothing and equipment which must be used when carrying out services. It includes the use of face masks when airbrushing.

Skin patch test
A test where a small amount of product is applied to the skin and left on for 24 hours to check that the client is unlikely to react badly.

Skin type
A way of classifying the skin according to the amount of oil it produces.

Stencilling
A make-up technique using a pre-cut or custom designed template to achieve sharp definition and/or continuity and consistency.

Sterilisation
The complete destruction of micro-organisms and their spores.

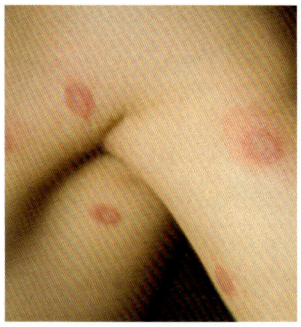

Tinea Corporis
Ringworm of the body. A contagious fungal infection where there are circles of red itchy skin, which heal from the centre.

> **Revision tip**
>
> Open questions are useful during consultation to gain opinions and ideas.

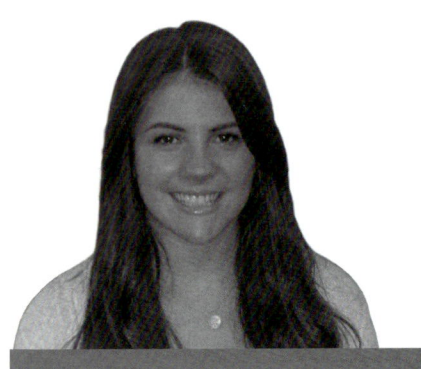

Follow in the footsteps of... *Danielle Smith*

Danielle has been studying Media Make-up at Cambridge Regional College for the past year. She finds face and body art particularly interesting as it involves varied and creative aspects such as special effects, painting and creating unusual pieces of costume. She loves having the freedom to explore her own ideas and create an overall look that will get people talking. Danielle recently competed at World Skills UK, which was a great introduction to the industry. Despite some fierce competition she won 1st place in the regional round. In the future Danielle's main ambition is to take her designs into film and television work, and to the fashion industry. Read on for Danielle's top tips!

What you must know
You must be able to:

1. Explain the importance of preparing and developing a design plan
2. Describe the environmental conditions suitable for face and body art design
3. Describe the different consultation techniques used to identify design objectives
4. Explain the importance of carrying out sensitivity tests
5. Describe how to select products, tools and equipment to suit the design objectives
6. Explain the contra-indications which may prevent or restrict face and body art design
7. Explain how to communicate and behave in a professional manner
8. Describe health and safety working practices
9. Explain the importance of positioning themselves and the client correctly throughout the treatment

Continues on next page

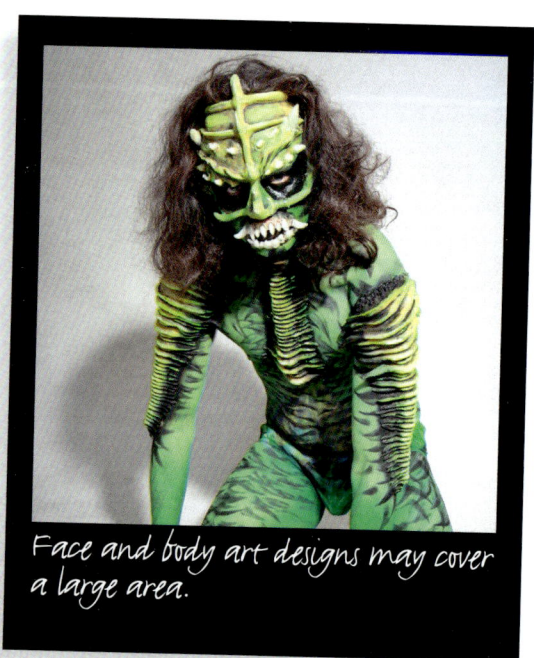

Face and body art designs may cover a large area.

Image courtesy of Jenni Lenard

10 Explain the importance of using products, tools, equipment and techniques to meet the design objectives, client skin type and condition

11 Describe how application can be adapted to suit the design plan, client skin type and condition

12 State the contra-actions that may occur during and following application and how to respond

13 Explain the importance of completing the make-up to meet the design

14 Explain the importance of recording and evaluating the results of the make-up design

15 Describe the aftercare advice that should be provided

16 Describe the structure and function of the skin

17 Describe the diseases and disorders of the skin

18 Describe skin types and conditions

> *When painting the body, paint the base colour with a sponge/airbrush gun to avoid any unwanted brush lines. When adding intricate detail or creating 3D effects, use a fine brush.*

Revision tip

Good ventilation is needed during body art to ensure the regular exchange of fresh and stale air, to help reduce odours and germs.

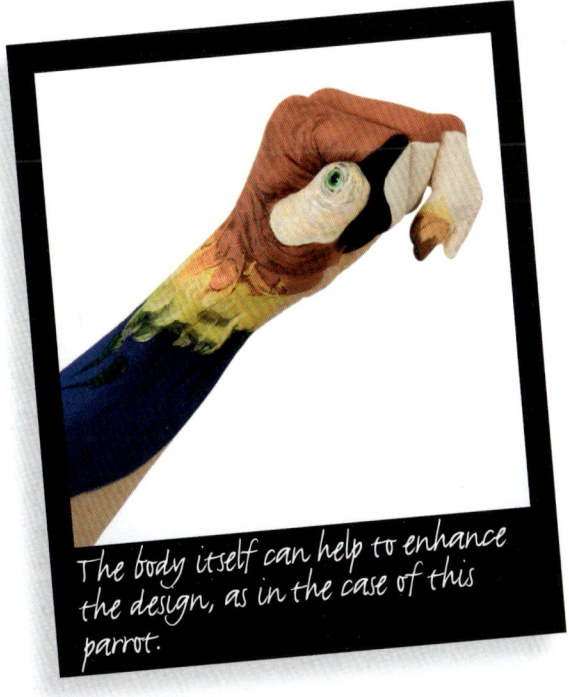

The body itself can help to enhance the design, as in the case of this parrot.

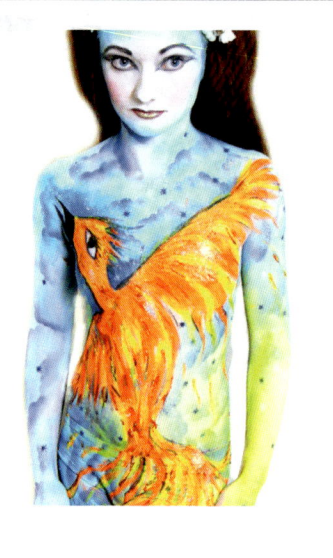

Correct positioning of the client is necessary to prevent injury such as back strain, as well as to achieve the best end result.

Face and

Consider the background and the model's pose when photographing your work.

A well thought out and detailed design plan will enable you to work in a logical sequence.

Give the aftercare advice clearly, including removal techniques, and check that the client has understood it.

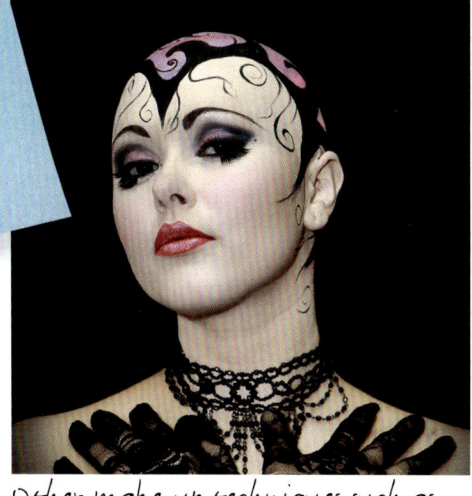

Other make-up techniques such as the use of a bald cap can enhance your design.

body art

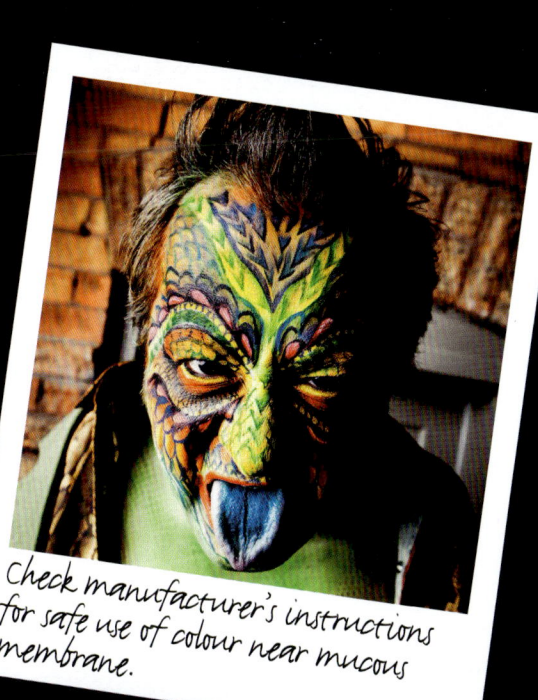

Check manufacturer's instructions for safe use of colour near mucous membrane.

"
Handmade stencils are a great way to save time if you're put in high pressure situations. After painting over the stencil be sure to fill in the finer detail to make the design stand out and enhance the overall appearance.

What you must do
Practical observations

This page shows what you need to do during your practical task. You can look at it beforehand, but you're **not** allowed to have it with you while carrying out your practical task. You must achieve **all** the criteria; you can achieve 1 mark, 2 marks or 3 marks for the criteria indicated with *.

Conversion chart

Grade	Marks
Pass	10–11
Merit	12–15
Distinction	16–18

○ Please tick when all pre-observation requirements have been met.

	Apply face and body art design		
1 Prepare yourself, the client and the work area for face and body art design	1		
2 Use suitable consultation techniques to identify design objectives *	1	2	3
3 Carry out a skin sensitivity test	1		
4 Position yourself and the client correctly throughout the treatment	1		
5 Select and use products, tools, equipment and techniques to suit the design objectives, client/model skin type and conditions *	1	2	3
6 Communicate and behave in a professional manner	1		
7 Follow health and safety working practices	1		
8 Complete the make-up to meet design objectives *	1	2	3
9 Record and evaluate the results of the application	1		
10 Provide suitable aftercare advice *	1	2	3
Total			
Grade			
Candidate signature and date			
Assessor signature and date			

Unit 323 Level 3 VRQ Beauty Therapy

What you must do
Practical observations descriptors table

This table shows what you need to do to achieve 1, 2 or 3 marks for the criteria indicated with * on the previous page.

	1 mark	2 marks	3 marks
2 Use suitable consultation techniques to identify design objectives	Basic consultation Examples: uses open and closed questions, checks for contra-indications, identifies the design objectives correctly.	Good consultation Examples: positive body language, uses open and closed questions to identify contra-indications, expectations and reasons/occasion for the design; identifies the design objectives and any factors that may limit or restrict the service.	Thorough consultation Examples: positive body language, uses open and closed questions to identify contra-indications, expectations and reasons/occasion for the design; identifies the design objectives and any factors that may limit or restrict the service, allows the client/model to ask any questions to confirm understanding.
5 Select and use products, tools, equipment and techniques to suit the design objectives, client/model skin type and conditions	Selects and uses appropriate products, tools and equipment to meet the design plan.	Selects and uses appropriate products, tools and equipment, in a logical sequence with creativity and confidence, to meet the design plan.	Selects and uses appropriate products, tools and equipment, in a logical sequence with creativity and confidence, to meet the design plan, adapts and modifies techniques as necessary and informs the client/model of the changes.
8 Complete the make-up to meet design objectives	The service is completed within the agreed time and brought to a satisfactory close, and meets the design objectives.	The service is completed within the agreed time and brought to a satisfactory close, and meets the design objectives, and the client is shown the result.	The service is completed within the agreed time and brought to a satisfactory close, make-up applied in a logical sequence with creativity and confidence to meet the design objectives, the client is shown the result.

Continues on next page

What you must do
Practical observations descriptors table (continued)

This table shows what you need to do to achieve 1, 2 or 3 marks for the criteria indicated with * on page 212.

	1 mark	2 marks	3 marks
10 Provide suitable aftercare advice	Basic aftercare advice is provided including possible contra-actions and how to deal with them.	Good level of aftercare advice is provided including possible contra-actions and how to deal with them, home care products, future services.	Excellent aftercare advice is provided including possible contra-actions and how to deal with them, home care products, future services, application and removal techniques and recommendations.

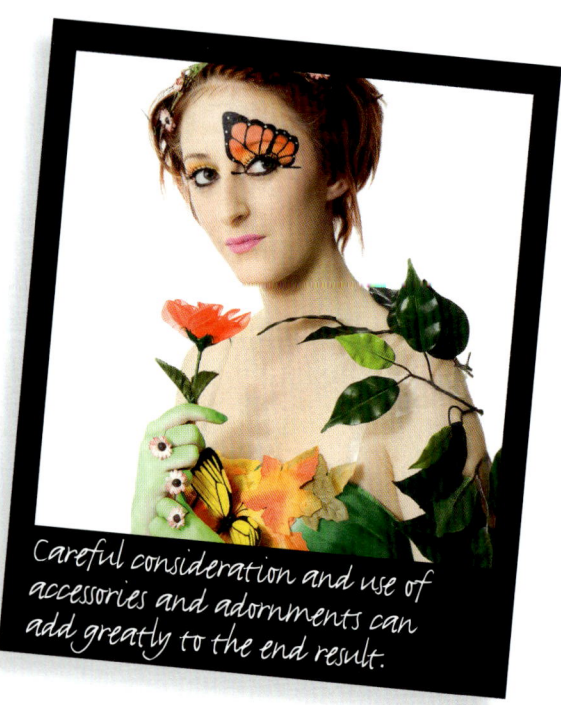

Careful consideration and use of accessories and adornments can add greatly to the end result.

> "If you want to include handmade prosthetic pieces in your design, make sure the edges are thin and smooth when creating them. This will make it easier to apply and disguise.

Image courtesy of www.peteralvey.co.uk

Comment form
Unit 323 Design and apply face and body art

This form can be used to record comments by you, your client, or your assessor.

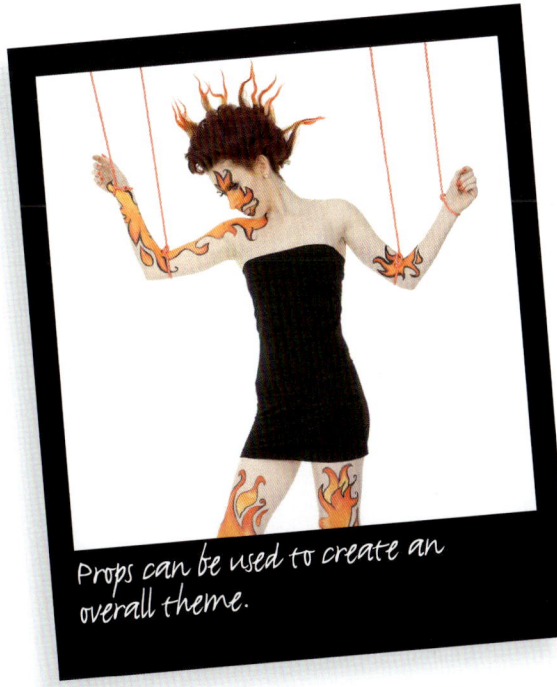

Props can be used to create an overall theme.

Image courtesy of www.peteralvey.co.uk

> To hide edges, use an orange stipple sponge as it gives a smooth and skin-like texture.

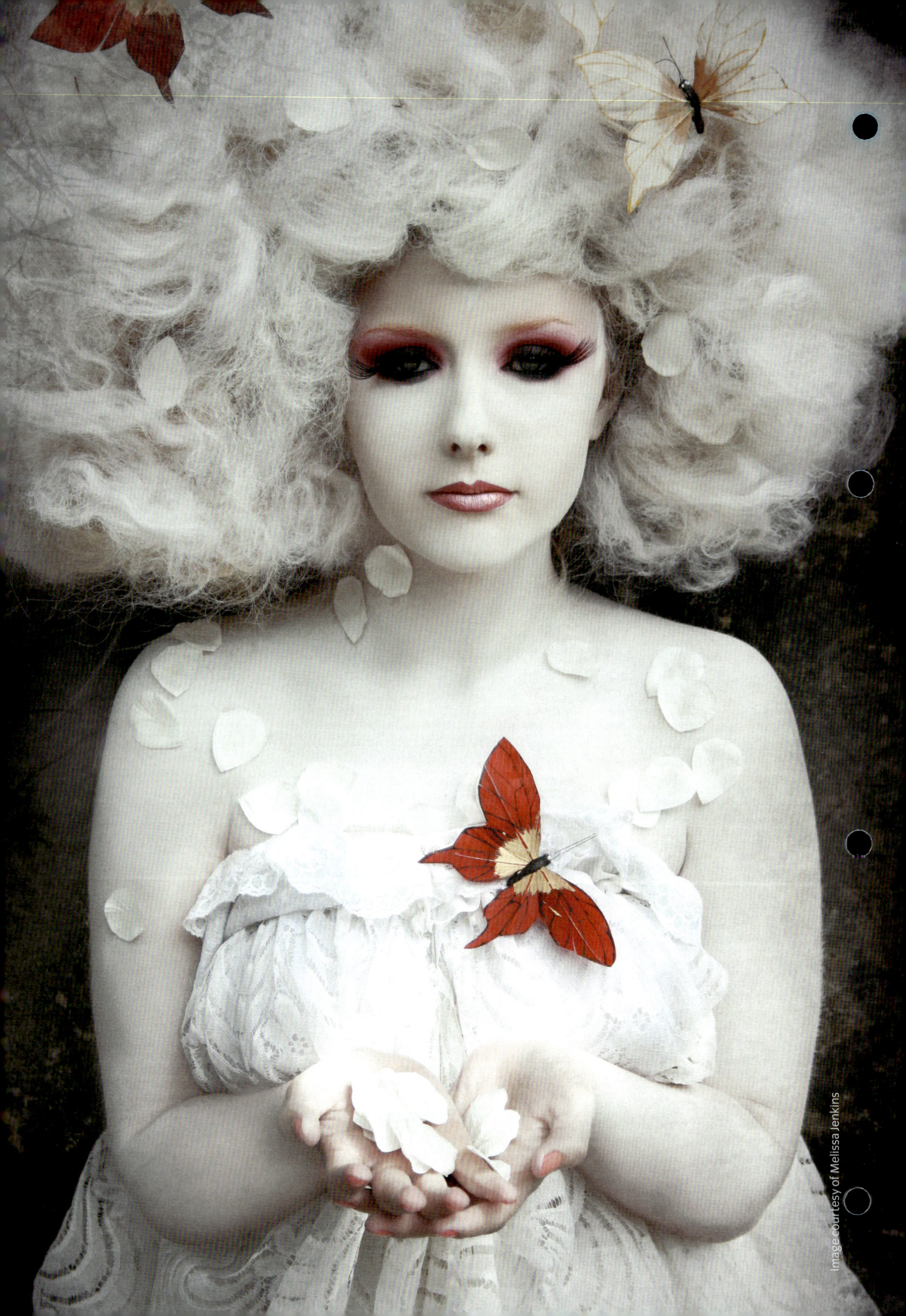

Image courtesy of Melissa Jenkins

324

Fashion and photographic make-up

Fashion is not only a glamorous industry; it is at the forefront of many trends and has a cultural impact on the way we live our lives. Working in this fast-paced industry as a make-up artist can be both exciting and nerve-racking. Whether covering catwalk shows or photographic shoots, you may find that you work under the direction of a chief designer, with a specific vision of how the make-up should look, or you may be in a position to plan, devise and apply the make-up yourself. This unit covers everything you need to know in order to create fashion and photographic make-up images. It also includes advice on creating accurate historical/period looks and images for black and white photography.

Assignment mark sheet
Unit 324 Fashion and photographic make-up

Your assessor will mark you on each of the practical tasks in this unit. This page is used to work out your overall grade for the unit. You must pass **all** parts of the tasks to be able to achieve a grade. For each completed practical task, a pass equals 1 point, a merit equals 2 points and a distinction equals 3 points.

What you must know	Tick when complete
Task 1a: produce an information sheet	
Task 1b: produce a fact sheet	
Task 1c: anatomy and physiology	
Or tick if covered by an online test	

What you must do	Grade	Points
Task 2a: Apply fashion make-up		
Task 2b: Apply photographic make-up		

Conversion chart

Grade	Points
Pass	1–1.5
Merit	1.6–2.5
Distinction	2.6–3

Total points for graded tasks	
Divided by	÷ 2
= Average grade for tasks	
Overall grade (see conversion chart)	

Candidate name:

Candidate signature: Date:

Assessor signature: Date:

Quality assurance co-ordinator signature (where applicable): Date:

External Verifier signature (where applicable): Date:

What does it mean?
Some useful words are explained below

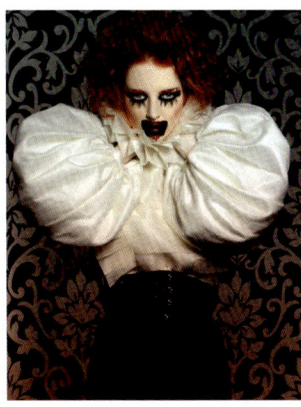

Avante-garde
People or works which are experimental or innovative, particularly in art and culture.

Body language
Gestures, facial expressions, eye contact and postures which are often used unconsciously.

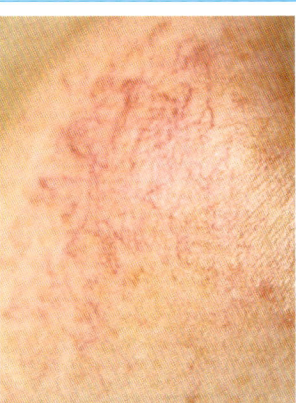

Broken capillaries
Tiny, red thread-like blood vessels which are visible on the surface of the skin.

Budget
The amount of money available to spend on a project.

Catwalk show
Usually performed on a runway, these feature models who are showcasing designer's clothes or new collections.

Client
The person who has commissioned the work. They might not always be present so careful planning and confirmation of design is needed.

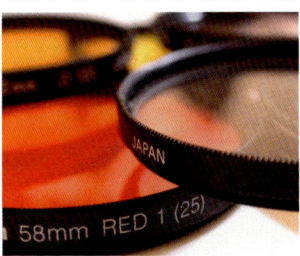

Coloured filters
Used in photography to change the look or mood of the end result.

Contra-indications
Conditions which restrict or prevent the make-up from taking place.

Dehydrated skin
This is a lack of water or moisture within the skin as opposed to a lack of oil, and can occur on any skin type.

Design objective
The aim or desired end result of the make-up.

Disinfection
Hygiene process which reduces the number of micro-organisms present.

Erythema
Redness of the skin resulting from dilation of blood vessels, due to stimulation, irritation or allergy.

Freelancer
Self-employed person who pursues a profession without a long-term commitment to any particular employer.

High fashion
Make-up which is applied to support the impact of unique, exclusive and trend-setting clothes, often showcased on the runway at international fashion shows.

Kabuki brush
Originating from Kabuki theatre in Japan, these are short and wide domed brushes. They are excellent for defining the cheeks and are considered by many to be the brush of choice for mineral make-up and bronzer application.

Normal skin
An unusual skin type which has an even colouring with regular pore size and no flakiness, oily patches or other blemishes.

Pancake
Invented by Max Factor in the 1930s to replace greasepaint, this is a thick, densely pigmented full-coverage base.

Continues on next page

What does it mean?
Some useful words are explained below (continued)

Papule
A hard red spot which does not contain pus and is often very painful.

Personal space
An invisible area surrounding a person. It varies between individuals, but invading it can lead to feelings of discomfort or anxiety.

Portfolio
A collection of your work to include photographs, sketches, design plans and testimonials from clients as well as any published work.

Professionalism
The formally agreed codes of conduct and behaviour within a job role, and the informal expectations of clients and colleagues of a person who holds that job.

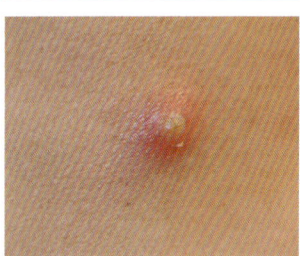

Pustule
A spot which contains pus.

Show reel
A short DVD of your work to show to potential clients.

Skin sensitivity tests
A small amount of product is applied to the skin and left on for 24 hours to check that the client is unlikely to react unfavourably.

Spirit gum
An adhesive solution made of gum (resin) and ether and used to fix a variety of items to the skin, eg glitter and sequins. It is a potential allergen, so it is vital to perform a skin sensitivity test before use.

Sterilisation
A hygiene process which destroys all micro-organisms and their spores, preventing cross infection.

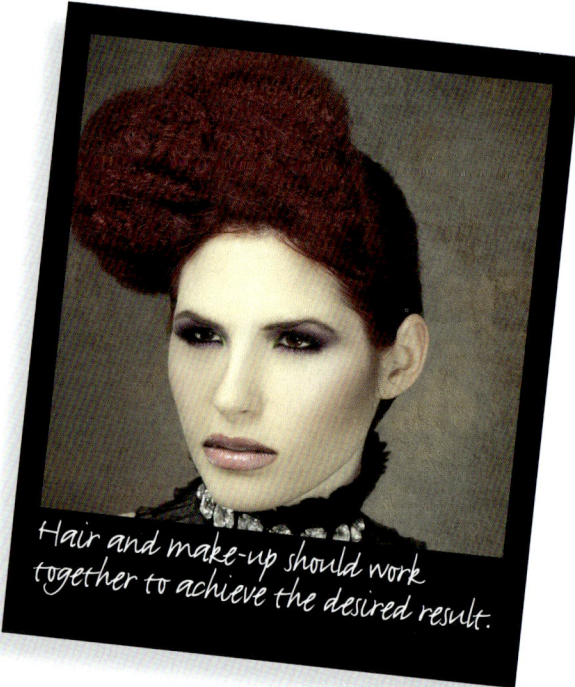

Hair and make-up should work together to achieve the desired result.

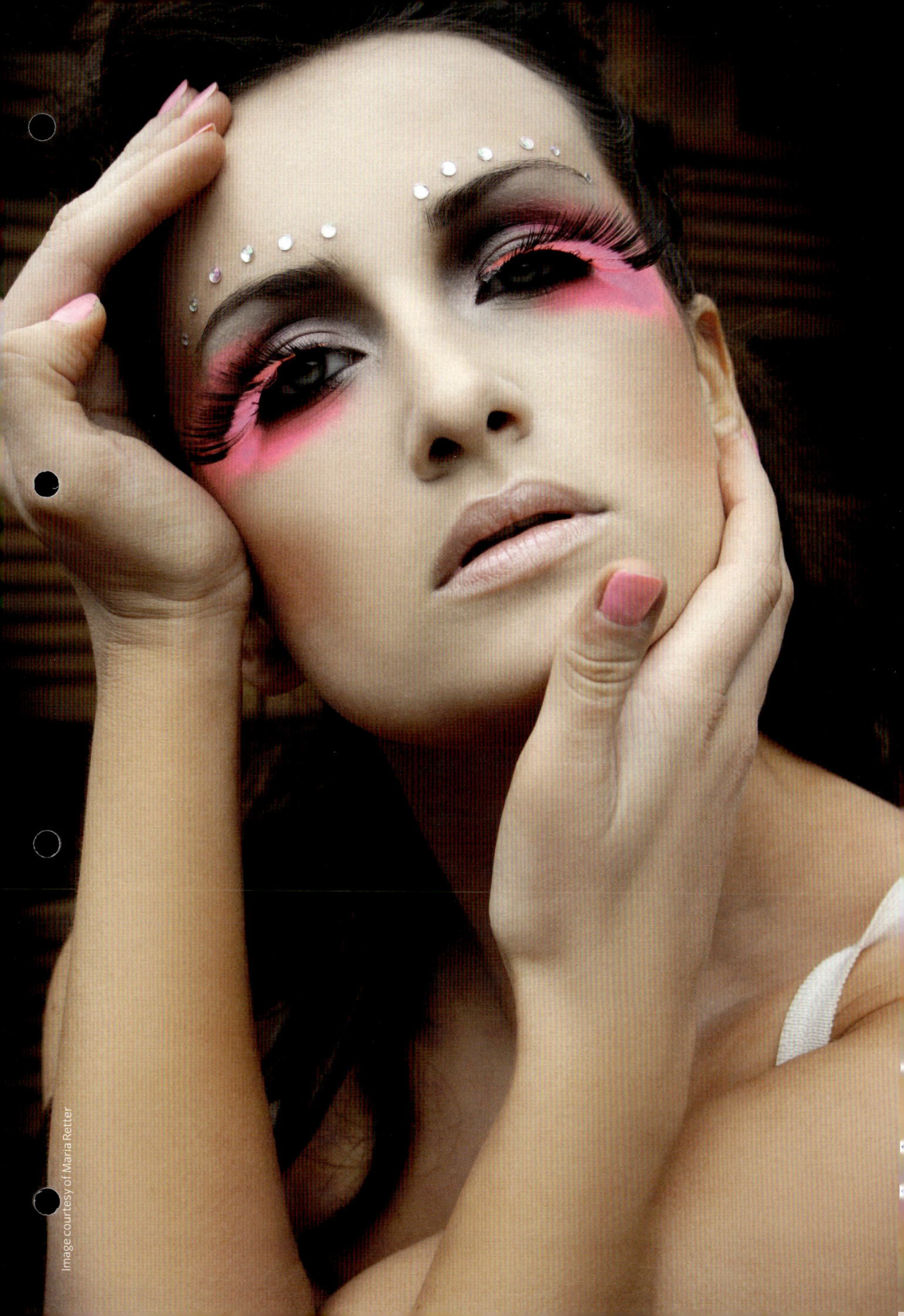

Image courtesy of Maria Retter

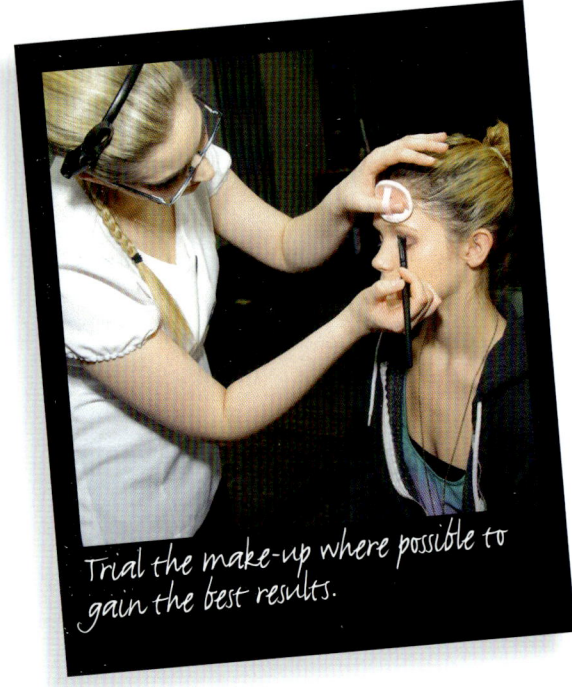

Trial the make-up where possible to gain the best results.

What you must know
You must be able to:

1 Describe the importance of working to a budget

2 Describe ways of effectively presenting a design plan

3 Explain the importance of preparing and developing a design plan

4 Describe the environmental conditions suitable for fashion and photographic make-up

5 Describe the consultation techniques used to identify design objectives

6 Explain the importance of carrying out skin sensitivity tests

7 Describe how to select products, tools and equipment to suit the design objectives

8 Explain the contra-indications that may prevent or restrict make-up application

9 Explain how to communicate and behave in a professional manner

10 Describe health and safety working practices

11 Explain the importance of positioning themselves and the client correctly throughout the design

Continues on next page

Revision tip

Fluorescent lighting will affect the make-up colour by taking away the warmth from the make-up.

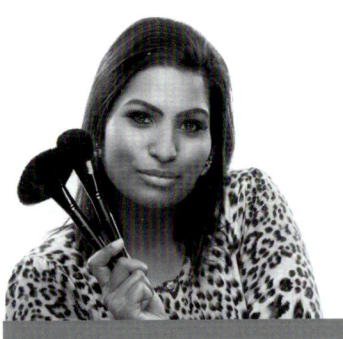

Follow in the footsteps of...
Sita Gill

After studying Media Studies, it was clear to Sita that the media and make-up world was where she wanted to be. She took several make-up courses and is now a professional, specialist make-up artist. Sita's career has included working for Elizabeth Arden and Dior as a Beauty Consultant. She has also worked for two magazines as a make-up columnist, giving tips and advice on make-up application. Sita is now a teacher, passing on her skills and knowledge to others who share her passion for make-up. **Look out for the blue quote marks for Sita's creative tips!**

12 Explain the importance of using products, tools, equipment and techniques to meet the design objectives, client skin type and condition

13 Describe how application can be adapted to suit the design plan, client skin type and condition

14 State the contra-actions that may occur during and following the application and how to respond

15 Explain the importance of completing the design application to meet the design objectives

16 Explain the importance of recording and evaluating the make-up design

17 Describe the aftercare advice that should be provided

18 Describe the structure and functions of the skin

19 Describe skin types, conditions, diseases and disorders

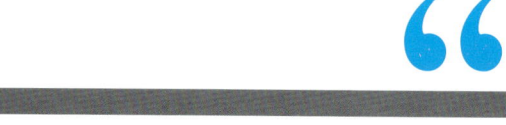

Try to do some model test shoots with photographers for experience. This will also help you to get bookings.

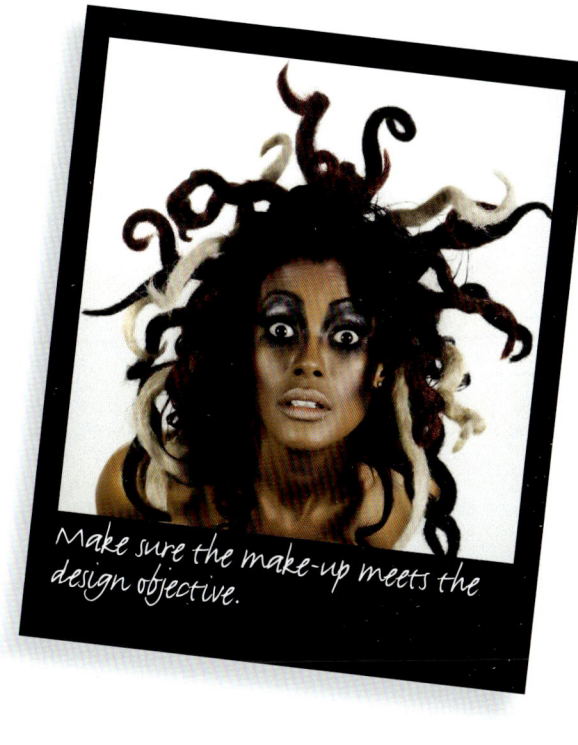

Make sure the make-up meets the design objective.

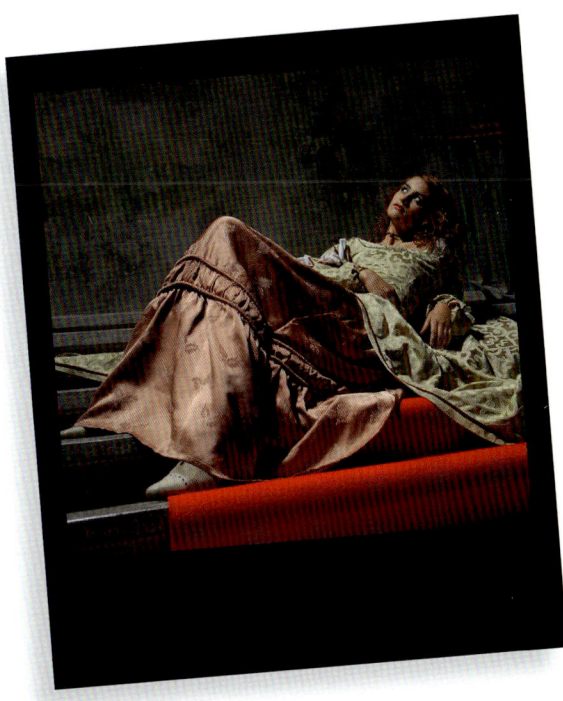

Revision tip

Blue toned lighting will neutralise pink/red shades and the make-up will appear greyer.

Fashion and photographic make-up Unit 324

Buy fashion magazines both for inspiration and to keep on top of what is on trend.

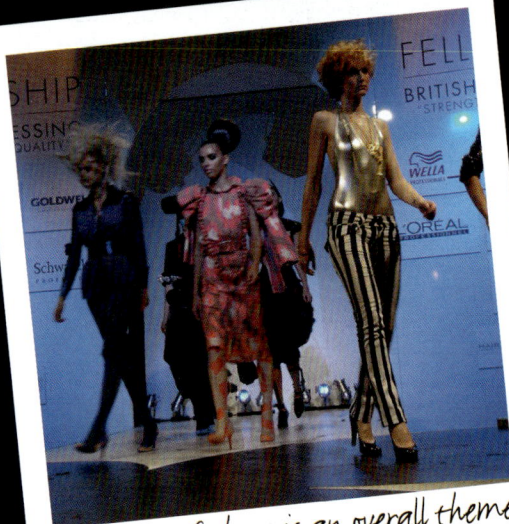

Find out if there is an overall theme to the runway show.

Fashion

Remember that the way a photograph is lit can create effects which are impossible to reproduce by make-up alone.

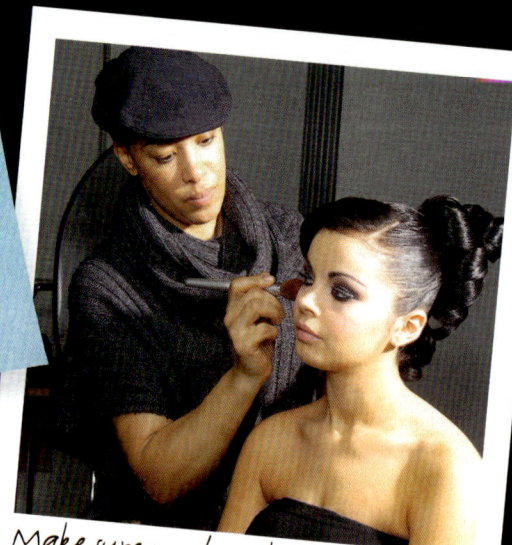

Make sure you have kept a record of make-up used in case 'touch ups' are necessary.

make-up

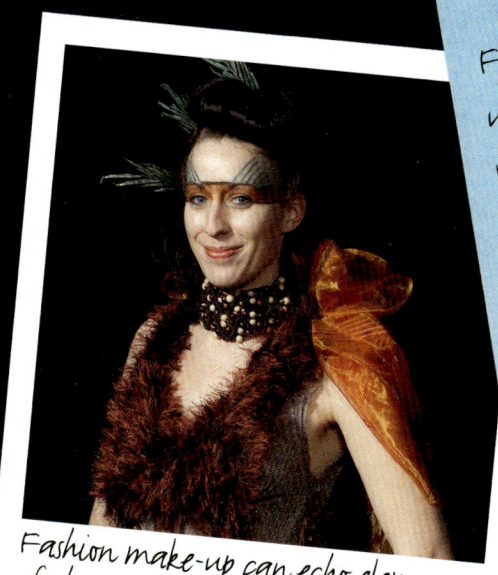

Fashion make-up can echo elements of the model's clothes.

Image courtesy of The Folkestone Academy

For innovative looks try using make-up in a new way — for example coloured eyeshadows for face shading.

Always check that any red pigmented make-up is safe to use close to the eyes.

> " *Always practise the make-up application if you have designed it for a themed shoot, as the make-up artist needs to ensure the model and theme work well together.*

What you must do
Practical observations

This page shows what you need to do during your practical task. You can look at it beforehand, but you're **not** allowed to have it with you while carrying out your practical task. You must achieve **all** the criteria; you can achieve 1 mark, 2 marks or 3 marks for the criteria indicated with *.

Conversion chart

Grade	Marks
Pass	10–11
Merit	12–15
Distinction	16–18

○ Please tick when all pre-observation requirements have been met.

	Apply make-up					
	a Fashion make-up			b Photographic make-up		
False lashes used	Y/N			Y/N		
1 Prepare yourself, the client/model and the work area for make-up application	1			1		
2 Use suitable consultation techniques to identify design objectives *	1	2	3	1	2	3
3 Carry out necessary tests	1			1		
4 Position yourself and the model correctly throughout the treatment	1			1		
5 Select and use products, tools, equipment and techniques to suit the design objectives, client/model skin type and conditions *	1	2	3	1	2	3
6 Communicate and behave in a professional manner	1			1		
7 Follow health and safety working practices	1			1		
8 Complete the service to meet the design objectives *	1	2	3	1	2	3
9 Record and evaluate the results of the application	1			1		
10 Provide suitable aftercare advice *	1	2	3	1	2	3

Total

Grade

Candidate signature and date

Assessor signature and date

What you must do
Practical observations descriptors table

This table shows what you need to do to achieve 1, 2 or 3 marks for the criteria indicated with * on the previous page.

	1 mark	2 marks	3 marks
2 Use suitable consultation techniques to identify design objectives	Basic consultation Examples: uses open and closed questions, checks for contra-indications, identifies the design objectives correctly.	Good consultation Examples: positive body language, uses open and closed questions to identify contra-indications, expectations and occasion; identifies the design objectives and any factors that may limit or restrict the service.	Thorough consultation Examples: positive body language, uses open and closed questions to identify contra-indications, expectations and occasion; identifies the design objectives and any factors that may limit or restrict the service, allows the model to ask any questions to confirm understanding.
5 Select and use products, tools, equipment and techniques to suit the design objectives, client model skin type and conditions	Selects and uses products, tools equipment and basic techniques to meet the design plan and the client/model's skin type and condition.	Selects and uses appropriate products, tools, equipment and a range of techniques in a logical sequence with creativity and confidence, to meet the design plan, the client/model's skin type and condition, and effect required.	Selects and uses appropriate products, tools, equipment and a range of techniques in a logical sequence with creativity and confidence, to meet the design plan, the client/model's skin type and condition, and effect required, adapts and modifies techniques as necessary and informs the model of the changes.
8 Complete the service to meet the design objectives	The service is completed within the agreed time and brought to a satisfactory close, meets the design objectives.	The service is completed within the agreed time and brought to a satisfactory close, meets the design objectives, the client/model is shown the result and the end result is agreed.	The service is completed within the agreed time and brought to a satisfactory close, make-up applied neatly and blended well to meet the design objectives, the client/model is shown the result, positive feedback is gained.

Continues on next page

What you must do
Practical observations descriptors table (continued)

This table shows what you need to do to achieve 1, 2 or 3 marks for the criteria indicated with * on page 226.

	1 mark	2 marks	3 marks
10 Provide suitable aftercare advice	Basic aftercare advice is provided including possible contra-actions and how to deal with them.	Good level of aftercare advice is provided including possible contra-actions and how to deal with them, home care products, future services.	Excellent aftercare advice is provided including possible contra-actions and how to deal with them, home care products, future services, advice on application and removal techniques.

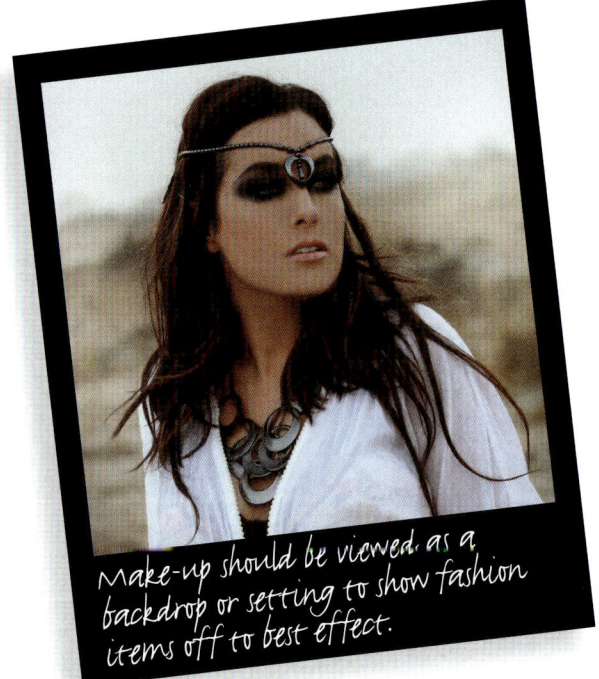

Make-up should be viewed as a backdrop or setting to show fashion items off to best effect.

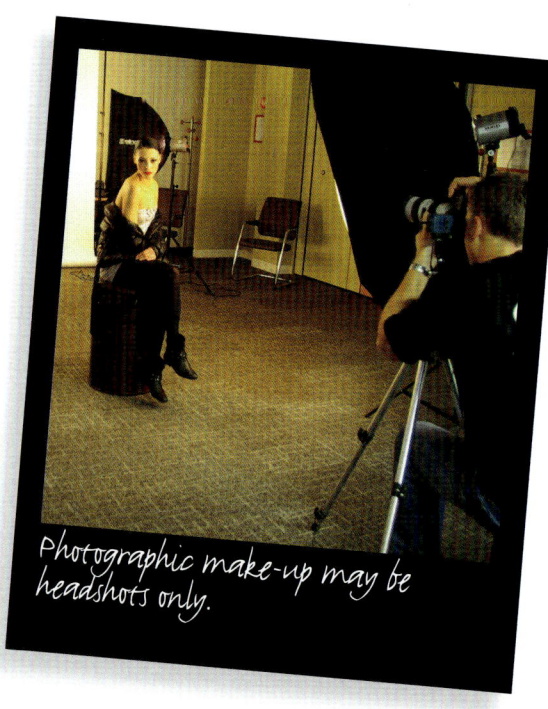

Photographic make-up may be headshots only.

Image courtesy of Melissa Jenkins

Comment form
Unit 324 Fashion and photographic make-up

This form can be used to record comments by you, your client, or your assessor.

_____

_____

_____

_____

_____

_____

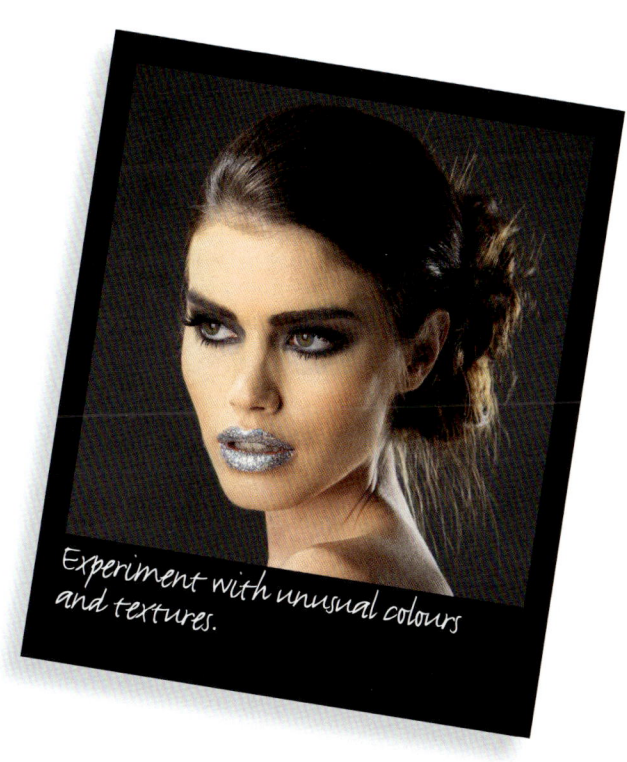

Experiment with unusual colours and textures.

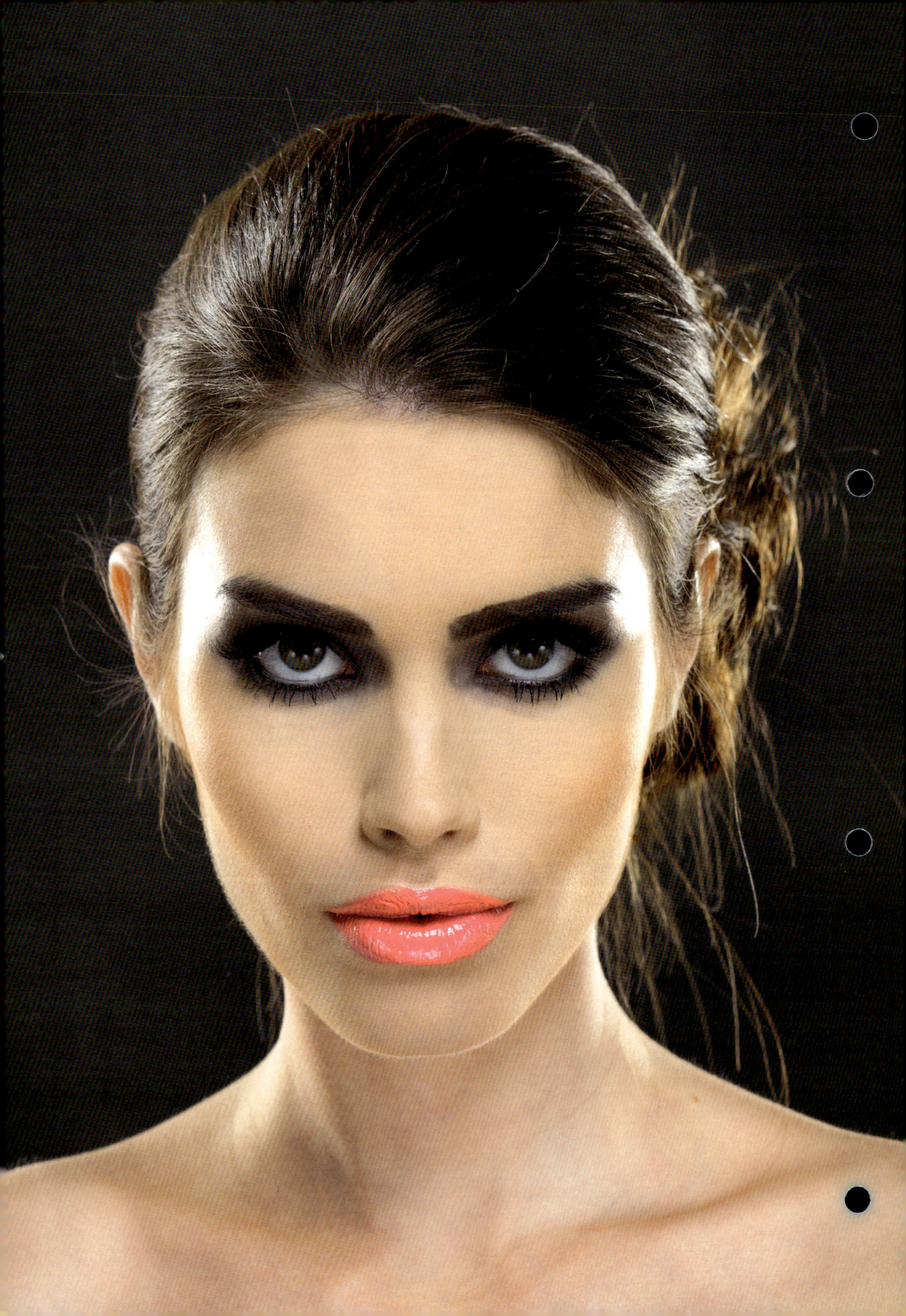

327

Apply airbrush make-up to the face

With the advances in digital media, airbrushed make-up is the finish of choice for a glowing and flawless face. Airbrushing is a liquid form of make-up sprayed on at very low pressure, leaving behind a seamless layer of colour. The high coverage but thin texture results in a natural, sheer end result. In this unit you will learn how to prepare and develop suitable make-up design plans, carry out a detailed skin analysis to choose the best products and carry out the make-up professionally to meet the design objective. The micro-fine surface that can be achieved is sought after by brides, and indeed anyone who needs a flawless finish, with the advantage that the end result will look the same in photographs as it does in real life.

Assignment mark sheet
Unit 327 Apply airbrush make-up to the face

Your assessor will mark you on each of the practical tasks in this unit. This page is used to work out your overall grade for the unit. You must pass **all** parts of the tasks to be able to achieve a grade. For the practical task a pass equals 1 point, a merit equals 2 points and a distinction equals 3 points.

What you must know	Tick when complete
Task 1a: produce an information sheet	
Task 1b: produce a fact sheet	
Task 1c: anatomy and physiology	
Or tick if covered by an online test	

What you must do	Grade	Points
Task 2: Apply airbrush make-up to the face		

Overall grade

Candidate name:

Candidate signature: Date:

Assessor signature: Date:

Quality assurance co-ordinator signature (where applicable):   Date:

External Verifier signature (where applicable):   Date:

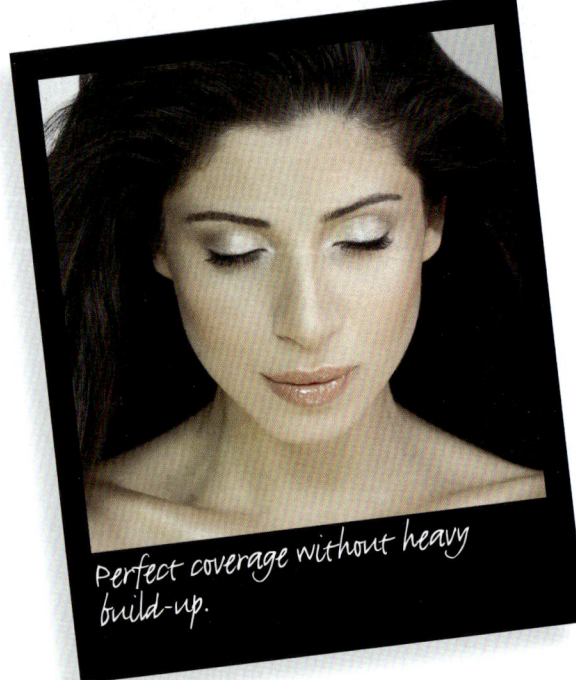

Perfect coverage without heavy build-up.

Image courtesy of Kett Cosmetics

What does it mean?
Some useful words are explained below

Acid mantle
The layer of sebum and sweat on the skin's surface that provides lubrication and protects against bacteria.

Adverse skin reactions
A response of the skin to a product such as irritation, itching, redness or swelling.

Airbrushing
Using a compressor to spray a fine mist of product onto a surface. Air brush tools consist of a trigger, compressor and reservoir.

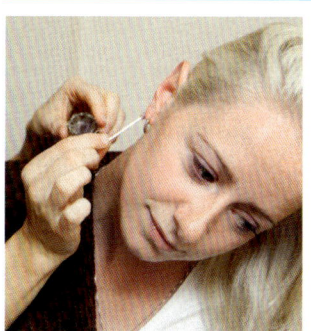

Compatibility tests
A small amount of product is applied to the skin and left on for 24 hours to check that the client is unlikely to react unfavourably.

Contra-indications
Conditions which restrict or prevent the make-up from taking place.

Dehydrated skin
A lack of water or moisture within the skin as opposed to a lack of oil, and can occur on any skin type.

Design objective
The aim or desired end result of the make-up.

Double action technique
Involves depressing the trigger on the top of the airbrush with the index finger to release air only, and drawing it back gradually to the make-up release threshold.

Freehand
Manipulation of the airbrush medium without shields or stencils.

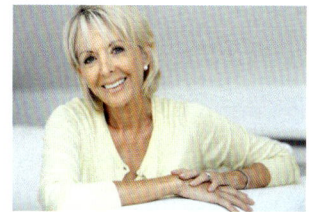

Mature skin
In beauty therapy terms this is any skin over the age of 25. However, the skin is generally not classed as being mature until the signs of ageing are apparent.

Media
The make-up products used to create the effect.

Normal skin
An uncommon skin type with small pores and a smooth texture, an even colouring, and no blemishes, flaky or oily patches present.

PSI
Pounds per square inch is a measurement of the amount of pressure put out by an airbrush. A higher PSI will produce a heavier result, while a low PSI will create a sheer finish.

Ringworm
A contagious fungal infection where there are circles of red, itchy skin which heal from the centre.

Sensitive skin
Skin which reacts readily to products, heat or pressure. Whilst it can occur on any skin type, it usually has a fine texture, thin epidermis and blood vessels very close to the surface, which can result in blotchiness, redness, flushing, increased warmth and irritation if stimulated.

Silicone-based make-up
Make-up which produces a fresh dewy look.

Single action technique
Derives its name from the fact that only one action is required for operation. The single action of depressing the trigger releases a fixed ratio of make-up to air gravity feed. The colour cup is on top of the brush.

Siphon feed
The colour cup or container is either on the bottom or side of the brush.

Continues on next page

What does it mean?
Some useful words are explained below (continued)

Skin analysis
A careful assessment of the skin to determine its type and condition, taking into account contributory factors.

Skin type
A way of classifying the skin according to the amount of oil it produces.

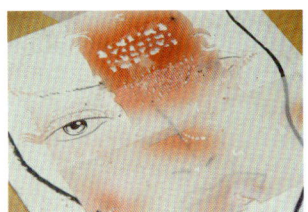

Stencilling
A make-up technique using a pre-cut or custom designed template to achieve sharp definition and/or continuity and consistency.

Water-based make-up
Dries to a natural matte finish that is neither drier nor shinier in appearance than skin is naturally.

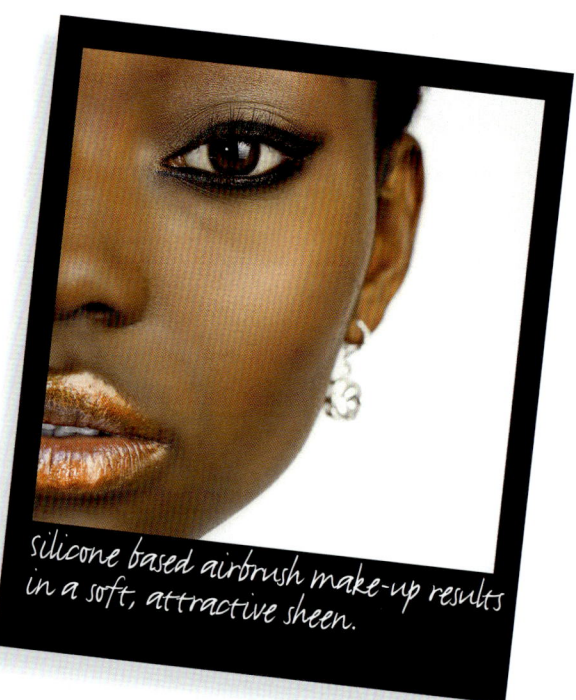

silicone based airbrush make-up results in a soft, attractive sheen.

Image courtesy of iStockphoto.com/quavondo

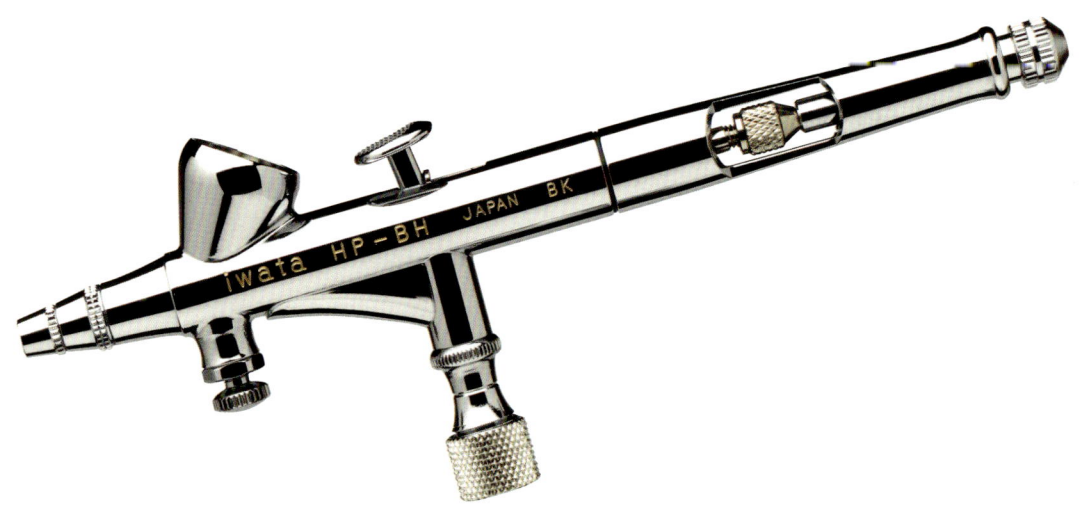

Image courtesy of The Airbrush Co. Ltd.

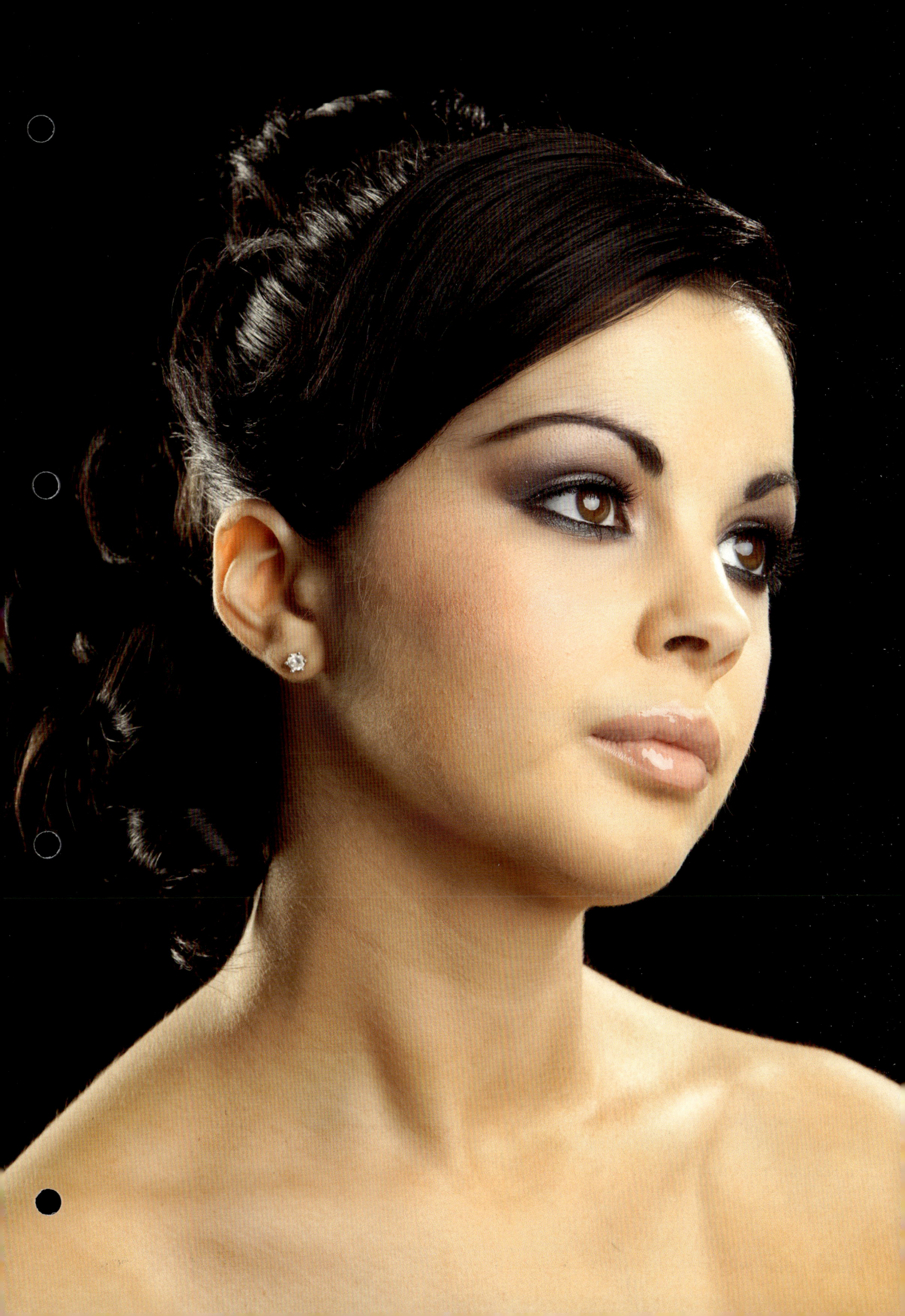

> **Revision tip**
>
> Ventilation refers to the flow of fresh air through an area, NOT the temperature!

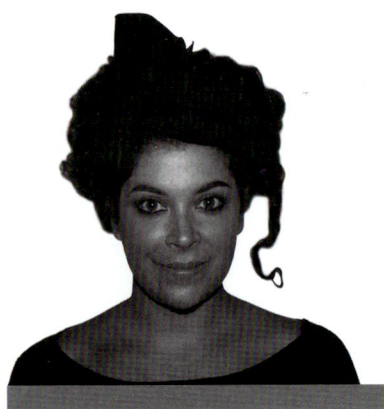

Follow in the footsteps of...
Carly Utting

"Carly decided she wanted to become a make-up artist when her grandparents returned from a "behind the scenes" theatre tour and had the opportunity of watching someone create beautiful theatrical make-up. As soon as she saw the photos she knew she wanted to be a make-up artist. The thought of being able to transform a human face or body into something beautiful was so inspiring she enrolled on a two year make-up course. After finishing the course she started working for M·A·C. It was at M·A·C that she first tried her hand at body painting and airbrushing. She loves the ability these techniques give her to help people look and feel better. Read on for Carly's fantastic airbrush make-up tips!

What you must know
You must be able to:

1 Explain the importance of preparing and developing airbrush make-up design plans

2 Describe salon requirements for preparing themselves, the client and work area

3 Describe the environmental conditions suitable for airbrush make-up treatment

4 Describe the different consultation techniques used to identify treatment objectives

5 Explain the importance of carrying out a detailed skin analysis and relevant tests

6 Describe how to select products, tools and equipment to suit client treatment needs, skin type and conditions

7 Explain the contra-indications that prevent or restrict airbrush make-up

8 Explain how to communicate and behave in a professional manner

9 Describe health and safety working practices

10 Explain the importance of positioning themselves and the client correctly throughout the treatment

Continues on next page

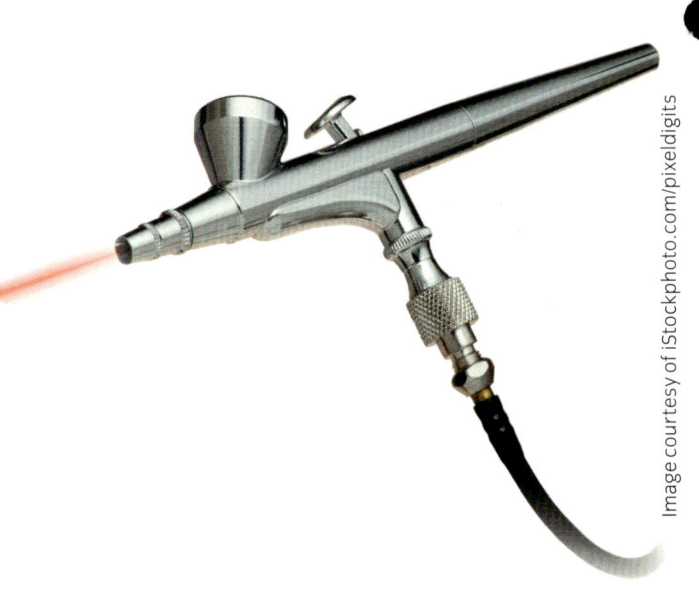

Image courtesy of iStockphoto.com/pixeldigits

11 Explain the importance of using products, tools, equipment and techniques to meet the design plan and to suit client's treatment needs, skin types and conditions

12 Describe how treatment can be adapted to suit client treatment needs

13 State the contra-actions that may occur during and following treatments and how to respond

14 Explain the importance of completing the treatment to the satisfaction of the client

15 Explain the importance of completing treatment records

16 Describe the methods of evaluating the effectiveness of the treatment

17 Describe the aftercare advice that should be provided

18 Describe the different skin types and conditions

19 Describe the structure and function of the skin

> *Delicately outline everything you paint with your airbrush. The make-up will stand out tenfold.*

Revision tip

Double-action airbrushes allow for finer control as the flow rate can be controlled by the trigger. This allows for gradual fade effects and blending.

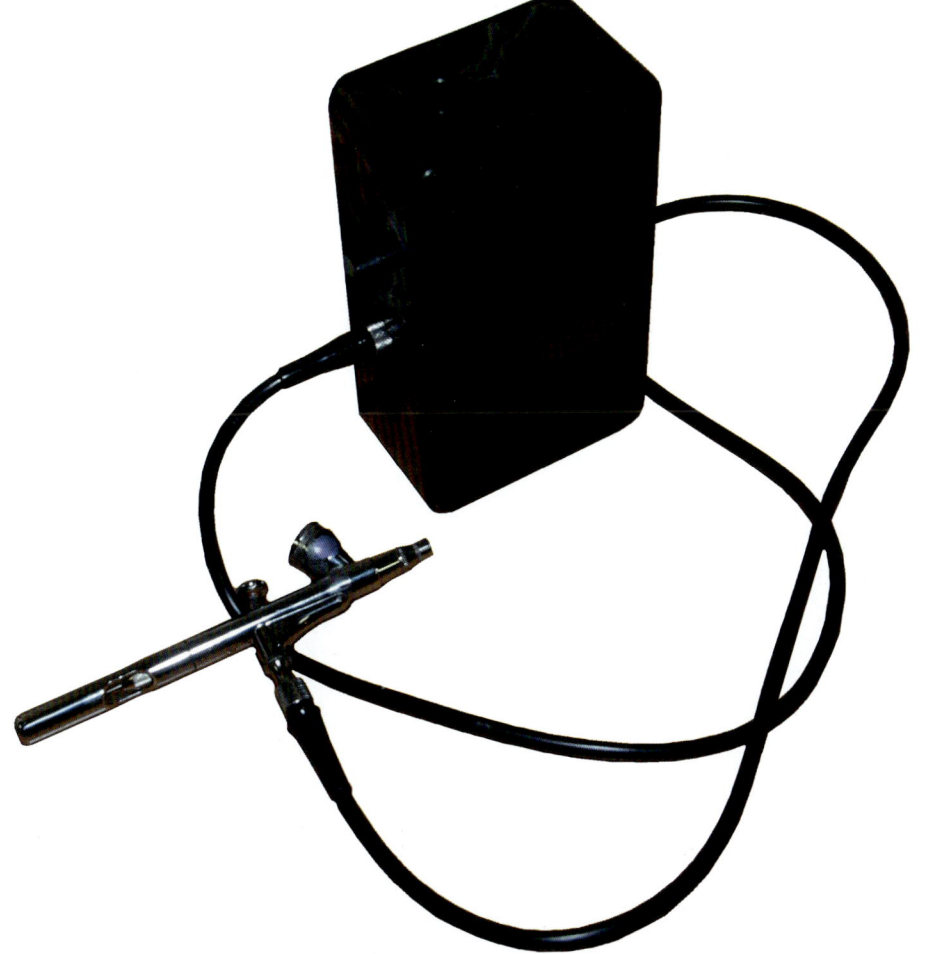

Apply airbrush make-up to the face Unit 327

Airb

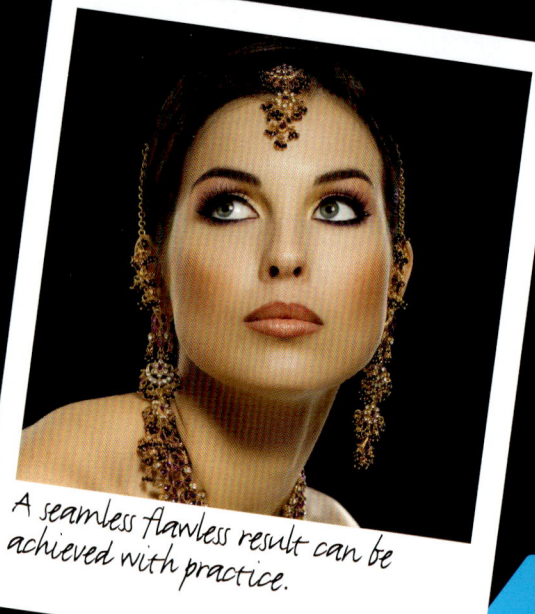

A seamless flawless result can be achieved with practice.

> " Some airbrush foundations can appear very matte. To avoid this apply M·A·C Strobe Liquid to the skin before airbrushing foundation.

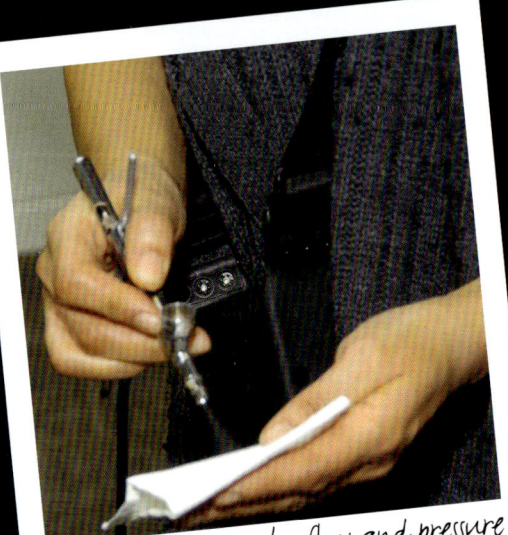

Use tissue to test the flow and pressure through the airbrush.

Use a water-based airbrush foundation for clients with a sensitive skin, as silicone and alcohol content may irritate.

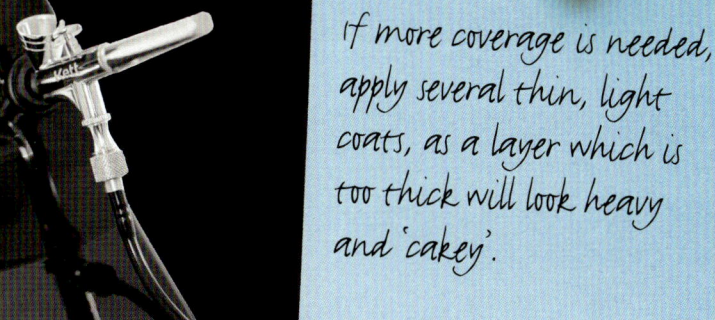

If more coverage is needed, apply several thin, light coats, as a layer which is too thick will look heavy and 'cakey'.

rush

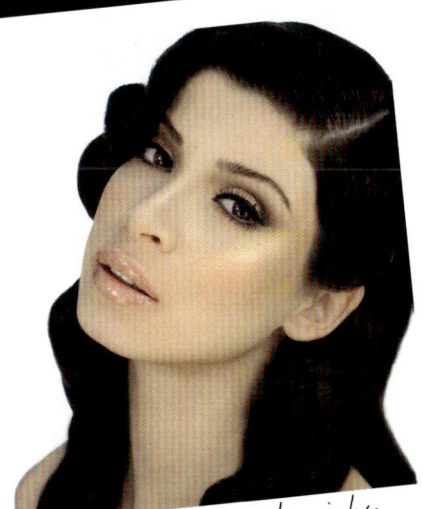

Make sure you choose the right product to suit your client's skin.

Choose the right formulation for your client's skin as digital media can cause an overly matte foundation to look very dry. Similarly, an overly dewy finish can appear greasy or oily in Hi-Def.

What you must do
Practical observations

This page shows what you need to do during your practical task. You can look at it beforehand, but you're **not** allowed to have it with you while carrying out your practical task. You must achieve **all** the criteria; you can achieve 1 mark, 2 marks or 3 marks for the criteria indicated with *.

Conversion chart

Grade	Marks
Pass	11–13
Merit	14–19
Distinction	20–23

○ Please tick when all pre-observation requirements have been met.

	Apply airbrush make-up to the face		
1 Prepare yourself, the client and the work area for airbrush make-up application	1		
2 Use suitable consultation techniques to identify treatment objectives *	1	2	3
3 Carry out a skin analysis *	1	2	3
4 Provide clear recommendations to the client *	1	2	3
5 Position yourself and the client correctly throughout the service	1		
6 Follow health and safety working practices	1		
7 Communicate and behave in a professional manner	1		
8 Select and use products, tools, equipment and techniques to meet design plan and to suit client/model's treatment needs, skin type and conditions *	1	2	3
9 Complete the service to the satisfaction of the client *	1	2	3
10 Record and evaluate the results of the service	1		
11 Provide suitable aftercare advice *	1	2	3
Total			
Grade			
Candidate signature and date			
Assessor signature and date			

What you must do
Practical observations descriptors table

This table shows what you need to do to achieve 1, 2 or 3 marks for the criteria indicated with * on the previous page.

	1 mark	2 marks	3 marks
2 Use suitable consultation techniques to identify treatment objectives	Basic consultation Examples: uses open and closed questions, checks for contra-indications, identifies the service objectives correctly.	Good consultation Examples: positive body language, uses open and closed questions to identify contra-indications, expectations and occasion; identifies the service objectives and any factors that may limit or restrict the service.	Thorough consultation Examples: positive body language, uses open and closed questions to identify contra-indications, expectations and occasion; identifies the service objectives and any factors that may limit or restrict the service, allows the client/model to ask any questions to confirm understanding.
3 Carry out a skin analysis	Skin cleansed, magnifier and light used. Some recording of skin characteristics.	Skin cleansed, magnifier and light used, good observations of skin characteristics recorded.	Skin is cleansed thoroughly, magnifier and light used, detailed observations of skin characteristics recorded.
4 Provide clear recommendations to the client	A basic treatment plan is recommended Example: objectives of the service identified.	A good treatment plan is recommended Examples: objectives of the service identified, taking into account skin type/conditions, and client/model's expectations.	A thorough treatment plan is recommended Examples: objectives of the service identified, taking into account skin type/conditions, client/model's expectations, general health, medication (if any), lifestyle, occasion established, colour preferences and desired look.

Continues on next page

What you must do
Practical observations descriptors table (continued)

This table shows what you need to do to achieve 1, 2 or 3 marks for the criteria indicated with * on page 240.

	1 mark	2 marks	3 marks
8 Select and use products, tools, equipment and techniques to meet design plan and to suit client/model's treatment needs, skin type and conditions	Selects and uses products, tools, equipment and basic techniques to meet the desired objective and the client/model's skin type and condition.	Selects and uses appropriate products, tools, equipment and a range of techniques in a logical sequence with creativity and confidence, to meet the desired objective, the client/model's skin type and condition, and effect required.	Selects and uses appropriate products, tools, equipment and a range of techniques in a logical sequence with creativity and confidence, to meet the desired objective, the client/model's skin type and condition, and effect required, adapts and modifies techniques as necessary and informs the client/model of the changes.
9 Complete the service to the satisfaction of the client	The service is completed within the agreed time, brought to a satisfactory close, and meets the design objectives.	The service is completed within the agreed time, brought to a satisfactory close, and meets the design objectives, the client/model is shown the result and the end result is agreed.	The service is completed within the agreed time, brought to a satisfactory close, and meets the design objectives, make-up applied neatly and blended well, the client/model is shown the result, positive feedback is gained.
11 Provide suitable aftercare advice	Basic aftercare advice is provided including possible contra-actions and how to deal with them.	Good level of aftercare advice is provided including possible contra-actions and how to deal with them, home care products, future services and treatment intervals.	Excellent aftercare advice is provided including possible contra-actions and how to deal with them, home care products, future services and treatment intervals, advice on application and removal techniques.

Comment form
Unit 327 Apply airbrush make-up to the face

This form can be used to record comments by you, your client, or your assessor.

___

___

___

___

___

___

___

Be careful about the prepping products you use before airbrushing make-up, as anything too emollient will affect the wear of the foundation.

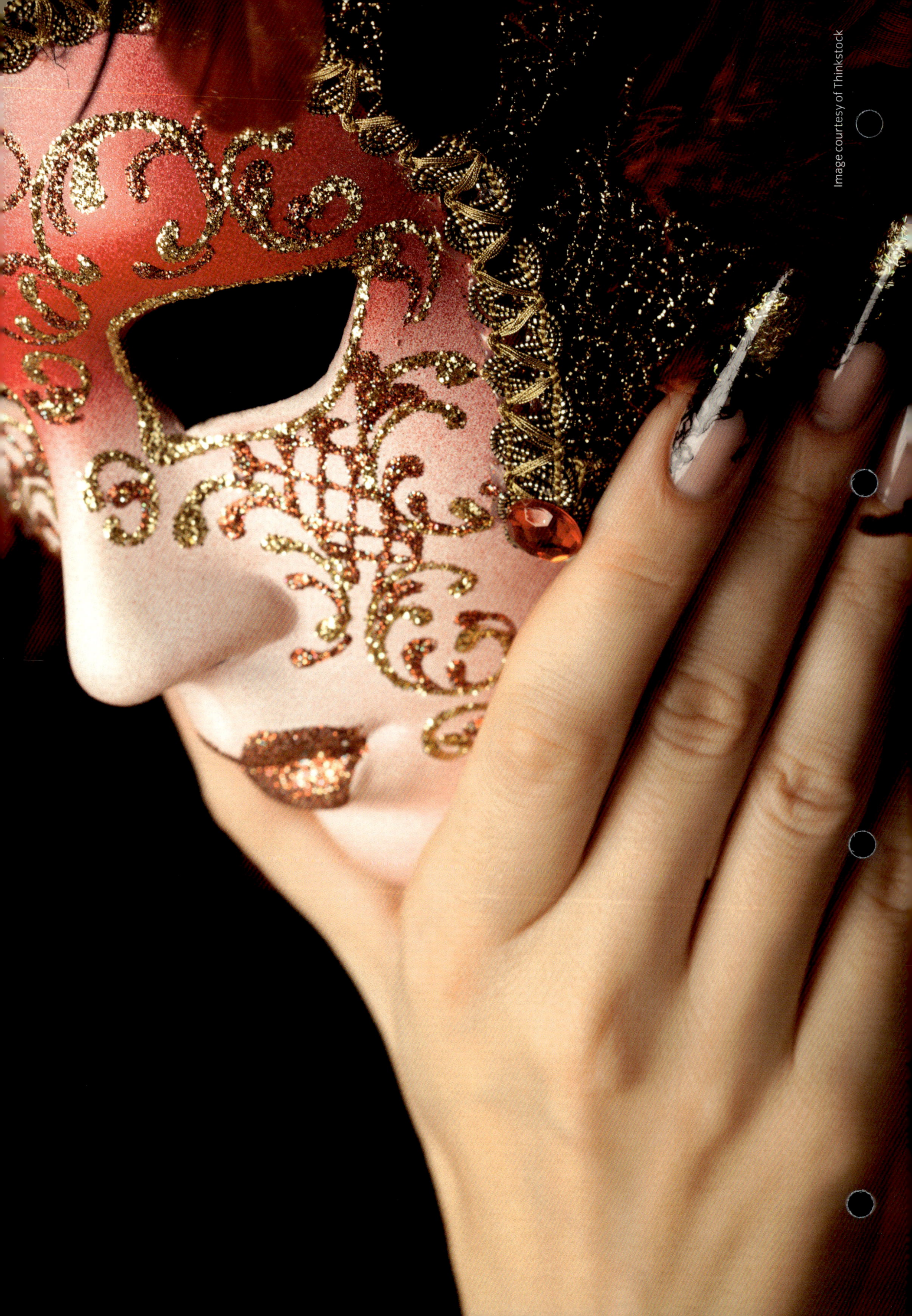

Image courtesy of Thinkstock

328

Airbrush design for the nails

Airbrushing can be used to create many amazing designs on nails using techniques such as freehand, stencilling or creating a colour fade. It is also fantastic for producing perfect French designs which can be completed using a stencil, creating a traditional rounded shape on the free edge or alternative shapes such as Chevron and French designs. You can make your own stencils from paper, lace and frisket. The designs can be easily removed when required and can be completed on natural nails and nail enhancements. It is important to know how to care for your airbrush to gain maximum benefit from it.

Assignment mark sheet
Unit 328 Airbrush design for the nails

Your assessor will mark you on each of the practical tasks in this unit. This page is used to work out your overall grade for the unit. You must pass **all** parts of the tasks to be able to achieve a grade. For the practical task a pass equals 1 point, a merit equals 2 points and a distinction equals 3 points.

What you must know	Tick when complete
Task 1a: produce an information sheet	
Task 1b: produce a fact sheet	
Task 1c: produce a fact sheet	
Task 1d: anatomy and physiology	
Or tick if covered by an online test	

What you must do	Grade	Points
Task 2: Airbrush design for nails		

Overall grade

Candidate name:

Candidate signature: Date:

Assessor signature: Date:

Quality assurance co-ordinator signature (where applicable): Date:

External Verifier signature (where applicable): Date:

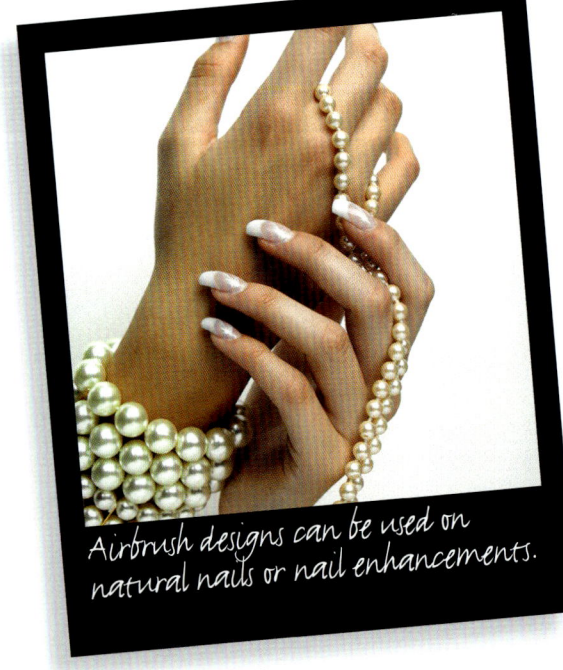

Airbrush designs can be used on natural nails or nail enhancements.

Image courtesy of Sterex

What does it mean?
Some useful words are explained below

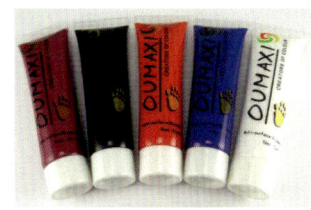

Acrylic-based paints
These contain water but have a high concentration of acrylic and high colour definition.

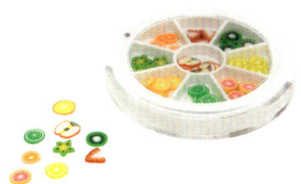

Additional media
Decals/embellishments that may be added to enhance a nail art design (such as feathers, lace, fabric, jewels, etc).

Airbrushing
A method of painted nail art. It uses a compressor and airbrush gun to deliver the paints onto the nail plate.

Avant-garde
This refers to a style used within nail art that is non-commercial. It is often used within the media industry and for competition work.

Colour fade
A technique used in airbrushing that fades two or more complementary colours into each other.

Compressor
The equipment used as the source of air supply when airbrushing nail art.

PSI
Pounds per square inch – this relates to the amount of air pressure expended from the airbrush compressor.

Stencil
A plastic type sheet which has pre-cut shapes within it that are used to create shapes when airbrushing.

Water-based paints
These contain acrylic for colour but have a high water content so the colour definition is not as strong; good for beginners.

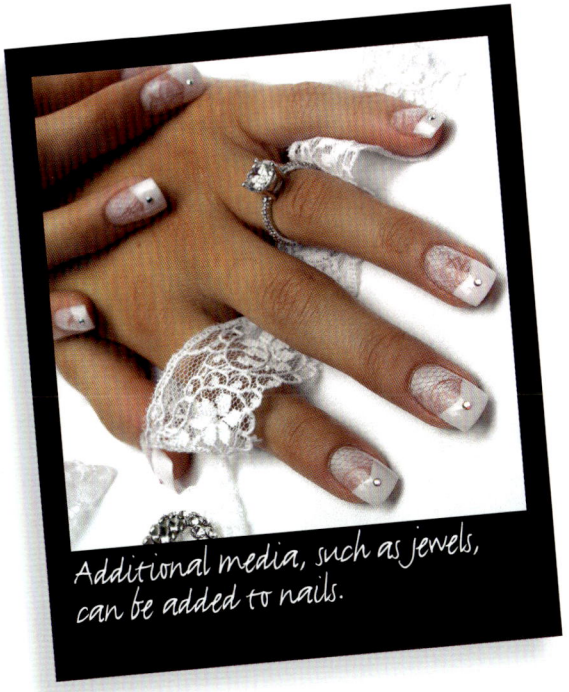

Additional media, such as jewels, can be added to nails.

> **Revision tip**
>
> Don't work too close to the nail when airbrushing as this can spoil the design by splattering the paint.

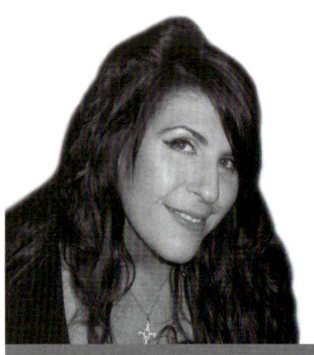

Follow in the footsteps of... *Beverley Braisdell*

Beverley studied her City & Guilds qualification in Hairdressing, Beauty Therapy, Theatrical and Media Make-up, and Holistic Therapies at Wigan and Leigh College. Beverley's passions are nails and make-up: she has worked as an educator delivering nails and make-up training in Athens, Greece, where she also judged a national nails competition. She has also worked as a make-up artist on films using special effects make-up. Beverley is currently a full-time lecturer at Wigan and Leigh College. She is also on the Habia nail services forum. Read on for Beverley's fantastic airbrushing nails quotes!

What you must know
You must be able to:

1. Explain the importance of developing nail art design plans
2. Describe salon requirements for preparing themselves, the client and work area
3. Describe the environmental conditions suitable for airbrush nail treatment
4. Describe the different consultation techniques used to identify treatment objective
5. Explain the importance of carrying out a detailed nail and skin analysis
6. Describe how to select products, tools and equipment to suit client treatment needs, skin and nail conditions
7. Explain the contra-indications that prevent or restrict airbrush nail treatment
8. Explain how to communicate and behave in a professional manner
9. Describe health and safety working practices
10. Explain the importance of positioning themselves and the client correctly throughout the treatment

Continues on next page

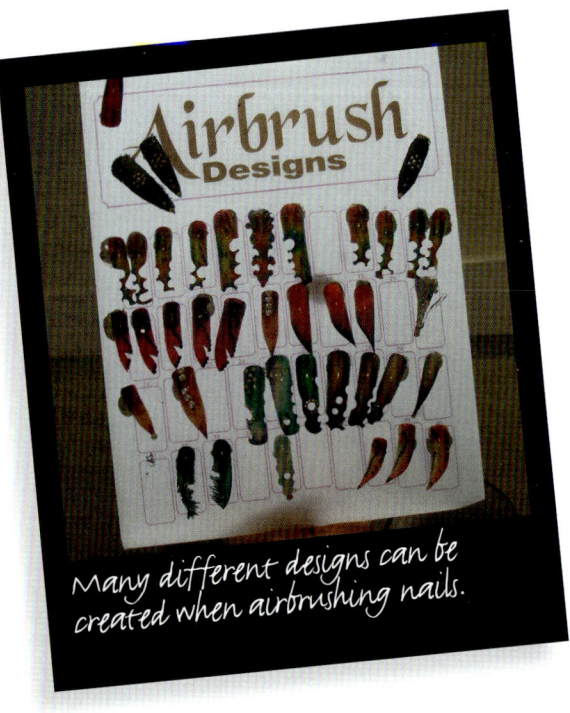

Many different designs can be created when airbrushing nails.

11 Explain the importance of using products, tools, equipment and techniques to meet design plan and to suit client's treatment needs, nail and skin conditions

12 Describe how treatment can be adapted to suit client treatment needs

13 State the contra-actions that may occur during and following treatments and how to respond

14 Explain the importance of completing the treatment to the satisfaction of the client

15 Explain the importance of completing treatment records

16 Describe the methods of evaluating the effectiveness of the treatment

17 Describe the aftercare advice that should be provided

18 Describe the structure and function of the nail and skin

19 Describe the different skin types and conditions

20 Describe the different natural nail shapes

Revision tip

Base coating the enhancements or natural nail plate prior to application of the airbrush design will help it to last longer. When the design is completed, apply topcoat to seal it, bring out the depth of colour and add shine.

> *You can gain maximum benefit from your airbrush compressor by using it for both nail art and make-up work.*

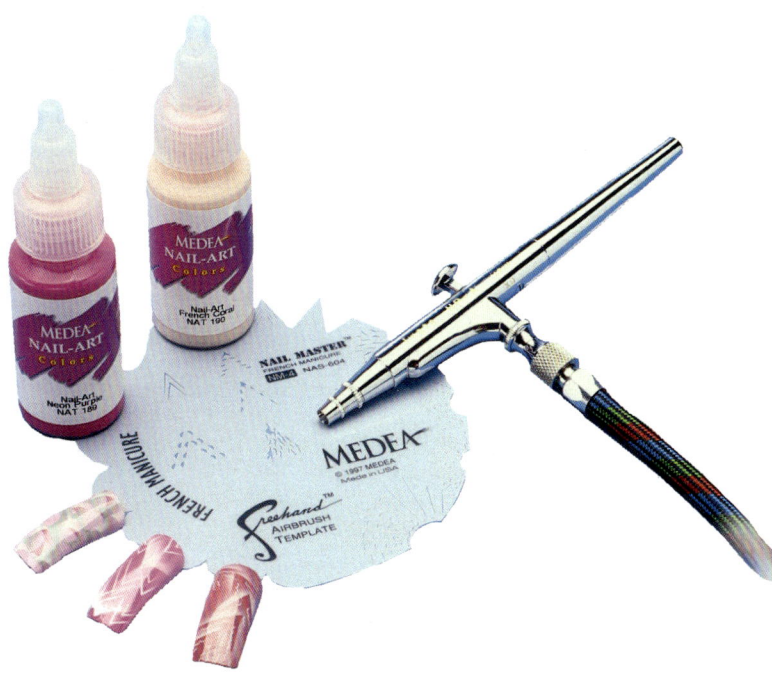

Image courtesy of The Airbrush Co Ltd.

Airbrush design for the nails Unit 328 249

Airbrush is fantastic for creating perfect French polish results. Alternative French polish shapes such as a chevron and fancy French designs can also be applied.

> **Colour fading is a fabulous effect that can easily be achieved with your airbrush.**

Airbru

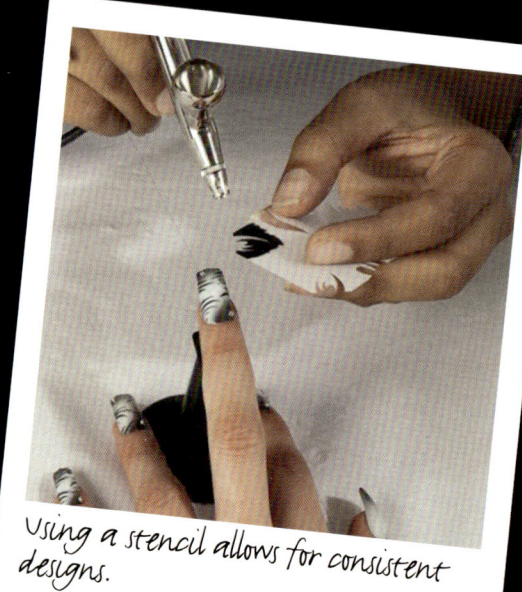

Using a stencil allows for consistent designs.

If the paint is wet as it hits the nail, try positioning the airbrush gun further away or, if using a dual action airbrush gun, pull back gently on the trigger to release less paint.

Image courtesy of Sterex

sh nails

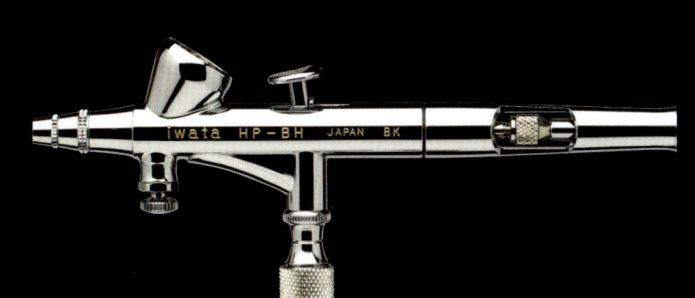

Image courtesy of The Airbrush Co Ltd.

Have your compressor serviced yearly to keep it in good working order.

Ensure that you thoroughly clean the airbrush gun at the end of each working day by stripping it down to remove any residue of paint.

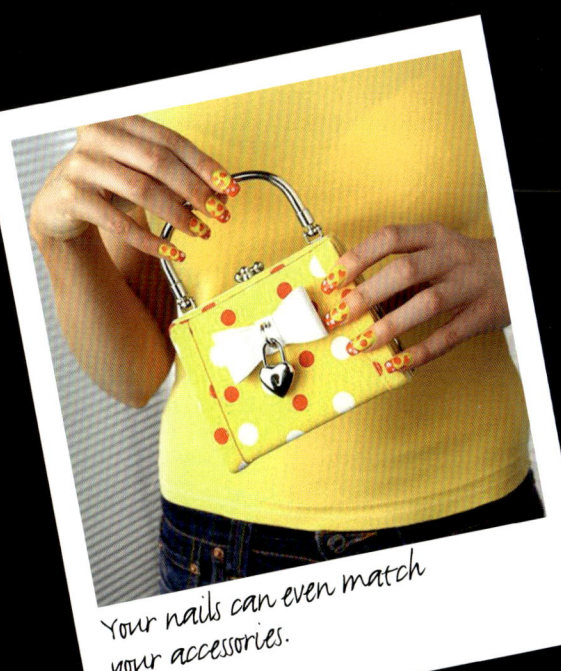

Your nails can even match your accessories.

Image courtesy of Sterex

What you must do
Practical observations

This page shows what you need to do during your practical task. You can look at it beforehand, but you're **not** allowed to have it with you while carrying out your practical task. You must achieve **all** the criteria; you can achieve 1 mark, 2 marks or 3 marks for the criteria indicated with *.

Conversion chart

Grade	Marks
Pass	10–12
Merit	13–17
Distinction	18–20

○ Please tick when all pre-observation requirements have been met.

	Airbrush design for nails		
1 Prepare yourself, the client and the work area for airbrush design for nails	1		
2 Use suitable consultation techniques to identify treatment objectives *	1	2	3
3 Carry out a nail and skin analysis	1		
4 Provide clear recommendations to the client *	1	2	3
5 Follow health and safety working practices	1		
6 Communicate and behave in a professional manner	1		
7 Select and use products, tools, equipment and techniques to suit client's treatment needs, skin and nail conditions *	1	2	3
8 Complete the treatment to the satisfaction of the client *	1	2	3
9 Record and evaluate the results of the treatment	1		
10 Provide suitable aftercare advice *	1	2	3
Total			
Grade			
Candidate signature and date			
Assessor signature and date			

What you must do
Practical observations descriptors table

This table shows what you need to do to achieve 1, 2 or 3 marks for the criteria indicated with * on the previous page.

	1 mark	2 marks	3 marks
2 Use suitable consultation techniques to identify service objectives	Basic consultation carried out Examples: closed questions used throughout, questioning covered contra-indications.	Good consultation carried out Examples: open and closed questions, positive body language, questioning covered contra-indications, general health, lifestyle and expectations.	Thorough consultation carried out Examples: open questions, effective use of body language, questioning covered contra-indications, general health, lifestyle and expectations. Candidate is able to accurately identify any treatment modification where necessary based on the nail and skin analysis.
4 Provide clear recommendations to the client	A basic treatment plan is recommended Examples: Contra-indications and objectives of the treatment identified.	A good treatment plan is recommended Examples: contra-indications and objectives of the treatment, taking into account condition of the nail, client lifestyle and expectations.	A thorough treatment plan is recommended Examples: objectives of the treatment identified, taking into account skin and nail conditions, general health, client lifestyle, expectations, contra-indications and treatment modifications.

Continues on next page

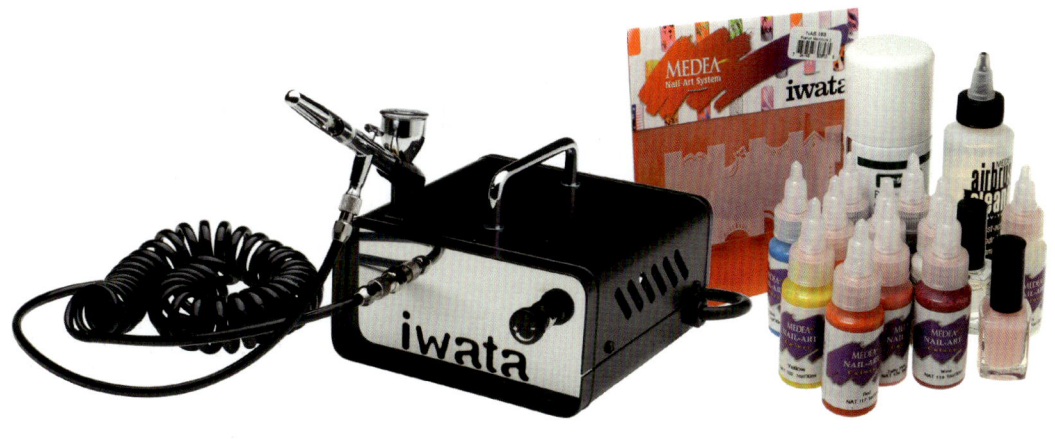

Image courtesy of The Airbrush Co Ltd.

Airbrush design for the nails Unit 328 253

What you must do
Practical observations descriptors table (continued)

This table shows what you need to do to achieve 1, 2 or 3 marks for the criteria indicated with * on page 252.

	1 mark	2 marks	3 marks
7 Select and use products, tools, equipment and techniques to suit client's treatment needs, skin and nail conditions	Correctly selects products, tools, equipment and PSI. Ensures relevant safety tests are carried out. Carries out the service correctly according to skin and nail condition, treatment objectives and client requirements. Design consistent on all nails.	Correctly selects products, tools, equipment and PSI. Ensures relevant safety tests are carried out. Carries out the service in a logical sequence with creativity and confidence according to skin and nail condition, treatment objectives and client requirements. Stencil is well positioned with good symmetry. Nail design is balanced and consistent on all nails.	Correctly selects products, tools, equipment and PSI. Ensures relevant safety tests are carried out. Carries out the service in a logical sequence with creativity and confidence according to skin and nail condition, treatment objectives and client requirements. Stencil is well positioned with good symmetry. Nail design is balanced and consistent on all nails, detail is well blended and clearly defined.
8 Complete the service to the satisfaction of the client	The treatment is completed within the agreed time, meets the design objectives. Cleans the surrounding skin to ensure any over-sprayed paint has been removed.	The treatment is completed within the agreed time, meets the design objectives. Cleans the surrounding skin to ensure any over-sprayed paint has been removed. The client is shown the result and the end result is agreed.	The treatment is completed within the agreed time, meets the design objectives. Cleans the surrounding skin to ensure any over-sprayed paint has been removed. The client is shown the result and the end result is agreed. Positive feedback is gained.

Continues on next page

	1 mark	2 marks	3 marks
10 Provide suitable aftercare advice	Basic aftercare advice is provided including possible contra-actions and how to deal with them.	Good level of aftercare advice including possible contra-actions and how to deal with them, home care products, removal of art work and further services.	Excellent aftercare advice to including possible contra-actions and how to deal with them, home care products, removal of art work, advice to prolong art work in between appointments as appropriate, further treatments/rebooking.

> *Be careful when positioning your stencil – your designs must be symmetrical.*

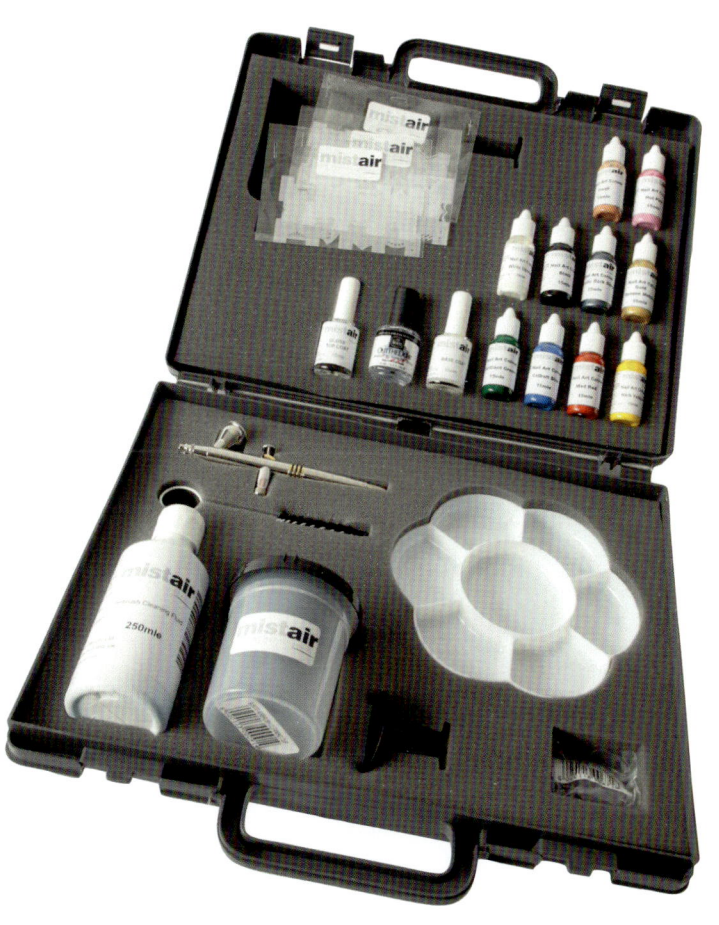

Image courtesy of Sterex

Airbrush design for the nails Unit 328

Comment form
Unit 328 Airbrush design for the nails

This form can be used to record comments by you, your client, or your assessor.

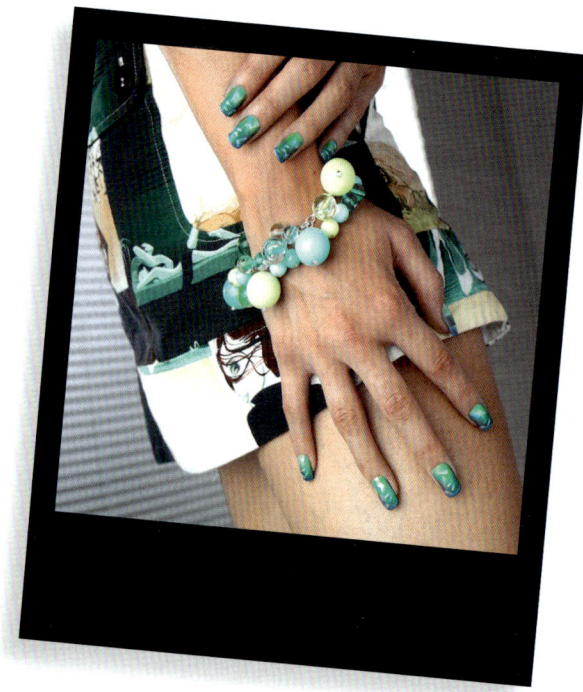

The airbrush paint should be dry as it hits the nail. If it isn't, check you're not spraying too close to the nail.

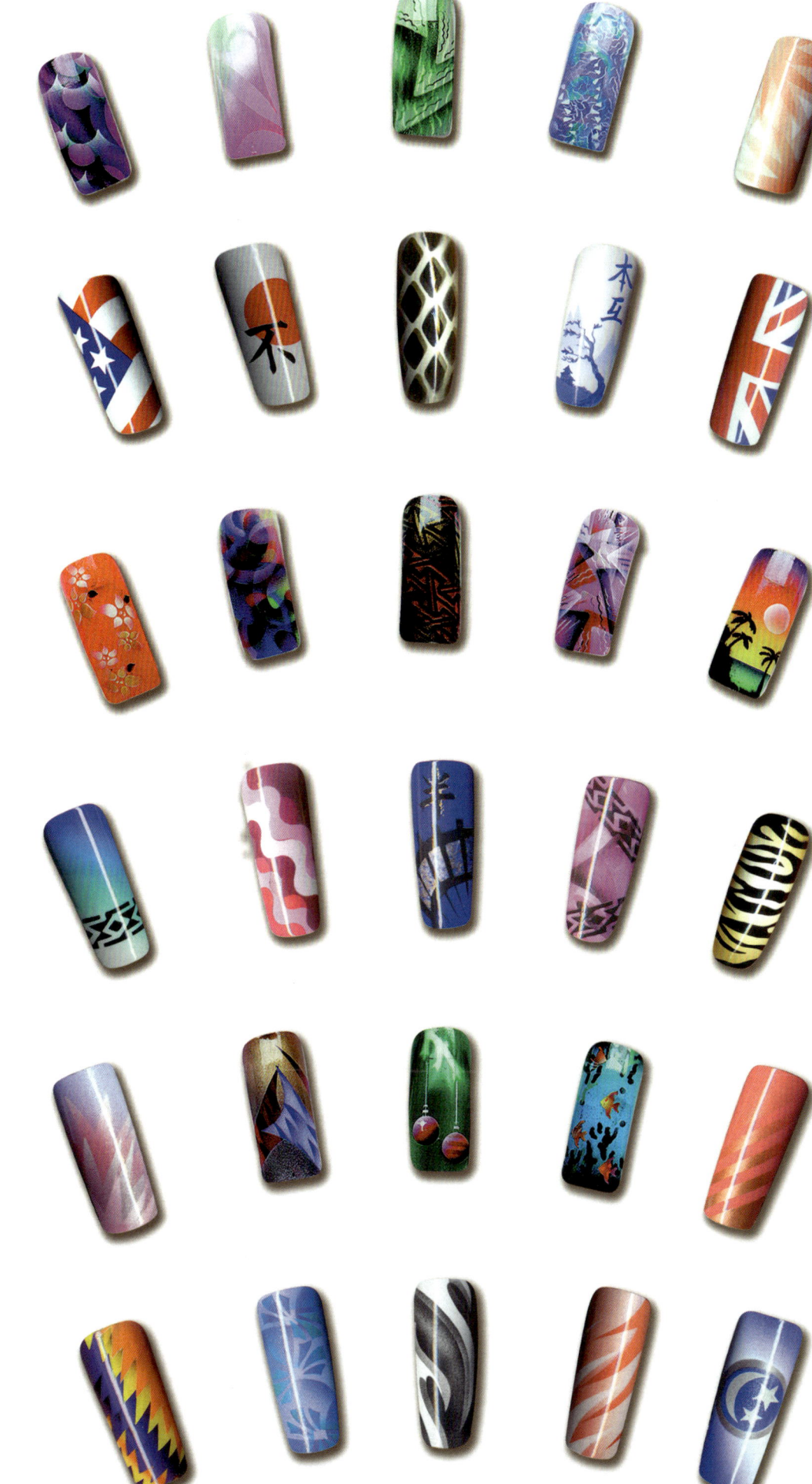

Image courtesy of The Airbrush Co. Ltd.

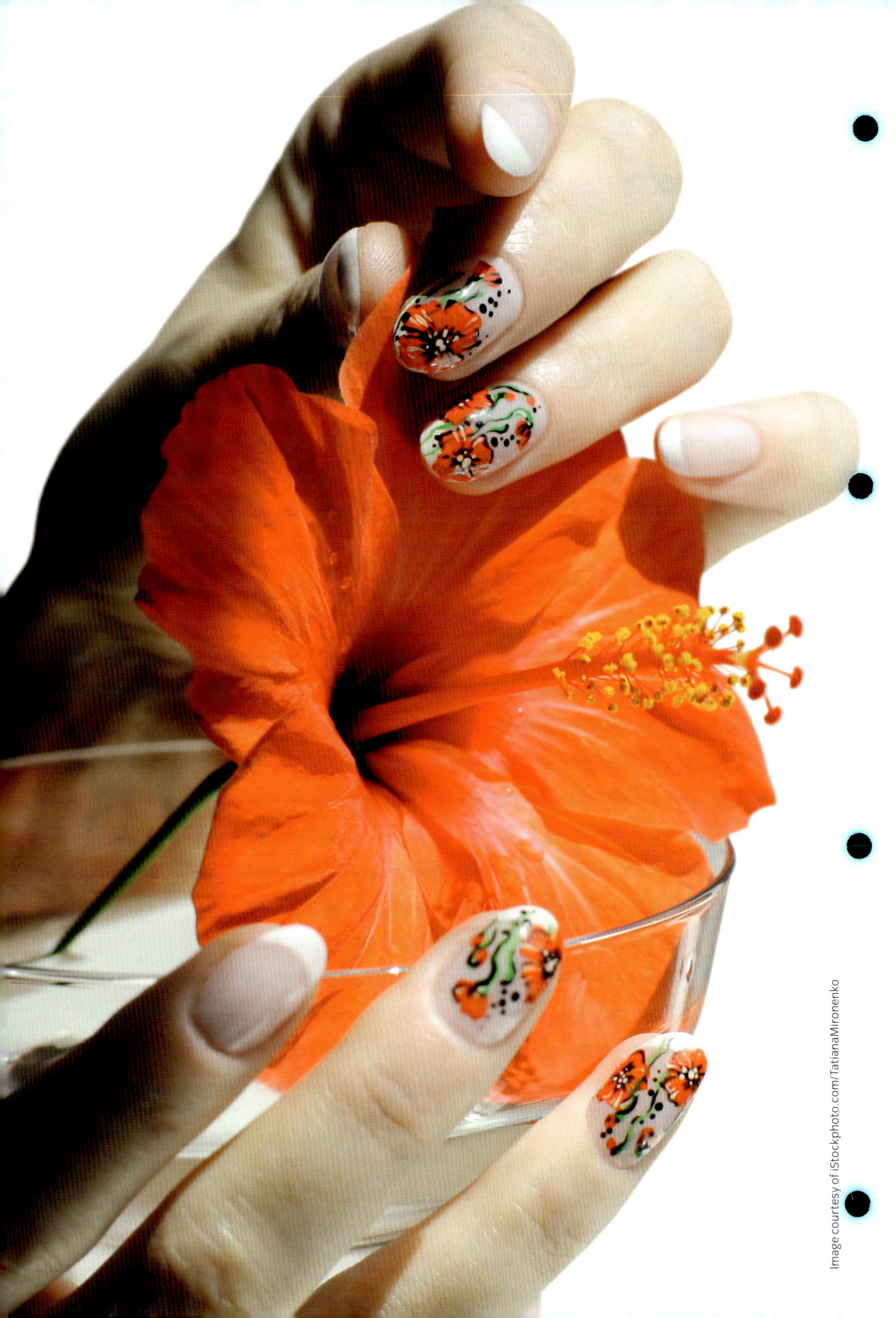

329

Design and apply nail art

This is a fabulous add-on service to offer, as personalising a design to suit your client's needs will keep them coming back to you time after time. Nail art can be created on the fingers and toes and can also be encased within the nail extension overlay. Glitters, crushed shells, gems, decals and dried flowers are a few examples of what can be embedded within the nail enhancement. As always it is very important to follow the manufacturer's instructions when using nail art products.

Assignment mark sheet
Unit 329 Design and apply nail art

Your assessor will mark you on each of the practical tasks in this unit. This page is used to work out your overall grade for the unit. You must pass **all** parts of the tasks to be able to achieve a grade. For the practical task a pass equals 1 point, a merit equals 2 points and a distinction equals 3 points.

What you must know	Tick when complete
Task 1a: produce an information sheet	
Task 1b: produce a fact sheet	
Task 1c: produce a fact sheet	
Task 1d: anatomy and physiology	
Or tick if covered by an online test	

What you must do	Grade	Points
Task 2: Nail art		
	Overall grade	

Candidate name:

Candidate signature: Date:

Assessor signature: Date:

Quality assurance co-ordinator signature (where applicable):   Date:

External Verifier signature (where applicable):   Date:

What does it mean?
Some useful words are explained below

3D
Nail art designs that are usually created using liquid and powder and which stand out from the nail plate.

Aftercare advice
The professional advice a client should follow after the treatment.

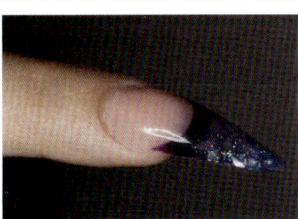

Cut out
A nail art technique that could involve an alternative tip shape such as the stiletto shape that have been cut away into the tip.

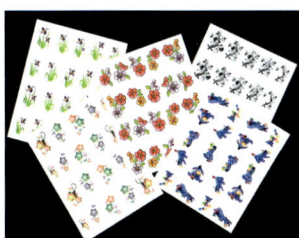

Decal
A transfer picture applied to the nail.

Embedding
A nail art technique that encases nail art designs within the overlay, making it more permanent.

Hooked/claw nail
A natural nail plate that curves downwards at the free edge.

Marbling
This technique involves swirling two or more colours together and can be done with paints, coloured gel or liquid and powder.

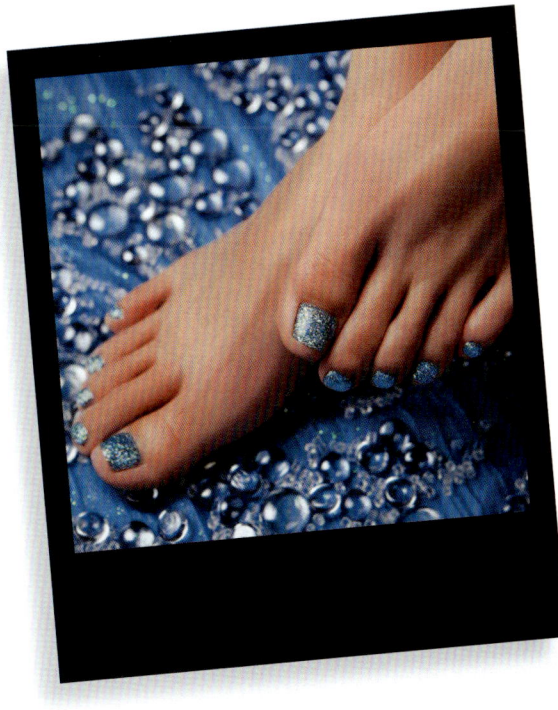

> **Revision tip**
> Precision is the key to perfect nail art, practice makes perfect.

What you must know
You must be able to:

1. Explain the importance of developing nail art design plans
2. Describe salon requirements for preparing themselves, the client and work area
3. Describe the environmental conditions suitable for nail art
4. Describe the different consultation techniques used to identify service objectives
5. Explain the importance of carrying out a nail and skin analysis
6. Describe how to select products, tools and equipment to suit client service needs, nail and skin conditions
7. Explain the contra-indications that prevent or restrict nail art
8. Explain how to communicate and behave in a professional manner
9. Describe health and safety working practices
10. Explain the importance of positioning themselves and the client correctly throughout the service

Continues on next page

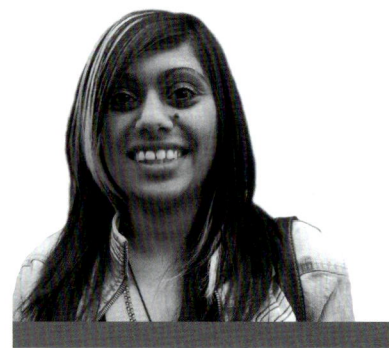

Follow in the footsteps of... *Bindu Patel*

Bindu is a former student of Wigan and Leigh College where she studied Hairdressing and Nail Services at Levels two and three. It was obvious from the beginning of her nail course that she was a very talented nail artist. She won a silver award in the national final UK Skills nail art competition and second place in the AHT national student nail art competition. Now she travels the world on board a cruise ship as a nail technician.

Read on for Bindu's fantastic tips!

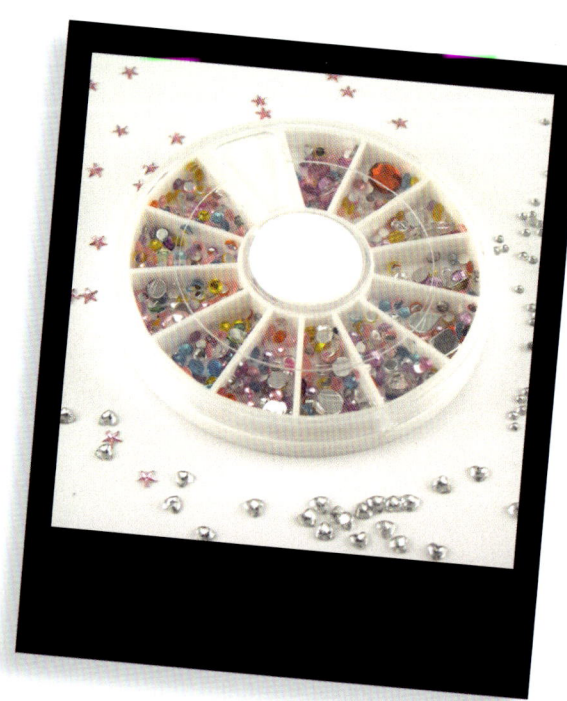

Image courtesy of Nail Delights (www.naildelights.com)

11 Explain the importance of using products, tools, equipment and techniques to meet design plan and to suit client's service needs, nail and skin conditions

12 Describe how the service can be adapted to suit client needs

13 State the contra-actions that may occur during and following services and how to respond

14 Explain the importance of completing the service to the satisfaction of the client

15 Explain the importance of completing service records

16 Describe the methods of evaluating the effectiveness of the service

17 Describe the aftercare advice that should be provided

18 Describe the structure and functions of the nail and skin

19 Describe the different skin and nail conditions

20 Describe the different natural nail shapes

> *Experiment with colours, glitters and paints to make your nail art service really individual.*

Revision tip

During the consultation, find out the client's occupation and any hobbies, as well as what occasion the nail art is to be worn for. This will ensure that the design will be appropriate.

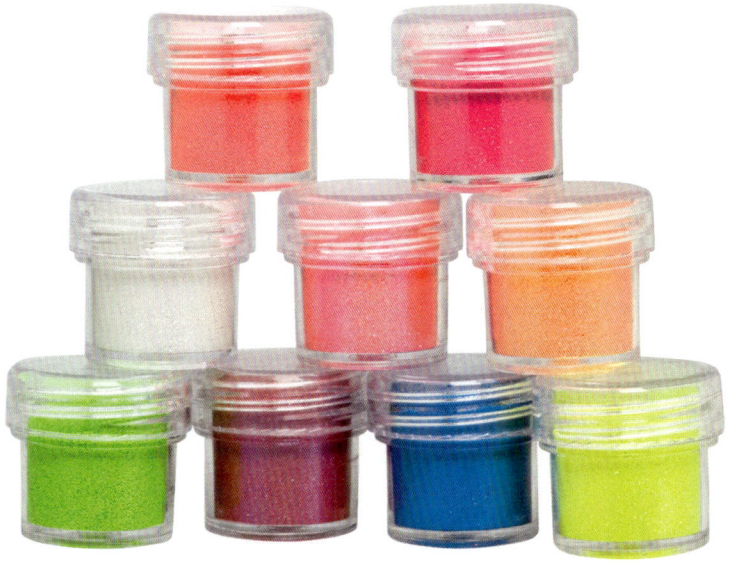

Image courtesy of NSI (UK) Ltd. (www.nsinails.co.uk).

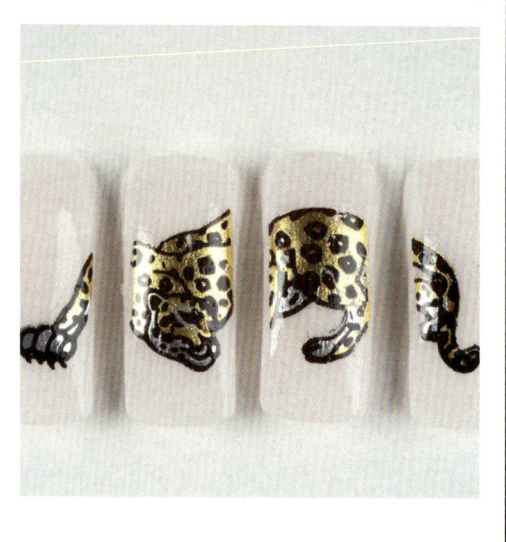

> You can add depth to your nail art designs by applying 3D painting techniques with an airbrush.

Image courtesy of Derby College

Design

Embedding nail art within the nail enhancements allows it to be worn until it is either removed or reapplied during the maintenance service.

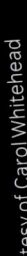

Image courtesy of Carol Whitehead

nail art

Coloured liquid and powder mixed with glitter can create a fantastic alternative to the French option without adding on any extra service time.

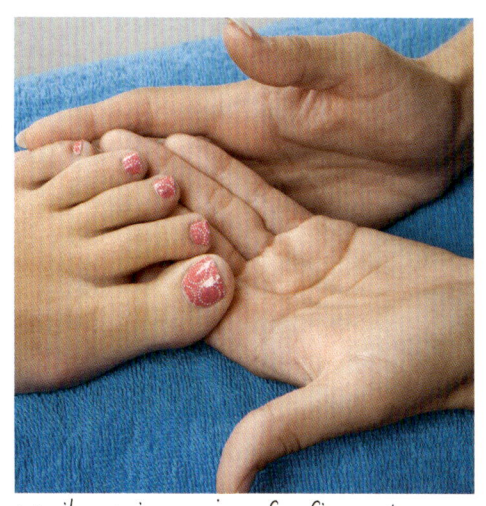

Nail art is not just for fingers!

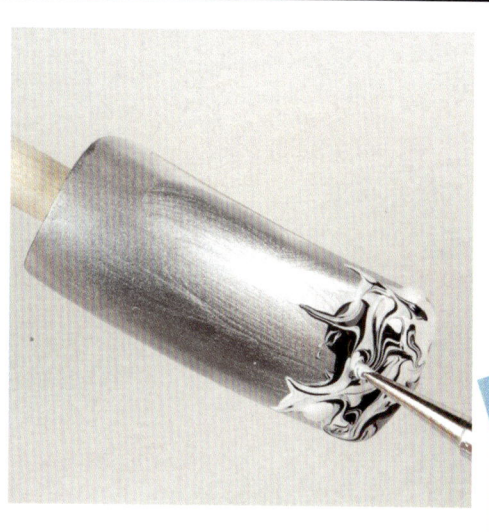

Nail art is a fantastic add-on service that can bring in extra revenue.

What you must do
Practical observations

This page shows what you need to do during your practical task. You can look at it beforehand, but you're **not** allowed to have it with you while carrying out your practical task. You must achieve **all** the criteria; you can achieve 1 mark, 2 marks or 3 marks for the criteria indicated with *.

Conversion chart

Grade	Marks
Pass	11–13
Merit	14–18
Distinction	19–21

○ Please tick when all pre-observation requirements have been met.

	Nail art		
1 Prepare yourself, the client and the work area for nail art	1		
2 Use suitable consultation techniques to identify service objectives *	1	2	3
3 Carry out a nail and skin analysis	1		
4 Provide clear recommendations to the client *	1	2	3
5 Follow health and safety working practices	1		
6 Communicate and behave in a professional manner	1		
7 Position yourself and the client correctly throughout the service	1		
8 Select and use products, tools, equipment and techniques to meet the design plan, suit client's service needs, and nail and skin conditions *	1	2	3
9 Complete the treatment to the satisfaction of the client *	1	2	3
10 Record and evaluate the results of the treatment	1		
11 Provide suitable aftercare advice *	1	2	3

Total

Grade

Candidate signature and date

Assessor signature and date

What you must do
Practical observations descriptors table

This table shows what you need to do to achieve 1, 2 or 3 marks for the criteria indicated with * on the previous page.

	1 mark	2 marks	3 marks
2 Use suitable consultation techniques to identify service objectives	Basic consultation Examples: uses open and closed questions, checks for contra-indications, identifies the service objectives correctly.	Good consultation Examples: positive body language, uses open and closed questions to identify contra-indications, expectations and occasion; identifies the service objectives and any factors that may limit or restrict the service.	Thorough consultation Examples: positive body language, uses open and closed questions to identify contra-indications, expectations and occasion; identifies the service objectives and any factors that may limit or restrict the service, allows the client to ask any questions to confirm understanding.
4 Provide clear recommendations to the client	A basic treatment plan is recommended Examples: explains service procedure and any adaptations to meet the client's service needs, equipment to be used.	A good treatment plan is recommended Examples: explains service procedure and any adaptations to meet the client's service needs, equipment to be used based on factors identified during consultation (lifestyle, natural nail shape, client wishes, results of skin and nail analysis, contra-indications), a choice of products to be used.	A thorough treatment plan is recommended Examples: explains service procedure and any adaptations to meet the client's service needs, equipment to be used based on factors identified during consultation (lifestyle, natural nail shape, client wishes, results of skin and nail analysis, contra-indications), explains effects and benefits of the type of products/techniques used and the adaptation/modification to suit client service needs, allows the client to ask questions about the treatment plan.

Continues on next page

What you must do
Practical observations descriptors table (continued)

This table shows what you need to do to achieve 1, 2 or 3 marks for the criteria indicated with * on page 266.

	1 mark	2 marks	3 marks
8 Select and use products, tools, equipment and techniques to meet the design plan, suit client's service needs, and nail and skin conditions	Selects and uses correct products, tools and equipment, taking into account the client's service needs, nail and skin conditions, all excess nail products are removed from the surrounding skin. The design meets the design plan. Nail design is consistent on all nails.	Selects and uses correct products, tools and equipment, taking into account the client's service needs, nail and skin conditions, all excess nail products are removed from the surrounding skin. The design meets the design plan. Nail design is balanced and consistent on all nails. Communicates with the client throughout to confirm satisfaction.	Selects and uses correct products, tools and equipment, taking into account the client's service needs, nail and skin conditions, all excess nail products are removed from the surrounding skin. The design meets the design plan. Nail design is balanced and consistent on all nails, well blended or clearly defined detail. Communicates with the client throughout to confirm satisfaction.
9 Complete the service to the satisfaction of the client	The service is completed within the agreed time and brought to a satisfactory close, the design meets the objectives.	The service is completed within the agreed time and brought to a satisfactory close, the design meets the objectives, the client is shown the result and the end result is agreed.	The service is completed within the agreed time and brought to a satisfactory close, the design meets the objectives, the client is shown the result, positive feedback is gained from the client.

Continues on next page

	1 mark	2 marks	3 marks
11 Provide suitable aftercare advice	Basic aftercare advice Examples: how to deal with possible contra-actions, product(s) to use, future service needs.	Good level of aftercare advice Examples: how to deal with possible contra-actions, product(s) to use, specific advice (ie what to avoid immediately after the service, lifestyle), future service needs.	Excellent aftercare advice Examples: how to deal with possible contra-actions, product(s) to use, specific advice (ie what to avoid immediately after the service, lifestyle), recommends future service programme (maintenance and removal, introduction of new/alternative services/treatments).

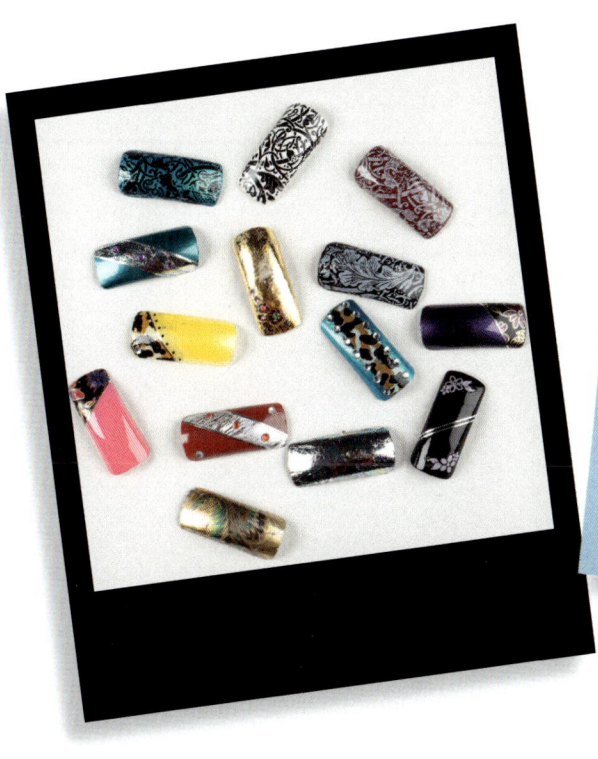

There are many wonderful nail art products available on the market, eg coloured glitters, crushed shells, dried flowers, polish secures and decals.

Design and apply nail art Unit 329

Comment form
Unit 329 Design and apply nail art

This form can be used to record comments by you, your client, or your assessor.

Applying a top-glossing/finishing gel over the top of the nail art design will bring out the colour and beauty of the design.

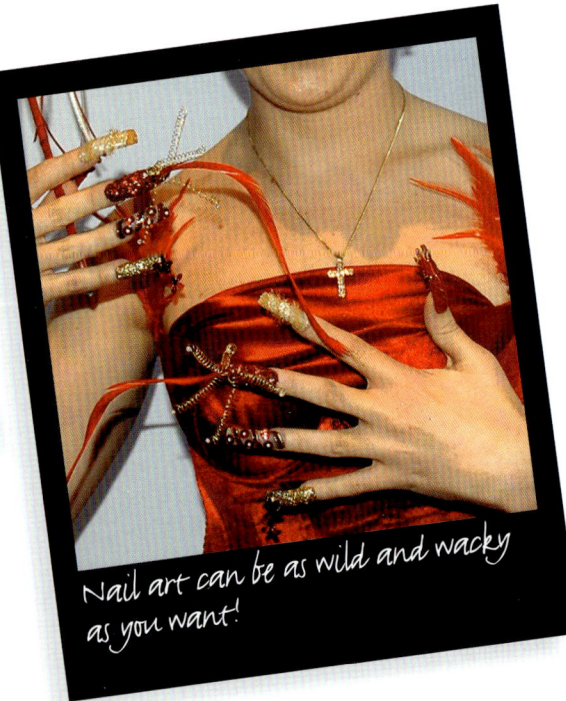

Nail art can be as wild and wacky as you want!

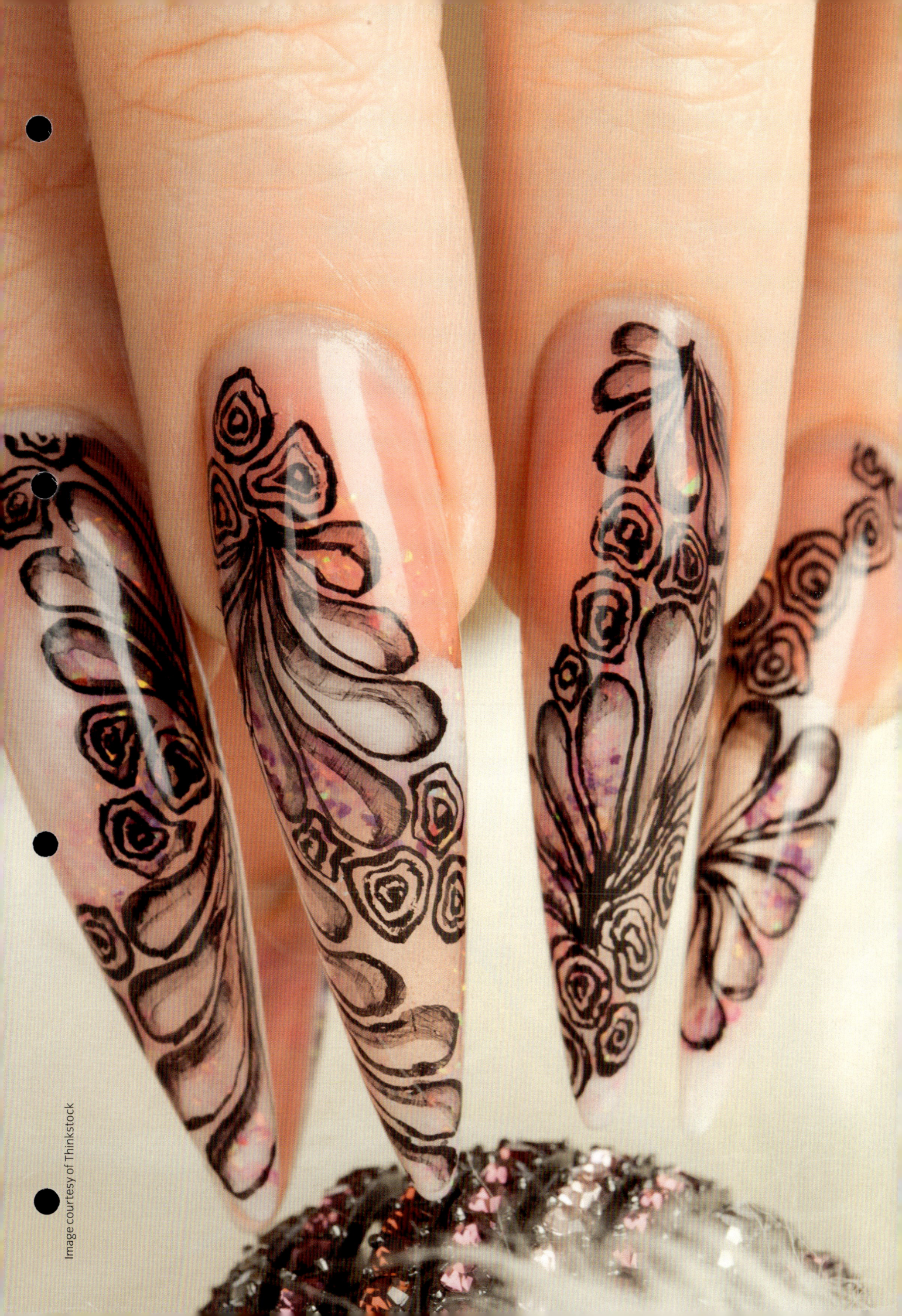

Image courtesy of Thinkstock

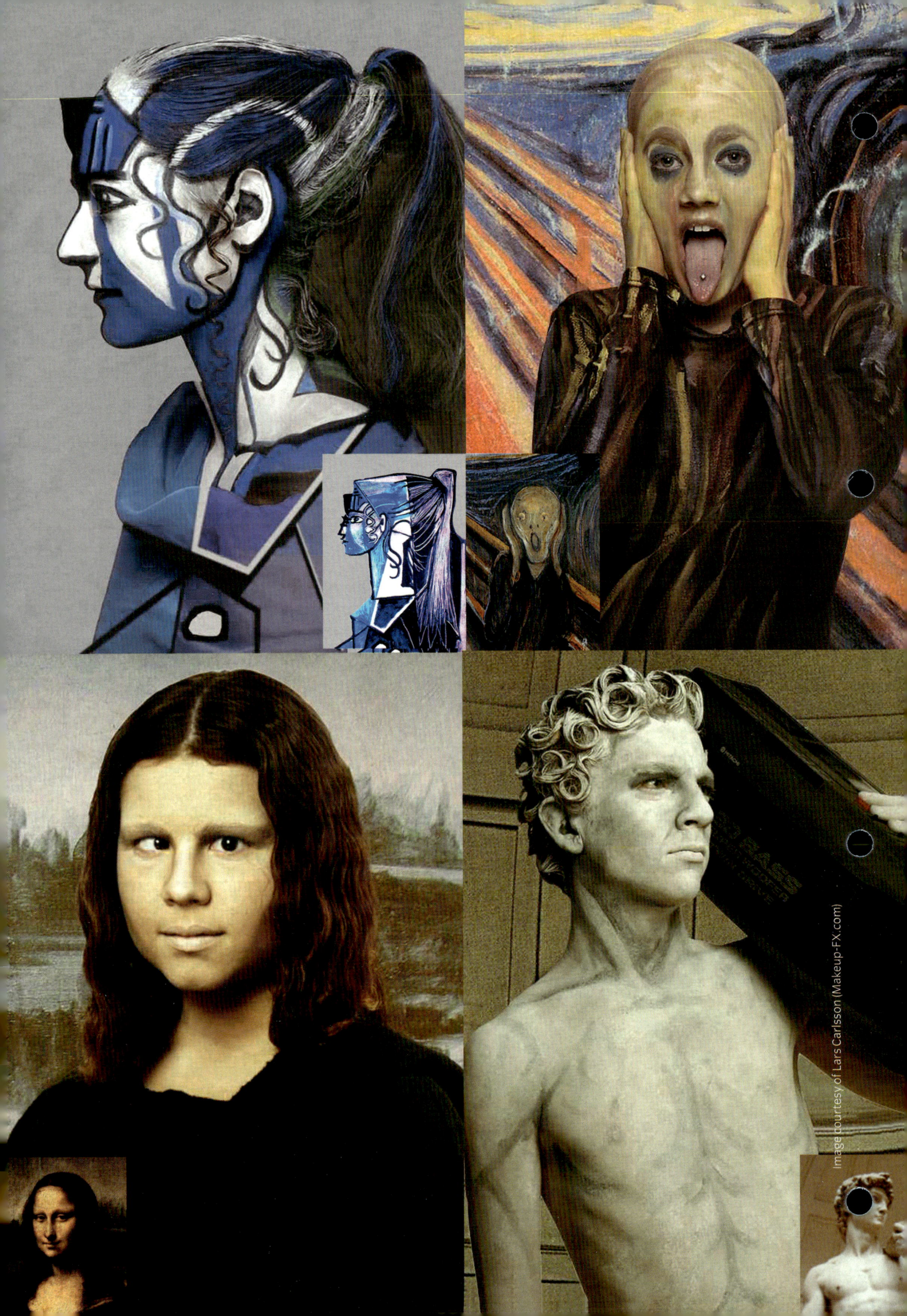

330

Media make-up

This unit covers the creation of 'casualty' type effects, including scars, burns and bruising. You will learn how to apply highlighting and shading techniques, along with other illusions, in order to effectively 'age' a performer. The application and seamless blending of small prosthetic pieces is also covered. In order to carry out this type of work successfully, careful research and development of ideas are important. Ways of accurately recording the process and the effectiveness of the end result will also need to be learned and followed.

Assignment mark sheet
Unit 330 Media make-up

Your assessor will mark you on each of the practical tasks in this unit. This page is used to work out your overall grade for the unit. You must pass **all** parts of the tasks to be able to achieve a grade. For the practical task a pass equals 1 point, a merit equals 2 points and a distinction equals 3 points.

What you must know	Tick when complete
Task 1a: produce an information sheet	
Task 1b: produce a chart	
Task 1c: produce a report	
Task 1d: produce a fact sheet	
Task 1e: produce a fact sheet	
Or tick if covered by an online test	

What you must do	Grade	Points
Task 2: Media make-up		

Overall grade

Candidate name:

Candidate signature: Date:

Assessor signature: Date:

Quality assurance co-ordinator signature   Date:
(where applicable):

External Verifier signature   Date:
(where applicable):

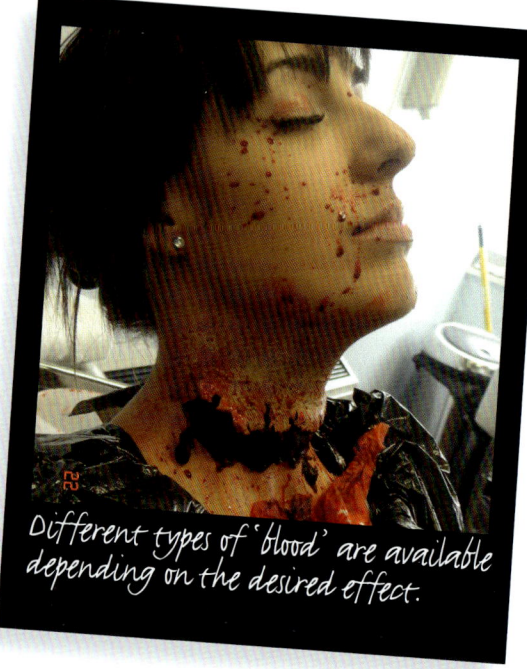

Different types of 'blood' are available depending on the desired effect.

Image courtesy of Jenni Lenard

What does it mean?
Some useful words are explained below

Adverse skin reactions
A response of the skin to a product such as irritation, itching, redness or swelling.

Character make-up
Changing a subject's physical appearance to suit the requirements of a script or part to be played. This may include changes in age, emphasis of particular facial features and so on.

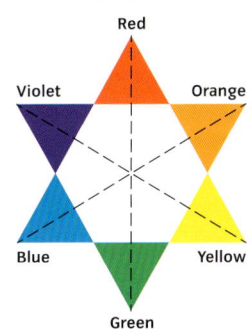

Colour wheel
A visual representation of colours arranged into a circle or wheel that shows relationships between primary, secondary and complementary colours, etc.

Compatibility tests
A small amount of product is applied to the skin and left on for 24 hours to check that the client is unlikely to react unfavourably.

Contra-indication
A condition which restricts or prevents the service from taking place.

Dilated capillaries
Tiny red, dilated blood vessels visible on the surface of the skin, often used when creating the ageing of a character.

Environmental factors
The conditions affecting the area you are working in, such as how it is lit, its temperature and the amount of ventilation.

Influencing factors
Issues, aspects or reasons for designing and carrying out a service in a particular way.

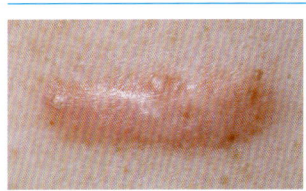

Keloid scar
A raised scar that grows above skin level. This can be created artificially using wax and liquid latex.

Liquid latex
Used to create artificial skin and scarring effects. When wet, the solution is in liquid form but it dries to a solid, flexible form.

Mood board
A collage of items such as images, photos, sketches, clippings, text, colours, textures and samples of objects used to inspire a design concept. They do not have to be limited to visual subjects, but serve as a visual tool to quickly inform others of the overall 'feel' of what is to be achieved.

Small prosthetics
Often made from silicone, these are 'false' noses, ear tips, chins and so on, which are applied and covered with make-up to blend in with the surrounding skin.

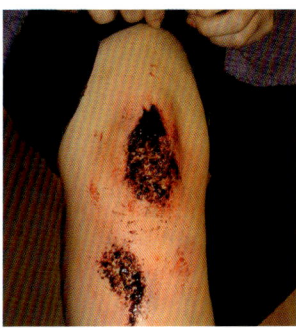

Special effects make-up
The creation of a look including wounds and injuries.

Spirit gum
An adhesive, made mostly of SD Alcohol 35-A (the solvent, or 'spirit') and resin (the adhesive, or 'gum'), used for applying and fixing prosthetics, wigs, beards and adornments such as gems.

Texturising materials
In media make-up these include any product or ingredient that adds texture, such as fabric and gems.

> **Revision tip**
>
> Make sure you understand the advantages and disadvantages of using open versus closed questions with different clients and in different situations.

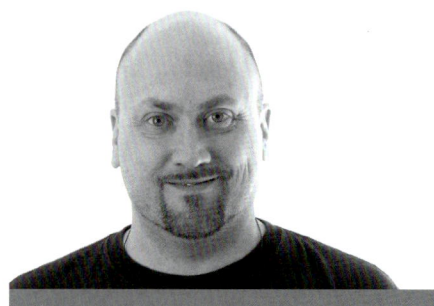

Follow in the footsteps of...
Lars Carlsson

At the age of 13 Lars started creating latex monster masks in his parents' basement. He devoted all his free time to practising his talent, and when he was 18 he was offered his first professional job in a theatre. He was given the opportunity to work there as an apprentice and was taught the skill of wig making. Over the last 20 years Lars has enjoyed working on several hundred theatre, opera, TV and film productions. Teaching is another big passion for Lars, which he does both in schools and through his website Makeup-FX.com. Read on for Lars' top tips on media make-up!

What you must know
You must be able to:

1 Describe requirements for client preparation, preparing themselves and the work area

2 Describe different consultation techniques used to identify service objectives

3 Describe the factors that need to be considered when selecting techniques, products and equipment

4 Explain the environmental conditions suitable for media make-up

5 Explain the safety considerations that must be taken into account when providing media make-up

6 Identify the range of tools and equipment used for media make-up

7 Identify products used and their key ingredients

8 Explain how to develop a mood board to include components of media/character/special effects make-up techniques

9 Describe the aims and limitations of media and special effects make-up

10 Explain the principles of colour theory

11 Describe the skin types and characteristics

12 Explain the importance of skin compatibility checks prior to using media and special effects make-up

Continues on next page

13 Describe how to carry out compatibility tests

14 Describe adverse skin reactions to products

15 Explain known contra-indications that prevent or restrict media make-up

16 Describe how to communicate and behave in a professional manner

17 Describe the importance of positioning themselves and the model correctly throughout the service

18 Explain safe and hygienic working practices

19 Explain contra-actions which might occur during and following the service and how to respond

20 Explain the advice on the removal of products that should be provided

21 Describe the importance of completing the service to the satisfaction of the client

22 Describe the methods of evaluating the effectiveness of the service

23 Explain how to carry out media and special effects make-up techniques to create characters using products

24 Describe how to apply, preserve, maintain and safely remove small ready made prosthetic pieces

25 Explain the importance of accurately recording the techniques and products used and of making a physical recording of the results

> *Make sure you protect yourself with the necessary personal protective equipment when working with products such as liquid latex.*

Revision tip

Different lighting will alter the appearance of the make-up. Make sure you are clear with regard to the conditions under which it is to be viewed.

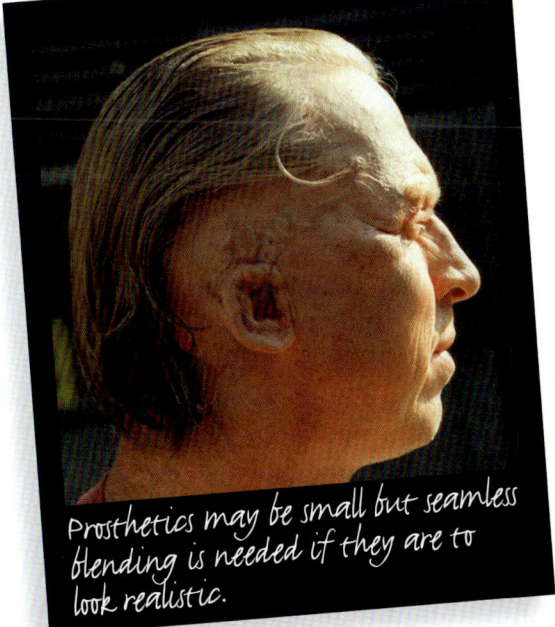

Prosthetics may be small but seamless blending is needed if they are to look realistic.

Media

> Always check that 'blood' which is to be held in the mouth or used very close to any orifices such as the eyes and nose is non-toxic.

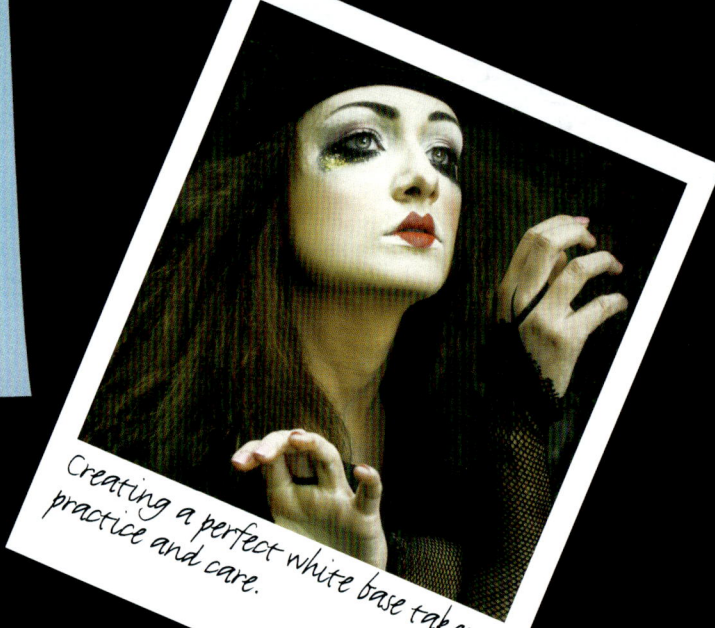

Creating a perfect white base takes practice and care.

Image courtesy of Maria Retter

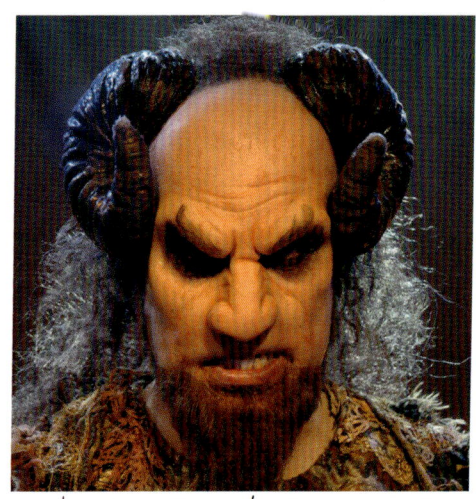

Make-up and prosthetics can produce some scary effects!

> When presenting your mood board, make sure you speak clearly and use a variety of different presentation methods. Check that everyone can both hear and see you clearly.

Makeup-FX.com

Image courtesy of Lars Carlsson (Makeup-FX.com)

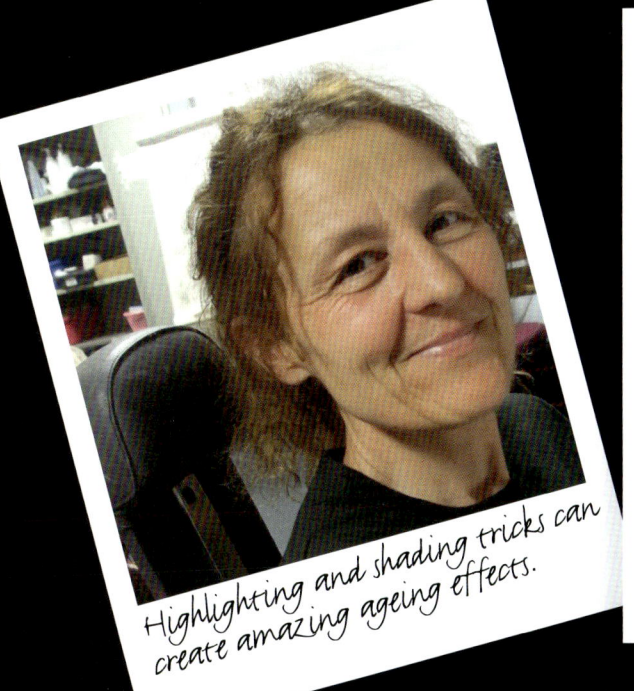
Highlighting and shading tricks can create amazing ageing effects.

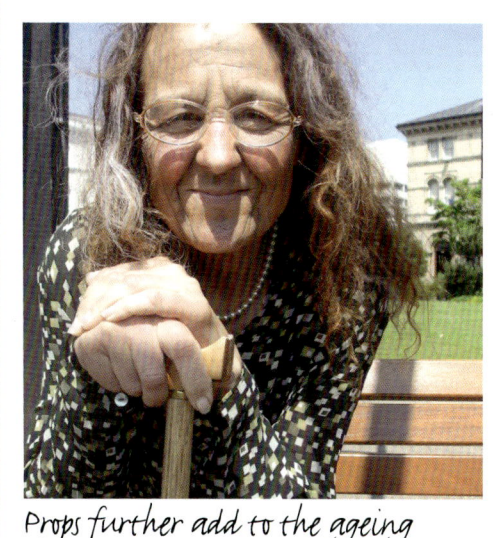
Props further add to the ageing illusion.

make-up

> "Never go to a job without practising the relevant skill first, even if you have done it a million times before. Your customer deserves to get the best!

It is important to provide suitable advice on how to deal with any contra-actions that may occur and how to effectively remove the products.

What you must do
Practical observations

This page shows what you need to do during your practical task. You can look at it beforehand, but you're **not** allowed to have it with you while carrying out your practical task. You must achieve **all** the criteria; you can achieve 1 mark, 2 marks or 3 marks for the criteria indicated with *.

Conversion chart

Grade	Marks
Pass	14–17
Merit	18–24
Distinction	25–28

○ Please tick when all pre-observation requirements have been met.

	Media make-up		
1 Present a mood board *	1	2	3
2 Prepare yourself, the model and the work area for media make-up application	1		
3 Use suitable consultation techniques to identify service objectives *	1	2	3
4 Identify influencing factors	1		
5 Provide clear recommendations based on factors *	1	2	3
6 Position yourself and the model correctly throughout the application	1		
7 Follow safe and hygienic working practices	1		
8 Communicate and behave in a professional manner	1		
9 Select and use products, tools and equipment taking into account identified factors *	1	2	3
10 Apply media and special effects make-up to age a character using components and prosthetic pieces *	1	2	3
11 Complete the service to the satisfaction of the client *	1	2	3
12 Provide suitable aftercare advice *	1	2	3
13 Record the techniques and products used	1		
14 Record and evaluate the results of the service	1		
Total			
Grade			
Candidate signature and date			
Assessor signature and date			

What you must do
Practical observations descriptors table

This table shows what you need to do to achieve 1, 2 or 3 marks for the criteria indicated with * on the previous page.

	1 mark	2 marks	3 marks
1 Present a mood board	The candidate presents a mood board using basic presentation techniques.	The candidate presents a mood board explaining in some detail how the ideas and techniques can be adapted to reflect the concept of components for media/character/special effect make-up techniques using a clear speaking voice and minimal resources.	The candidate presents a mood board explaining in depth the detail on how the ideas and techniques can be adapted to reflect the concept of components for media/character/special effect make-up techniques using a clear speaking voice adapted to suit the audience and using a variety of resources.
3 Use suitable consultation techniques to identify service objectives	Basic consultation Examples: uses open and closed questions, checks for contra-indications, identifies the service objectives correctly.	Good consultation Examples: positive body language, uses open and closed questions to identify contra-indications, expectations; identifies service objectives and any factors that may limit or restrict the service.	Thorough consultation Examples: positive body language, uses open and closed questions to identify contra-indications, expectations; identifies service objectives and any factors that may limit or restrict the service, allows the model to ask any questions to confirm understanding.

Continues on next page

Learn to use Photoshop. Today you need to be able to show directors digital make-up designs.

What you must do
Practical observations descriptors table (continued)

This table shows what you need to do to achieve 1, 2 or 3 marks for the criteria indicated with * on page 280.

	1 mark	2 marks	3 marks
5 Provide clear recommendations based on factors	A basic treatment plan is recommended. Examples: explains service procedure, and any adaptations to meet the service needs, based on factors.	A good treatment plan is recommended. Examples: explains service procedure and any adaptations to meet client treatment needs based on factors identified during consultation, contra-indications and choice of products.	A thorough treatment plan is recommended. Examples: explains service procedure and any adaptations to meet client treatment needs based on factors identified during consultation, contra-indications and choice of products, adaptation of techniques to suit service objectives, allows the client to ask questions about the media make-up.
9 Select and use products, tools and equipment taking into account identified factors	Selects and uses products, tools, equipment and basic techniques taking into account factors identified during consultation.	Selects and uses products, tools, equipment and a range of techniques taking into account factors identified during consultation in a logical sequence with creativity and confidence, to meet the service objectives and effect required.	Selects and uses products, tools, equipment and a range of techniques taking into account factors identified during consultation in a logical sequence with creativity and confidence, to meet the service objectives and effect required, adapts and modifies techniques as necessary and informs the model of the changes.
10 Apply media and special effects make-up to age a character using components and prosthetic pieces	Applies the media and special effects make-up to age a character using limited components and prosthetic pieces, showing evidence of some basic blending techniques.	Applies the media and special effects make-up to age a character using a range of components and prosthetic pieces, showing evidence of good blending techniques.	Applies the media and special effects make-up to age a character using a wide range of components and prosthetic pieces, showing evidence of excellent blending techniques.

Continues on next page

	1 mark	2 marks	3 marks
11 Complete the service to the satisfaction of the client	The service is completed within the agreed time and brought to a satisfactory close, meets the service objectives.	The service is completed within the agreed time and brought to a satisfactory close, meets the service objectives, the model is shown the result and the end result is agreed.	The service is completed within the agreed time and brought to a satisfactory close, media make-up and special effects are applied neatly and blended well to meet the service objectives, the model is shown the result, positive feedback is gained.
12 Provide suitable aftercare advice	Basic aftercare advice is provided including possible contra-actions and how to deal with them.	Good level of aftercare advice is provided including possible contra-actions and how to deal with them, and basic removal advice.	Excellent aftercare advice is provided including possible contra-actions and how to deal with them, advice on application and removal techniques and products.

> *Remember that you are helping to portray a character. You and your make-up are not the star of the show.*

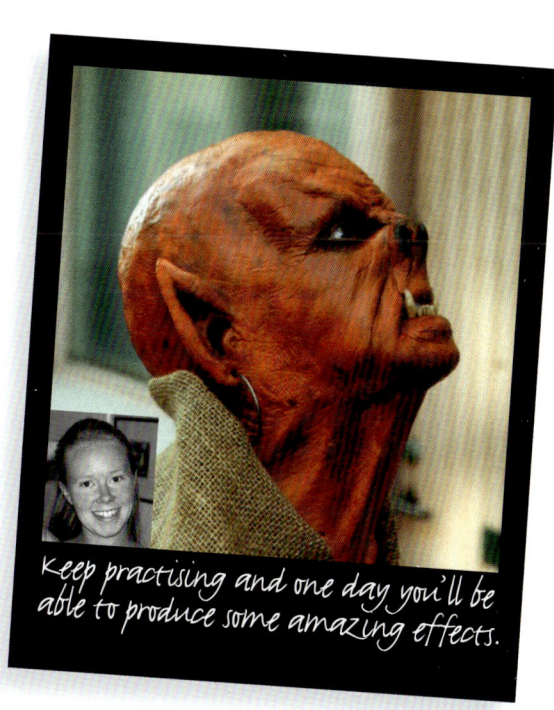

Keep practising and one day you'll be able to produce some amazing effects.

Image courtesy of Lars Carlsson (Makeup-FX.com)

Comment form
Unit 330 Media make-up

This form can be used to record comments by you, your client, or your assessor.

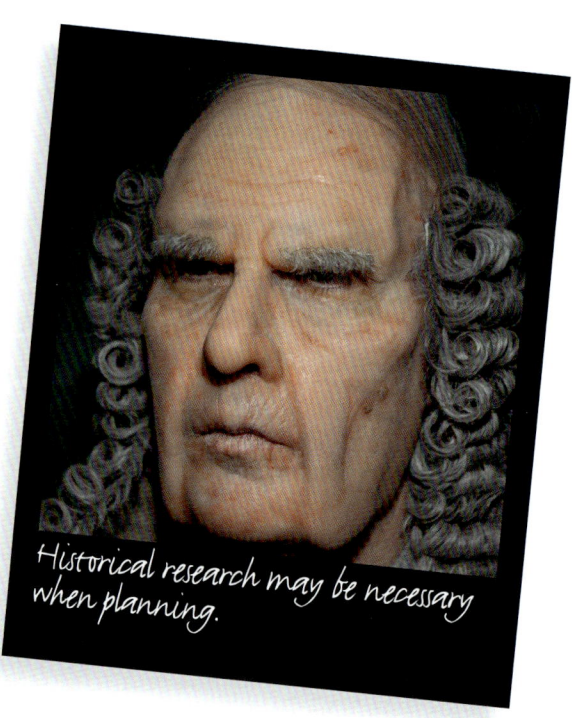

Historical research may be necessary when planning.

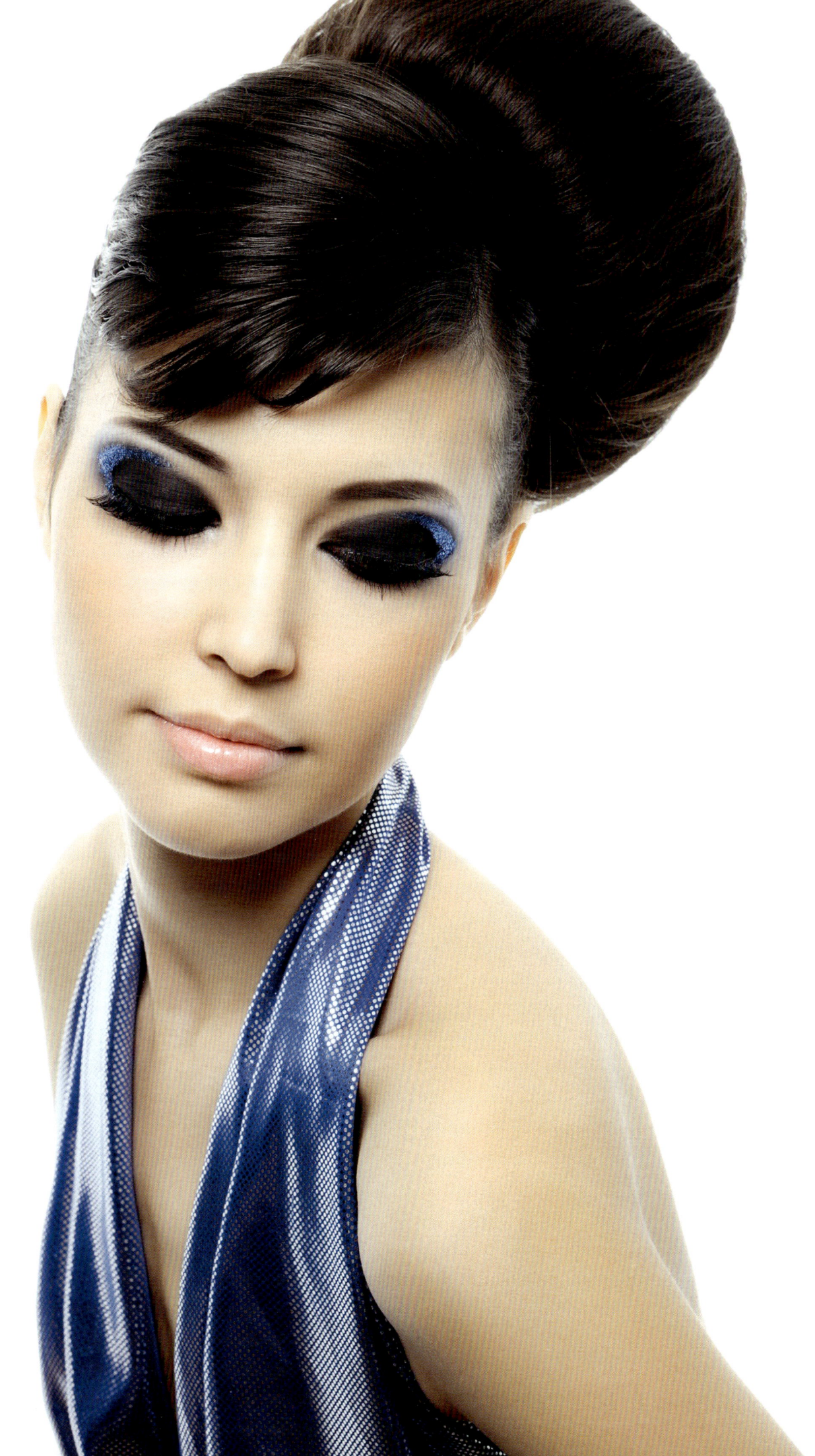

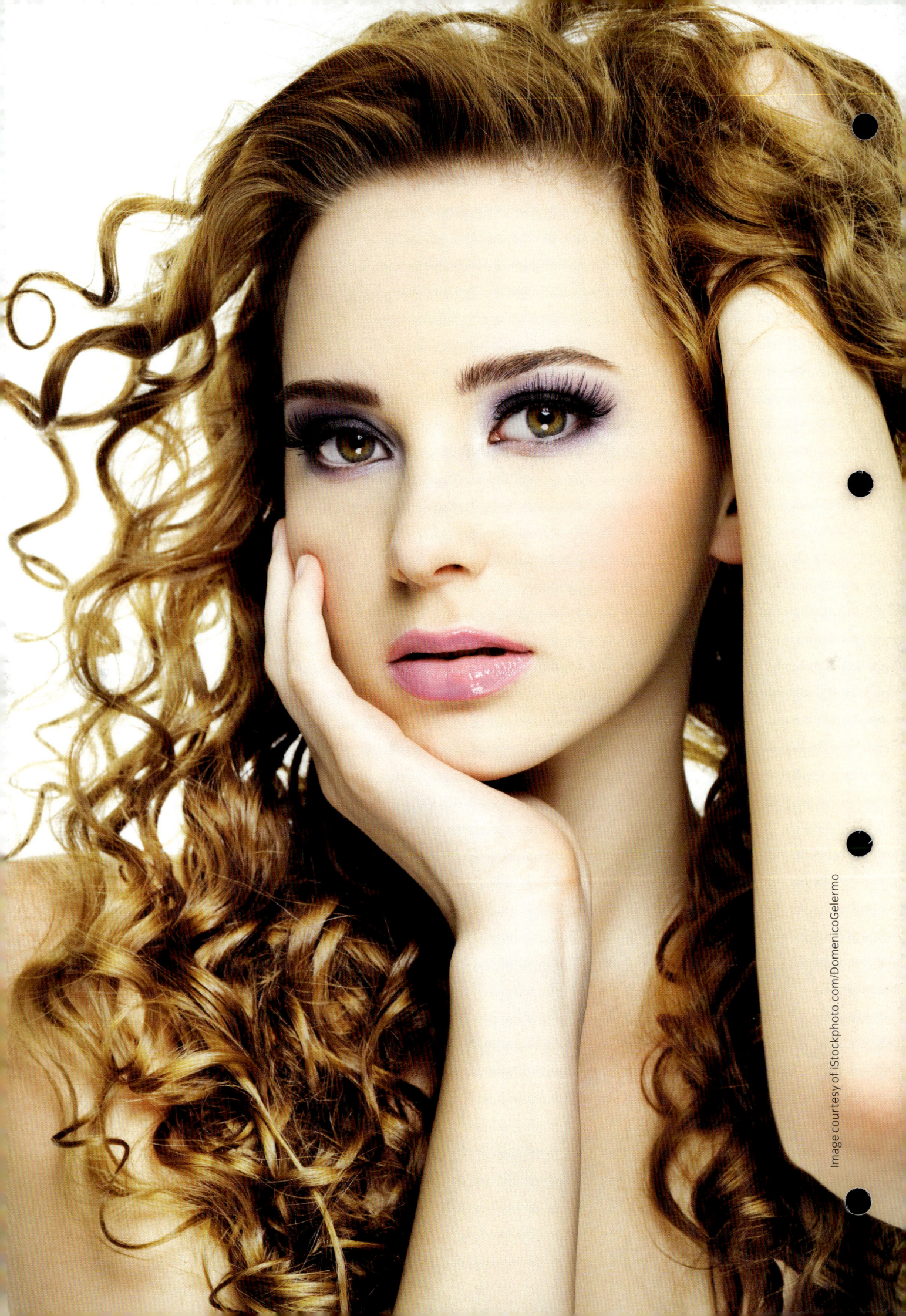

Image courtesy of iStockphoto.com/DomenicoGelermo

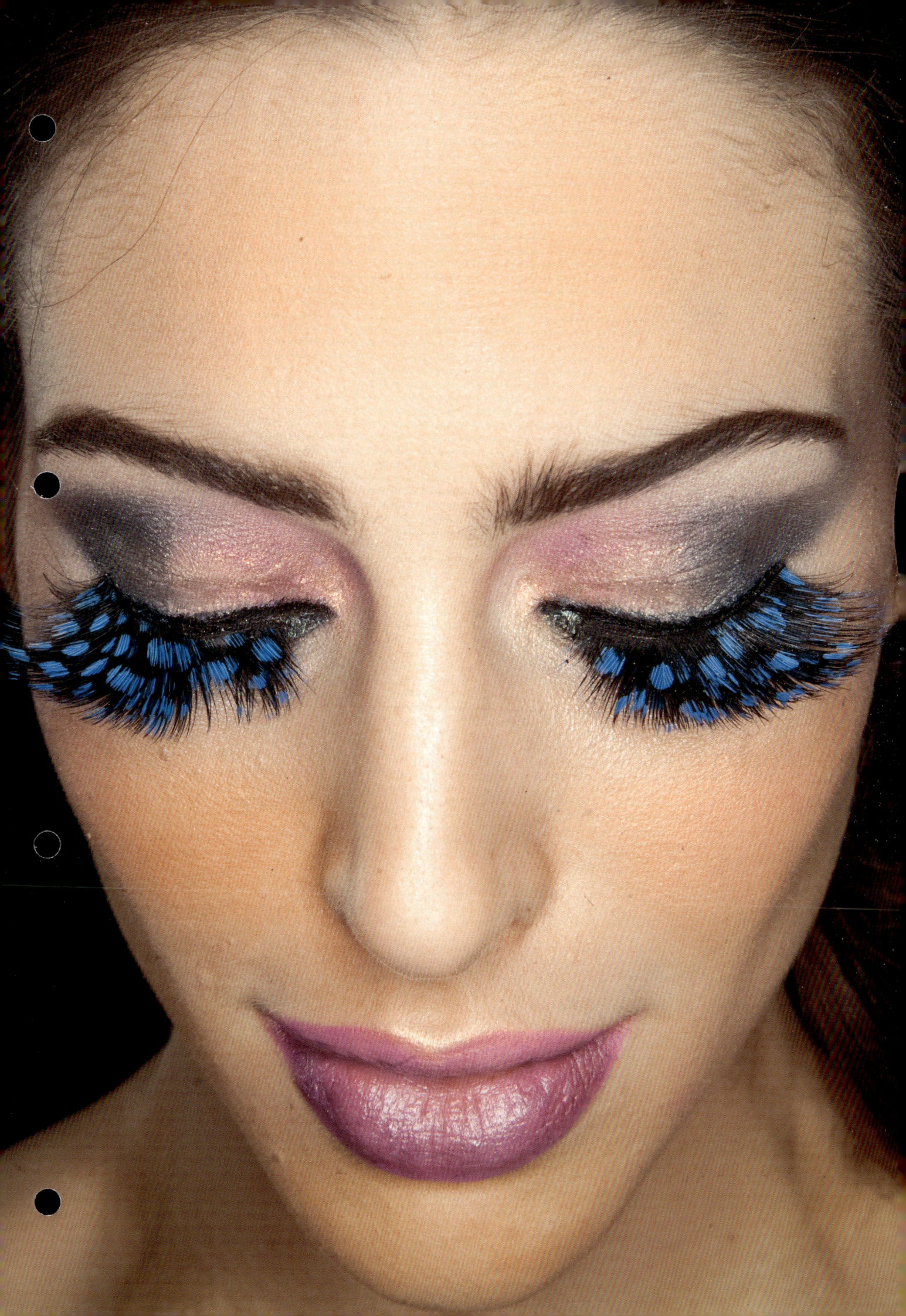

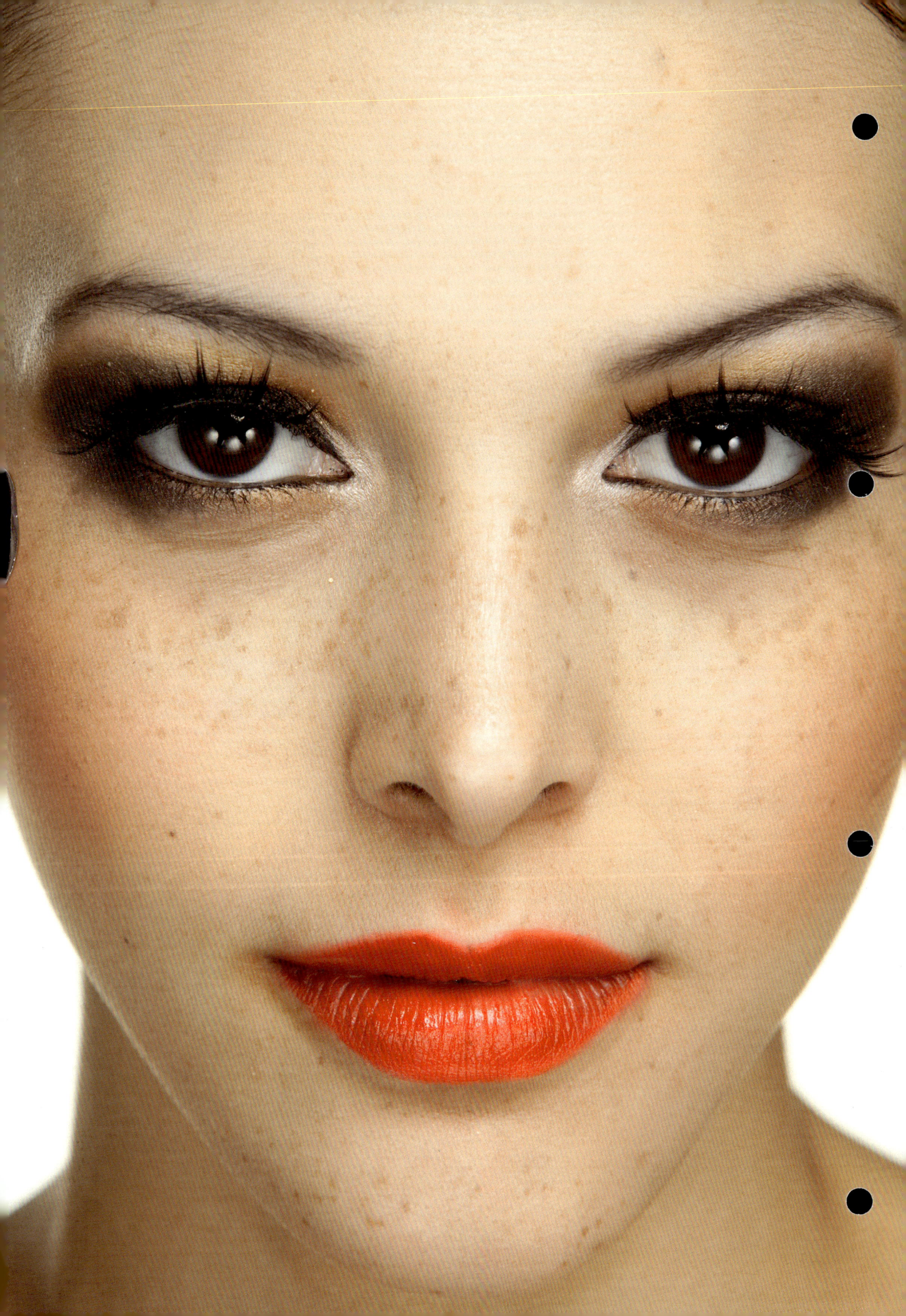

125004784
TL033003

ISBN 978-0-85193-217-0

9 780851 932170